DATE DUE

APR 9 '95			
APR 24 '95			
APR 10 1997			
040103			
DEC 21 2005			

HIV Epidemiology
Models and Methods

Workshop Participants

Robert J. Biggar
Bill Cameron*
Jordi Casabona
Don C. Des Jarlais
Roger Detels
Ferdinando Dianzani
Gaetano Maria Fara
Samuel R. Friedman
Mitchell H. Gail
Massimo Galli
M. Elizabeth Halloran
Anne M. Johnson
Marie Laga
Adriano Lazzarin
Andrew R. Moss
Alvaro Muñoz
Massimo Musicco
Alfredo Nicolosi
Nancy S. Padian
Peter Piot
Pierre J. Plourde
Giovanni Rezza
Alan M. Schultz
Zena Stein†
Mervyn Susser
Anastasios A. Tsiatis
Marti Vall
Anneke van den Hoek
Stefano Vella
Sten H. Vermund
David Vlahov

---

*AIDS Clinic, Ottawa General Hospital, Ottawa, Ontario, Canada, and †Columbia University School of Public Health, New York, New York, USA

HIV Epidemiology
Models and Methods

Editor

Alfredo Nicolosi, M.D., Ph.D.

Department of Epidemiology and Medical Informatics
Institute of Advanced Biomedical Technologies
National Research Council, Milan, Italy; and the
Gertrude H. Sergievsky Center, School of Public Health
Columbia University, New York, New York

RAVEN PRESS NEW YORK

Raven Press, Ltd., 1185 Avenue of the Americas, New York, New York 10036

Made in the United States of America

Library of Congress Cataloging-in-Publication Data
HIV epidemiology : models and methods / editor, Alfredo Nicolosi.
p. cm.
Based on the workshop promoted by the Italian National Research Council, held in Sept. 1992.
Includes bibliographical references and index.
ISBN 0–7817–0118–X
1. HIV infections—Epidemiology—Congresses. I. Nicolosi, Alfredo. II. Consiglio nazionale delle ricerche (Italy)
[DNLM: 1. HIV Infections—epidemiology—congresses. 2. Data Interpretation, Statistical—congresses. 3. Epidemiologic Methods—congresses. WD 308 H6751 1992]
RA644.A25H585 1994
614.5′993—dc20
DNLM/DLC
for Library of Congress 93-30218
CIP

9 8 7 6 5 4 3 2 1

Contents

V. Vaccine Trials Against HIV Infection

VI. Statistical Data Analysis and Interpretation

VII. Natural History

Contributors

Maria Grazia Agresti
Laboratory of Virology
Istituto Superiore di Sanità
Rome, Italy

Fernando Aiuti
Clinica Immunologica
Università "La Sapienza"
Rome, Italy

Barbara Alliegro
HIV–ISS
Centro Operativo AIDS—Istituto Superiore di Sanità
Rome, Italy

Gioacchino Angarano
Clinica delle Malattie Infettive
Università degli Studi
Bari, Italy

Helena Bacellar
Department of Epidemiology
The Johns Hopkins School of Public Health
Baltimore, Maryland, USA

Mauro Barbanera
Divisione di Malattie Infettive
University of Genoa, Italy

Robert J. Biggar
International AIDS Coordinator
Viral Epidemiology Section
Rockville, Maryland, USA

R. Bucciardini
Laboratory of Epidemiology
Istituto Superiore di Sanità
Rome, Italy

Andrea Canessa
Clinica di Malattie Infettive
University of Genoa, Italy

Manuel Carballo
Program on Substance Abuse
World Health Organization
Geneva, Switzerland

Jordi Casabona
AIDS Prevention and Control Programme
Department of Health
Generalitat de Catalunya
Barcelona, Catalonia, Spain
Preventive Medicine and Public Health Department
Autonomous University of Barcelona
Hospital de la Santa Creu i de Sant Pau
Barcelona, Catalonia, Spain

Francesco Castelli
Clinica di Malattie Infettive
University of Brescia, Italy

Kachit Choopanya
Health Department
Bangkok Metropolitan Administration (BMA)
Bangkok, Thailand

Maria Léa Corrêa Leite
Department of Epidemiology and Medical Informatics
Institute of Advanced Biomedical Technologies
National Research Council
Milan, Italy

Roel Coutinho
Municipal Health Service
Department of Public Health and Environment
Amsterdam, The Netherlands

Don C. Des Jarlais
Beth Israel Medical Center
New York, New York, USA

Roger Detels
Department of Epidemiology
University of California Los Angeles School of Public Health
Los Angeles, California, USA

Ferdinando Dianzani
Istituto di Virologia
Università "La Sapienza"
Rome, Italy

Marina Dorrucci
HIV–ISS
Centro Operativo AIDS—Istituto Superiore di Sanità
Rome, Italy

Gaetano Maria Fara
Istituto di Igiene "G. Sanarelli"
Università "La Sapienza"
Rome, Italy

Marco Floridia
Laboratory of Virology
Istituto Superiore di Sanità
Rome, Italy

Samuel R. Friedman
National Development and Research Institutes, Inc.
New York, New York, USA

Sergio Gafà
Divisione di Malattie Infettive
Ospedale di Reggio Emilio, Italy

Mitchell H. Gail
Epidemiologic Methods Section
National Cancer Institute
Bethesda, Maryland, USA

Massimo Galli
Institute of Infectious Diseases
University of Milan
Milan, Italy
Ospedale L. Sacco
Milan, Italy

Maddalena Gasparini
Institute of Advanced Biomedical Technologies
National Research Council
Department of Epidemiology and Medical Informatics
Milan, Italy

M. Giuliano
Laboratory of Virology
Istituto Superiore di Sanità
Rome, Italy

Marjorie Goldstein
National Development and Research Institutes, Inc.
New York, New York, USA

M. Elizabeth Halloran
Emory University School of Public Health
Atlanta, Georgia, USA

Anne M. Johnson
Academic Department of Genito Urinary Medicine
University College London Medical School
London, United Kingdom

Benny Jose
National Development and Research Institutes, Inc.
New York, New York, USA

Lawrence A. Kingsley
School of Public Health
University of Pittsburgh
Pittsburgh, Pennsylvania, USA

Marie Laga
Department of Infection and Immunity
Institute of Tropical Medicine
Antwerp, Belgium

Adriano Lazzarin
Institute of Infectious Diseases
University of Milan
Milan, Italy

Bruce Levin
Department of Biostatistics
School of Public Health
Columbia University
New York, New York, USA

Sergio Mariotti
Laboratory of Epidemiology
Istituto Superiore di Sanità
Rome, Italy

Andrew R. Moss
Department of Epidemiology and Biostatistics
University of California
San Francisco, California, USA

Alvaro Muñoz
Department of Epidemiology
The Johns Hopkins School of Public Health
Baltimore, Maryland, USA

Massimo Musicco
Department of Epidemiology and Medical Informatics
Institute of Advanced Biomedical Technologies
National Research Council
Milan, Italy

Alan Neaigus
National Development and Research Institutes, Inc.
New York, New York, USA

Alfredo Nicolosi
Department of Epidemiology and Medical Informatics
Institute of Advanced Biomedical Technologies
National Research Council
Milan, Italy
G. H. Sergievsky Center
School of Public Health
Columbia University
New York, New York, USA

Luigi Ortona
Clinica di Malattie Infettive
Catholic University
Rome, Italy

Alberto Osella
Department of Epidemiology and Medical Informatics
Institute of Advanced Biomedical Technologies
National Research Council
Milan, Italy

Nancy S. Padian
Department of Epidemiology and Biostatistics
University of California
San Francisco, California, USA

Patrizio Pezzotti
HIV–ISS
Centro Operativo AIDS—Istituto Superiore di Sanità
Rome, Italy

John P. Phair
School of Medicine
Northwestern University
Chicago, Illinois, USA

Peter Piot
WHO Collaborating Centre on AIDS
Institute of Tropical Medicine
Antwerp, Belgium

Pierre J. Plourde
Departments of International Medicine and Medical Microbiology
University of Manitoba
Winnipeg, Manitoba, Canada

Francis A. Plummer
WHO Centre for Research and Training on Sexually Transmitted Diseases
Department of Medical Microbiology
University of Nairobi
Kenya

Raffaele Pristerà
HIV–ISS
Centro Operativo AIDS—Istituto Superiore di Sanità
Rome, Italy

Giovanni Rezza
HIV–ISS
Centro Operativo AIDS—Istituto Superiore di Sanità
Rome, Italy

E. Ricchi
HIV–ISS
Centro Operativo AIDS—Istituto Superiore di Sanità
Rome, Italy

P. S. Rosenberg
Epidemiologic Methods Section
National Cancer Institute
Bethesda, Maryland, USA

Alfred J. Saah
Department of Epidemiology
The Johns Hopkins School of Public Health
Baltimore, Maryland, USA

Bernardino Salassa
Divisione di Malattie Infettive
Ospedale Amedeo di Savoia
Turin, Italy

Alberto Saracco
Institute of Infectious Diseases
Scientific Institute "Ospedale S. Raffaele"
Milan, Italy

Lewis K. Schrager
Epidemiology Branch
Division of AIDS
National Institute of Allergy and Infectious Diseases
Bethesda, Maryland, USA

Alan M. Schultz
Vaccine Research and Development Branch
Division of AIDS, BRDP, NIAID, NIH
Bethesda, Maryland, USA

Daniela Seminara
Division of Cancer Etiology
National Cancer Institute
Bethesda, Maryland, USA

Stephen C. Shiboski
Department of Epidemiology and Biostatistics
University of California
San Francisco, California, USA

Alessandro Sinicco
Clinica di Malattie Infettive
University of Turin, Italy

Jo L. Sotheran
National Development and Research Institutes, Inc.
New York, New York, USA

Ilene Speizer
Department of Epidemiology
The Johns Hopkins School of Public Health
Baltimore, Maryland, USA

Mervyn Susser
Gertrude H. Sergievsky Center
Columbia University Faculty of Medicine
New York, New York, USA

Umberto Tirelli
Centro Regionale Oncologico
Aviano, Italy

Anastasios A. Tsiatis
Department of Biostatistics
Harvard School of Public Health
Boston, Massachusetts, USA

Marti Vall
AIDS Prevention and Control Programme
Department of Health
Generalitat de Catalunya
Barcelona, Catalonia, Spain

Anneke van den Hoek
Municipal Health Service
Department of Public Health and Environment
Amsterdam, The Netherlands

Suphak Vanichseni
Health Department
Bangkok Metropolitan Administration (BMA)
Bangkok, Thailand

Stefano Vella
Laboratory of Virology
Istituto Superiore di Sanità
Rome, Italy

Sten H. Vermund
Division of AIDS
Epidemiology Branch
Vaccine Trials and National Institute of Allergy and Infectious Diseases
Bethesda, Maryland, USA

Pierluigi Viale
Divisione di Malattie Infettive
Ospedale di Piacenza, Italy

David Vlahov
Department of Epidemiology
The Johns Hopkins School of Hygiene and Public Health
Baltimore, Maryland, USA

Jane Wadsworth
Academic Department of Public Health
St. Mary's Hospital Medical School
London, United Kingdom

John Wenston
National Development and Research Institutes, Inc.
New York, New York, USA

Mauro Zaccarelli
Drug Treatment Center
USL Rm 10
Rome, Italy

Roberto Zerboni
CAVE
Milan, Italy

Acknowledgments

I thank the Members of the Scientific Committee—Carlo Brancati, Paolo Cerretelli, Don C. Des Jarlais, Ferdinando Dianzani, Gianfranco Donelli, Gaetano M. Fara, Enrico Garaci, W. Allen Hauser, Adriano Lazzarin, Mauro Moroni, Augusto Panà, Giovanni Rezza, Giorgio Ricci, Giovanni Rocchi, and Giovanni Battista Rossi—who contributed to the definition of the Workshop's scientific program, and Eleonora Kastelec who was responsible for the Workshop's organization.

Preface

Twelve years after the description of the first cases of acquired immunodeficiency syndrome (AIDS), epidemiologic studies of AIDS and human immunodeficiency virus (HIV) infection have evolved to a first degree of maturity. The modes of HIV transmission have been established, the most important risk factors identified, the natural history of the disease partially studied, a number of markers of progression described, and the effects of antiviral agents evaluated. We have also reached a summary conceptualization of the social, behavioral, epidemiologic, and biologic processes by which HIV transmission takes place and by which prevention can be made effective.

A number of well-established studies have contributed to a basic understanding of the epidemiology and natural history of HIV infection among different populations and settings. These studies have also refined the statistical methods used in study design and data analysis. The very complexity of HIV infection requires that the epidemiologic methods traditionally used in the study of degenerative diseases be combined with those used in the study of infectious diseases. However, although advances in epidemiologic knowledge concerning HIV infection have allowed researchers to recognize and overcome some of the biases inherent in early studies, there still are many unclear or controversial issues, which are complicated by the different epidemic patterns of HIV in industrialized and developing countries. Finally, there are new challenges to be faced in terms of the prevention of HIV infection, including the development and testing of a preventive vaccine.

In order to provide an opportunity to reflect on the current achievements of HIV epidemiologic research, to compare the methodologies used in different studies, and discuss future improvements, the Italian National Research Council promoted a workshop entitled "Models and Methods of Epidemiologic Research on HIV Infection," held in September 1992. The participants included many of the most experienced researchers in the field of HIV epidemiology, who presented their studies and discussed the methodologic problems arising from their work. Statistical and sociological contributions further helped to clarify possible sources of bias, problems of measurement, and methodologic issues.

This book collects the papers presented by the participants and records the discussions that followed the presentations. The topics include HIV infection among intravenous drug users, heterosexual and homosexual transmission, natural history, the effect of treatments, issues of statistical analysis and confounding, and vaccine development and trials. Many of the papers report original results; others are critical reviews of special topics, original statistical contributions to the methodologic problems facing HIV epidemiologic studies, or reports on the development and epidemiologic outlook in the field of vaccines. The discussions—for which a great deal of time was reserved in the Workshop—contain sharp analyses, criticisms, and comments, and cover a wide range of topics.

This book will be useful not only to readers already involved in epidemiologic studies on HIV but also to those who are beginning to participate in or conduct such studies. They will find the description and the results of important current studies and be sensitized to a number of the methodologic problems involved in HIV epidemiologic research.

Alfredo Nicolosi

HIV Epidemiology: Models and Methods,
edited by Alfredo Nicolosi. Raven Press, Ltd.,
New York © 1994.

1

The Amsterdam Cohort Study on HIV Infection Among Drug Users

Evaluation of Prevention Programs

Anneke van den Hoek and Roel Coutinho

Municipal Health Service, Department of Public Health and Environment, P.O. Box 20244, 1000 HE Amsterdam, The Netherlands

BACKGROUND INFORMATION ON AMSTERDAM DRUG POLICY

Of the estimated 20,000 Dutch drug users, 7,000 to 8,000 are living in Amsterdam. This estimate of the number of hard drug users in Amsterdam is based on a capture-recapture method and is a year prevalence. The estimated number of drug users staying on a regular day in Amsterdam is lower, approximately 5,500. This smaller number is due to the large number of foreign drug users who only stay a few days in Amsterdam.

It is estimated that about 40% of the drug users in Amsterdam inject their drugs. The current prevalence of the injection of drugs among drug users differs according to country of origin: About 40% of the Dutch drug users inject their drugs, compared to about 70% of drug users of foreign origin (mainly German and Southern European) and about 5% of the ethnic drug users (from Surinam, the Netherlands Antilles, Morocco, and Turkey).

The assistance system for drug users in Amsterdam can be described in three phases: getting in contact, harm reduction, and treatment. Contact with drug users is made by (a) street-corner workers, (b) physicians visiting arrested drug users in police cells, and (c) social nurses visiting all hospitalized drug patients.

Through regular contact, appropriate medical and social care can be given, which is considered beneficial for both drug users and society at large. This policy is called the harm reduction approach. The main instrument for harm reduction (as long as the drug user is not able or willing to stop his or her drug use) is the large-scale methadone program with a low level of threshold. In 1981, the low-threshold methadone program put in operation two mobile methadone buses, which visit six locations daily, and four outpatient methadone clinics. The idea is to contact drug users through the buses, and the aim of the program is to regulate their addiction and to give medical care. Continuation of injecting drug use while being on such a program is tolerated. As soon as a rather stable situation is reached, the client's general practitioner is asked to take over the methadone prescription. Referral to drug-free treatment programs is always possible. It is estimated that approximately 70% of the drug users are in touch with this assistance system.

Another activity of the harm reduction approach is the needle and syringe exchange program, aimed at the reduction of the harm by injecting. This program was initially started in 1984 through an initiative of the drug users' organization, the "Junkiebond." This program was initially started to prevent hepatitis B, but was soon overshadowed by the more important goal of AIDS prevention. In 1985, 100,000 needles and syringes were handed out, and this number has gradually risen to around 700,000 in 1988 and to approximately one million in 1990 and 1991. Participation in the program, which in 1991 operated in approximately 15 locations, does not require identification or registration. For this reason, no information is available on the number of participants or on their demographic characteristics.

When Amsterdam became aware of the AIDS epidemic, a rather unique situation for HIV prevention existed: being in contact with the majority of drug users and the operation of a needle and syringe program, which only needed to be expanded. In addition, a publicity campaign about AIDS and its prevention was started in 1986, and condoms were distributed among addicted prostitutes.

THE AMSTERDAM COHORT STUDY ON HIV INFECTION AND AIDS AMONG DRUG USERS

This study was started at the end of 1985. At that time only one drug user with AIDS had been reported in the Netherlands. An important reason for starting a study among drug users in Amsterdam was that the assistance system for drug users here operates in a different way than in other countries and enables contact to be established with the majority of the drug users.

The aims of the study are

a. to study the prevalence and incidence of HIV infection and AIDS in relation to (changes in) drug use and sexual behavior.
b. to evaluate the impact of various HIV-prevention programs for drug users.
c. to study determinants of risky injecting and sexual behavior.
d. to study the natural history of HIV infection.

METHODS

Participants are recruited at methadone outposts and the weekly sexually transmitted disease (STD) clinic for drug-using prostitutes. Both injecting and noninjecting drug users are invited to participate. Participation is voluntary and, after extensive information has been given, informed consent is obtained. Blood samples for serology, virology, and immunology are taken and participants interviewed using a standard questionnaire which includes questions concerning clinical symptoms, medical history, lifestyle, use of oral and intravenous drugs (methadone included), and prostitution. Participants are asked to return for a follow-up visit every 4 months. On each occasion, the same interview is conducted and blood samples are collected. Twenty-five Dutch guilders are paid per follow-up visit to encourage continued participation. After April, 1989, all participants are physically examined by a physician at each visit, and at varying intervals additional questions on specific psychosocial or behavioral issues are added to the basic questionnaire.

Prevalence and Incidence of HIV Infection

Between December, 1985, and January, 1992, 884 drug users (all without AIDS-related disease) entered the study. The recruitment of new participants was interrupted for 1 year between September, 1990, and September, 1991. In the first year of the study (1986), HIV prevalence among drug users with a history of injecting drug use was approximately 30% (1) and remained more or less stable among new intakes in this group in the following years (2). The HIV incidence rate per 100 person-years among HIV-negative, injecting drug users in the cohort for 1986 up to 1991 was 9.5, 4.9, 5.3, 4.2, 4.3 and 3.3, respectively (2,3). By January, 1992, a total of 43 seroconversions and 23 cases of AIDS had been observed among the participants.

Risk factors for the prevalence of HIV infection in injecting drug users (IDU) were a higher frequency of borrowing used needles and syringes, date of first injecting drug use longer ago, recent injecting drug use, relatively prolonged time living in Amsterdam, West German nationality, and injecting of heroin and cocaine together (1,4). Risk factors for incident HIV infection were duration of time living in Amsterdam and recent onset of injecting. Injecting mainly at home was related to a decreased incidence (3). Among noninjecting drug users, only a few HIV infections were found among males who had homosexual contacts (1). So far, the heterosexual spread of HIV among the population of drug users in Amsterdam seems to be limited.

Risk Reduction and Evaluation of Prevention Programs

During follow-up, a strong reduction in borrowing and lending of used needles and syringes was observed, and this behavioral change was not dependent on being informed of HIV serostatus (5). Over time, the use of the needle and syringe exchange program increased. However, reduction in needle sharing was not seen among new entrants to the study. Therefore, we concluded that the risk reduction observed during follow-up was mainly an effect of the study, with the exchange program only having a limited impact. Despite this risk reduction, the number of new HIV infections declined less than among homosexual men (2,3). The relatively high incidence of new HIV infections reflects the fact that, despite the previously described risk reduction, risky injecting behavior among seronegative drug users is still highly prevalent.

As mentioned before, in Amsterdam a special approach towards drug users, called harm reduction, has been developed. The goal of harm reduction is "to create a situation that greatly reduces the risk of addicts harming themselves or their environment." As part of this approach, low-threshold methadone programs and a large-scale needle and syringe exchange program have been implemented. Therefore, we were interested to see if we could find evidence that participation in the low-threshold methadone programs and the exchange program reduces the spread of HIV among injecting drug users.

The first study (4) concerns all drug users who had a history of injecting drug use and who enrolled in the study through low-threshold methadone clinics from December, 1985, until March, 1989. Long-term, regular participants in low-threshold methadone programs (LTM users) were compared to short-term or irregular participants. Long-term, regular methadone users were defined as IDU who started using methadone at least 5 years preceding the interview and who reported daily methadone use in the 5 years preceding the interview. The non-LTM users were defined as IDU who started using methadone in the 5 years preceding the interview and IDU who reported irregular use of methadone during these 5 years.

One hundred ninety-four IDU (50%) met the criteria for LTM use, and 189 (49%) fell in the non-LTM group (three IDU had missing data). Compared with non-LTM users on demographic and drug-use variables, LTM users are older, more often male, more often Dutch, and have lived longer in Amsterdam; they started injecting longer ago, and inject mainly heroin less often and cocaine, either by itself or with heroin, significantly more often. LTM users inject daily as often as non-LTM users. Frequency of borrowing and reuse of own needles and syringes are similar among LTM and non-LTM users. LTM users have a higher HIV prevalence (37%) than non-LTM users (20%; OR = 2.42, 95%CI = 1.54-3.83). There is a positive correlation between the number of years since the first methadone prescription and being HIV positive ($p = .005$). After controlling for possible confounders (demographic and drug-use variables), LTM-users had a slightly increased risk of HIV infection, which was not statistically significant (OR = 1.60, 95%CI = 0.93-2.74).

These results do not support the view that long-term, regular participation—as compared with short-term and irregular participation—in low-threshold methadone programs in Amsterdam is associated with less risky injecting behavior or with a decreased risk of HIV infection. This finding was confirmed in a study assessing risk factors for seroconversion to HIV (3). The behaviors of 31 seroconverters were compared with those of 202 seronegative injecting drug users (controls). Three independent risk factors for seroconversion were found in logistic regression: (a) living more than ten years in Amsterdam (OR = 2.45, 95%CI = 1.09-5.53); (b) first injecting less than or equal to 2 years ago (OR = 3.45, 95%CI = 1.20-9.81); and (c) injecting mainly at home (OR = 0.39, 95%CI = 0.18-0.88).

No evidence was found that receiving daily methadone at methadone posts reduced the chance of becoming infected with HIV. Neither did this study find evidence of a protective effect of obtaining needles and syringes via the exchange program, but data suggest that exchanging needles and syringes may have been protective at the start of the program. This latter finding is in agreement with an earlier study on the impact of the needle and syringe exchange program in Amsterdam on injecting behavior (6).

DISCUSSION OF SOME METHODOLOGICAL ASPECTS

Generally, one may say that little is known about the representativeness of the study samples of drug users and that the self-reports on injecting and sexual behavior may be unreliable (due to memory problems and answering biases, as people may have the tendency to respond in a socially desirable way) and are difficult to validate.

To assess the generalizability of the HIV prevalence in our study group, we conducted two other (anonymous) HIV prevalence studies among drug users in Amsterdam. In one study, IDU who had injected drugs recently were recruited 'on the streets,' and in the other study we recruited among clients of two methadone buses and one neighborhood methadone post of the drugs department of the Municipal Health Service in Amsterdam. It appeared that the prevalence found among participants of these two studies was not significantly different from the prevalence found among the participants of the cohort study. Also, the risk factors associated with HIV seropositivity in these two studies were very much comparable with the ones found in the cohort study.

The rather stable HIV seroprevalence that we found over the years, both for the crude prevalences and after attempting to correct for the influence of selection biases following from our sampling procedures, is difficult to interpret. Measuring the impact of behavior change by monitoring seroprevalence is especially difficult, because many factors that affect the general IDU population and are generally not well recorded have to be taken into account, for example, loss of seropositives for various reasons (mortality, hospitalization, moving, cessation of drug use, among others) and entrance of new seronegative injectors. It also appears from our data that a stable seroprevalence is still compatible with a rather high incidence.

Self-selection may also have occurred with respect to participation in the follow-up study. If taking part in the follow-up study is of more interest to those seronegative IDU that (continue to) behave riskfully and therefore run a higher risk of becoming infected with HIV, we may be overestimating the HIV incidence in IDU in Amsterdam when generalizing from this group. On the other hand, we have evidence that behavioral change did occur, especially in those drug users who took part in the follow-up study (2).

To evaluate the impact of prevention programs, a true experiment with random allocation of drug users to attendance or nonattendance of a program would be the best study design. However, this allocation would be in conflict with the harm reduction policy which includes accessibility of programs for all drug users. So, to evaluate the impact of the programs on risk reduction, we decided to compare self-selected attenders of a program with nonattenders. A problem with this design is that, in the beginning of a program, highly motivated drug users may attend. This may, when evaluating the program at that moment, result in the conclusion that the program is effective. However, the longer (low-threshold) programs exist, the more drug users may attend programs for other reasons than risk reduction. At the same time, health education messages may have reached drug users who then do not want to use the needle and syringe exchange program to obtain clean needles and syringes (highly motivated nonexchangers) but prefer to buy their needles and syringes at pharmacies and certain shops. These considerations may imply that the impact of a prevention program cannot be assessed by studying differences in risk behavior between attenders and nonattenders (neither in prevalence nor in incidence studies).

Part of the problems described above are not specific and therefore not limited to studies among drug users. However, there are some problems which are closely linked to the study group: compared with (longitudinal) studies among homosexual men, the data collection in studies among drug users is much less consistent. Follow-up visits of drug users are less regular, appointments are hardly kept, home addresses may change very frequently (if they have one), and participants are, for shorter or longer periods, often lost for follow-up, either because they are in (drug-free) treatment, or are in prison or, in the case of foreign drug users, have gone back to their own country. An allowance per follow-up visit is essential to encourage continued participation. Furthermore, close cooperation with the various assistance systems is also needed to trace the participants.

ACKNOWLEDGMENTS

The cohort study represents a collaborative effort between the Department of Public Health and Environment of the Municipal Health Service of Amsterdam, R.A. Coutinho and J.A.R. van den Hoek, project leaders; Department of Virology of the Academic Medical Center, University of Amsterdam, J. Goudsmit, project leader; Department of Clinical Viro-Immunology of the Central Laboratory of the Netherlands Red Cross Blood Transfusion Service and Laboratory for Experimental and Clinical Immunology, University of Amsterdam, F. Miedema, project leader. The cohort study is supported by the Netherlands Foundation for Preventive Medicine and the Ministry of Welfare, Health and Culture (WVC, Praeventiefonds).

REFERENCES

1. van den Hoek JAR, Coutinho RA, van Haastrecht HJA, van Zadelhoff AW, Goudsmit J. Prevalence and risk factors of HIV infections among drug users and drug-using prostitutes in Amsterdam. *AIDS* 1988;2(1):55–60.
2. van Haastrecht HJA, van den Hoek JAR, Bardoux C, Leentvaar-Kuijpers A, Coutinho RA. The course of the HIV epidemic among intravenous drug users in Amsterdam, The Netherlands. *Am J Public Health* 1991;81:59–62.
3. van Ameijden EJC, van den Hoek JAR, van Haastrecht HJA, Coutinho RA. The harm reduction approach and risk factors for HIV seroconversion in injecting drug users, Amsterdam. *Am J Epidemiol* 1992:156:236–243.
4. Hartgers C, van den Hoek JAR, Krijnen P, Coutinho RA. HIV prevalence and risk behavior among injecting drug users who participate in "low threshold" methadone programs in Amsterdam. *Am J Public Health* 1992;82:547–551.
5. van den Hoek JAR, van Haastrecht HJA, Coutinho RA. Risk reduction among intravenous drug users in Amsterdam under the influence of AIDS. *Am J Public Health* 1989;79:1355–1357.
6. Hartgers C, Buning EC, van Santen GW, Verster AD, Coutinho RA. The impact of the needle and syringe programme in Amsterdam on injecting behavior. *Aids* 1989;3:571–576.

DISCUSSION

Dr. Padian: One of your predictors was, "first injection less than 2 years ago." I'd like to know about more than 2 years ago.

Dr. van den Hoek: We took "less than 2 years ago" because we were interested in people who had started recently. We found that people who had started to inject less than 2 years previously had an increased risk for HIV infection, as has also been found in other studies.

Dr. Susser: Could you say more about the way you designated your intervention group versus controls in both studies? I am not clear about the differences in the characteristics of those who felt they were being fully exposed to treatment, and those who did not.

Dr. van den Hoek: The prevalence study compared long-term and shorter-term methadone users: Long-term methadone users had to report regular daily methadone use for the preceding 5 years; the other group consisted of those who had either been taking methadone for less than 5 years or who had been taking it irregularly over the 5 years. The data all came from self-reports, and we did not validate the methadone doses.

In the incidence study, we compared seroconverters with those who remained negative by looking at the behavior reported for the two previous periods: the mean frequency of exchanging needles (100%, 50% to 90%, and less than 50%), and daily versus nondaily methadone use.

Dr. Susser: So you exercised no other control, such as the date of entry into the program?

Dr. van den Hoek: We made comparisons in terms of the date of entry into the study, not the date of entry into the methadone program.

Dr. Biggar: Were any multivariate studies done and, if so, what were the results?

Dr. van den Hoek: Yes, multivariate studies were done. I showed you one from the prevalence study: the adjusted odds ratio for long-term methadone use, controlled for age, gender, nationality, the period of time spent living in Amsterdam, and the duration of injecting drug use. The same was also done in the second study. Only three variables were independently predictive of HIV seroconversion. We forced the exchange of needles and syringes, as well as the methadone program, into the model but we didn't find any effect.

Dr. Musicco: If I remember correctly, the odds ratio for methadone therapy in the first study was higher than one.

Dr. van den Hoek: It was 1.6.

Dr. Vlahov: In the study on methadone, was the outcome prevalent infection or seroconversion?

Dr. van den Hoek: In the first study it was prevalence data; in the second, incidence data.

Dr. Detels: I wonder if you may not have done yourself a disservice by saying that you didn't see an effect. It struck me that some of the differences in some of your groups were quite large. I wonder to what extent you actually had the power to be able to discern a difference. It might be useful to estimate the power that you had; if you didn't have the power, I don't think you can say there was no difference, just that you were unable to demonstrate it.

Dr. van den Hoek: Do you think that's also true for the first study?

Dr. Detels: Well, you showed that in non-Dutch subjects, the risk was 50% that of Dutch subjects; that's a two-fold difference. If you can't see it, that suggests that your power was very low.

Dr. Halloran: Could you speculate on what the factors "more than 10 years in Amsterdam" and "less than 2 years injecting" are surrogates for, and what is really going on in terms of dynamics? Why do you think that there is a higher incidence in people with less than 2 years injecting; is it that they use needles more or have different partners?

Dr. van den Hoek: Like others, we think that people who start injecting are often helped by other people, and so the chance of exchanging needles and syringes is much higher than in those who remain negative while they continue to inject. These people know how to do it and are less likely to borrow needles.

We are not completely sure of the meaning of the difference caused by living longer in Amsterdam, but we think that these people are probably much more involved with the scene of long-term drug usage, where the prevalence of HIV infection is quite high (40% to 50% in the long term). The people who have just entered the scene have less contact with the core of highly infective, long-term injecting drug users.

Dr. Moss: Over the last 5 years in San Francisco, we have done a seroconversion study in relation to the methadone maintenance treatment system. If you separate the people who had had more than a year's experience of methadone maintenance treatment at the time of recruitment from the others, there are major differences in their seroconversion rates. The seroconversion rate of the people on long-term maintenance treatment was 1% per year; taken as a whole, it was 4% per year in the others. I was surprised to find that a long-term history in the maintenance program provided such a strong protective effect.

Dr. van den Hoek: But you probably also found a difference in injecting behavior, which we didn't.

Dr. Moss: No, we found no difference in self-reported injecting behavior, or in other self-reported risk behaviors.

Dr. Friedman: It seems to me that one of the questions we should be thinking about at a methods-focused meeting is the extent to which the standard kinds of risk behavior, or the instruments we usually use, may not be fully capable of capturing what we are looking for. In New York, we are trying to study network variables, including trying to get sero-data to find out who's injecting with whom and so on (which is very difficult data to get). When we begin to consider why it is that new injectors in certain areas seem to seroconvert more than those in other geographic areas with different histories of the epidemic, we should be thinking about how we study social networks, and about other kinds of social behaviors, as well as mixing patterns and population dynamics (not to mention the questions we ask, like "how often do you . . . ?").

Dr. Musicco: You have presented some apparently disappointing data (for example, you did not find any relationship between syringe sharing and a sexual partner who was an intravenous drug user), but you did find that mainly injecting at home was a protective factor, perhaps implying that you have less opportunity of exchanging a syringe with a seropositive person. Some of your results may be due to the limited sensitivity of your questionnaire or the questions you asked.

Secondly, do you think that some of the results (particularly in your longitudinal study) may be explained by the fact that seropositivity at ascertainment was more intense in people who regularly followed the program? Or, because you are comparing people who attend your program in any case, is it that the contrast between regular and infrequent attenders is insufficient to demonstrate a difference? As Andrew Moss has said, when you compare attenders with nonattenders, a difference does exist.

Dr. van den Hoek: We didn't find that borrowing was a risk for seroconversion: 13 of our seroconverters didn't report borrowing needles. Of course, that may be answering bias, but it is also possible that they were telling the truth and that there may have been sexual transmission. Of these 13, 9 were women who reported having had sexual contacts. When we looked at the difference between new injecting partners and steady injecting partners, we did not find any association with HIV infection, although it may be that the answers to our questions are unreliable.

As far as attenders and nonattenders are concerned, most of the drug users in Amsterdam have attended a program for a longer or shorter period of time. So the only thing we could do was to compare regular with nonregular attenders, or people saying they had used methadone daily over a certain period with those who said that they hadn't.

Dr. Musicco: Isn't there a possibility that regular attenders were more investigated for seroconversion?

Dr. van den Hoek: No, I don't think so. The study was completely separate from the methadone program.

Dr. Nicolosi: Some of your findings are disappointing only in terms of the efficacy of needle exchange and the methadone program, and then only if they are looked at in comparison with other situations. But in intravenous drug user studies, there are remarkable differences from place to place. I noticed that, at the beginning of the program, there was evidence for a mildly protective effect in attenders as against nonattenders. What should perhaps be taken into consideration is that, at the beginning, there was a larger difference in behavior between attenders and nonattenders in Amsterdam; once word spread as to how the infection is transmitted, drug users became sensitized. Since it is easy for nonattenders to the needle exchange program to buy a new syringe in Amsterdam, it is possible that also they decreased the frequency of syringe sharing when they became aware of the risk of acquiring HIV infection. In Amsterdam you would expect to see a less dramatic effect of needle-exchange programs than in places where nonattenders cannot buy a new syringe without a prescription.

Another point is, you are talking about a low-threshold methadone program, but do you have any higher dose programs that you can use as a comparison?

Dr. van den Hoek: There are also high-threshold methadone programs in Amsterdam, in which the continuation of drug-using behavior is controlled by means of urine examinations. But all of our subjects were attending low-threshold programs, and they all continued to inject with the same frequency as people who were not on methadone.

Dr. Stein: I know you had only 31 incident cases, but 13 of them were women and 9 of them said they never borrowed. What was the male comparison? You know that they had sexual relations, but you don't know if they had sexual relations with drug users. It isn't at all unlikely that the pattern of getting sexually transmitted HIV is changing faster for women than for men, and so the greater number of conversions among women may have been due to noninjection factors.

Dr. van den Hoek: That's true, especially because 9 of the 13 people who said that they hadn't borrowed were women.

Dr. Stein: So, if you divide your converters into men and women, what was the proportion of nonborrowing men? Because the suggestion is that women are being increasingly affected by sexual transmission.

Dr. van den Hoek: I'd have to check that, but both papers have been published, so you could get more details there.

Dr. Gail: First I'd like to agree with what Roger Detels said about the sample size, because, with about 31 or 32 events, you might be able to pick up a three-fold relative risk, which was proving to be significant in your study.

Secondly, you mentioned the possibility that the high-risk people were differentially lost to follow-up or not lost to follow-up in the sero-incidence study. Have you tried to see whether high-risk people on long-term methadone maintenance were more or less likely to stay in continuous follow-up than those in the short-term methadone maintenance group? In other words, have you studied the factors influencing the completeness of follow-up in the two comparison groups?

Dr. van den Hoek: We haven't done that as yet, but it's a good point.

Dr. Vlahov: The point that was brought up by Nicolosi concerning low-dose versus high-dose [methadone programs] is interesting. There was a study by Diana Hartell at Columbia University in which she found quite a difference between high-dose and low-dose methadone.

Dr. van den Hoek: Can I add that a study on needle exchange has been done in England, and that they also found an initial protective effect which later disappeared?

Dr. Muñoz: Two factors are very powerful in your data, the constancy of both the prevalence and incidence rates. What were the changes over time of the percentage of those on short-term treatment; is it also constant?

Dr. van den Hoek: I don't know.

Dr. Friedman: To summarize, one issue is that, particularly in small population studies, you need to consider statistical power when you are evaluating something and you don't find the anticipated result.

Secondly, the validity of behavioral data is not a constant. At intake, we have considerable data indicating that it is pretty good with drug users; it's by no means perfect (it would flunk a lab test), but it's usable data. However, as people continue to have contact with studies, increased bias may develop; people in third or fourth follow-ups may try to change what they are saying for one reason or another. We have to find a way of measuring that.

The third issue involves "lost to follow-up" effects in cohort studies. The people from Abt Associates had a poster in Amsterdam in which they considered this in terms of some United States studies and showed that it is something which has to be taken very seriously, although their methods may not have been as good as the fact that they raised the question.

Fourthly, unmeasured variables. It seems to me that here we have a problem concerning the sexual and drug-use variables which aren't asked. For example, one risk factor we (and the Dutch) have discussed is this practice called frontloading, backloading, or drug sharing, where the drug passes through the syringe at some point in the measurement or mixing process. This simply wasn't measured. Other kinds of unmeasured variables are all of those related to the social network. It is always difficult to do incidence studies without becoming vulnerable to the problem of unmeasured variables. We simply have to learn which variables can be taken out of the questionnaires because they are not important, and which ones we should add.

The final point to be raised is the question of the unit of analysis. Many of our interventions are not really individual interventions only, but have a community impact. If it's possible, and if after a certain period of attendance you don't want to use syringe exchange, you may open up an easy way and get it at your pharmacy. What we really need to do is to find ways in which we can carry out studies in which the community is the unit of analysis. The other thing is that certain people will be in saturated networks, and certain people won't. We may never be able to find ways of measuring that, but if you get enough communities in a series of studies and follow them over time, and then see which ones stabilize where, as a function of what is going on inside those communities. . . . We'll probably never have it at a 0.05 level, given the resources that we get, but we can still learn an awful lot.

HIV Epidemiology: Models and Methods, edited by Alfredo Nicolosi. Raven Press, Ltd., New York © 1994.

2

The NISDA Study

Methods and Results of a Longitudinal Study of HIV Seroconversion

*†Alfredo Nicolosi, *Maria Léa Corrêa Leite, *Alberto Osella, and ‡Adriano Lazzarin

**Department of Epidemiology and Medical Informatics, Institute of Advanced Biomedical Technologies, National Research Council, 20131 Milan, Italy; †G.H. Sergievsky Center, Columbia University, New York 10032; ‡Institute of Infectious Diseases, University of Milan, IRCCS Ospedale S. Raffaele, 20100 Milan, Italy*

This paper is structured in two parts. I shall first present and discuss the main results of the Northern Italian Seronegative Drug Addicts (NISDA) study. Then, we will see the comparison of different models of analysis of longitudinal studies in the presence of time-dependent variables, as applied to this NISDA data.

The contribution of epidemiology to the understanding of HIV infection has been crucial ever since the detection of the epidemic. At the beginning, it led to the search for a virus; after the etiologic agent was discovered, it described—and still does—the natural history of the disease; and it has identified the mechanisms of transmission and risk-associated behaviors. The methodology applied to HIV infection presents peculiar features, in that the complexity of the disease requires the application of epidemiologic tools used in the study of degenerative diseases as well as those used in the study of infectious diseases. During the process of research, several problems have emerged, and potential biases from a number of possible sources have been identified.

AIDS was recognized in 1981 to 1982, and HIV was isolated and linked to AIDS in 1983 to 1984 (that is, less than 10 years ago). The first wave of epidemiologic research was obviously limited by the fact that we had only prevalent cases and limited follow-up times. There are now longitudinal studies on incident cases, which have partially confirmed and partially corrected the results of previous studies carried out on prevalent cases.

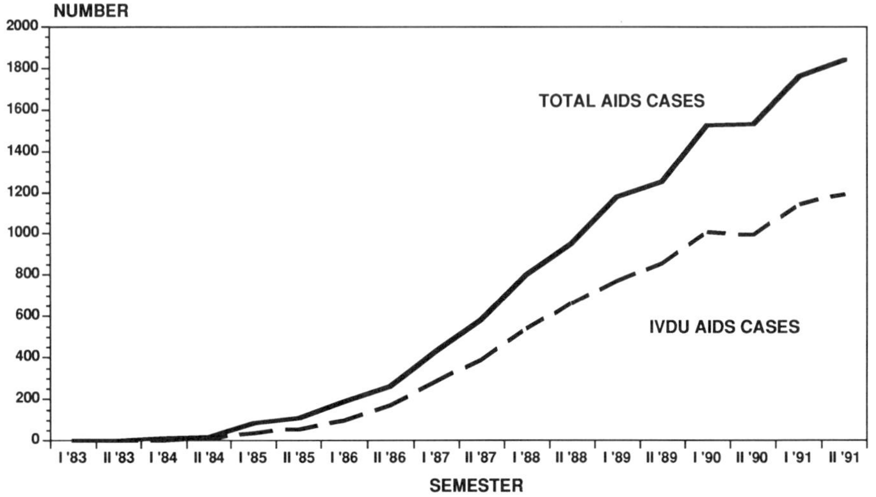

FIG. 1. The AIDS epidemic in Italy: total cases (————) and cases associated with intravenous drug use (-----).

The first case of AIDS in an intravenous drug user (IVDU) in Italy was diagnosed in the second half of 1983 (Fig. 1). It became clear that IVDUs represented the population most affected by AIDS in 1985. Now, IVDUs account for 70% of the AIDS cases. The number of IVDUs attending drug-dependence treatment centers increased from 13,905 in 1985 to 61,976 in 1990. New clients increased from 2,449 in 1985 to 18,209 in 1990. The number of deaths due to overdose increased from 196 in 1985 to 973 in 1990. The temporal patterns of other indices (the number of individuals arrested on drug-related charges and the number of young men not accepted into the Armed Forces because of IVDU) also show an increasing trend.

THE NISDA STUDY

The NISDA study is a prospective study involving HIV-negative IVDUs attending drug-dependence treatment centers, who are being followed to study the incidence and risk factors of HIV infection. The study covers the city of Milan and a number of other geographic areas in Northern Italy, where the prevalence of HIV infection among IVDUs varies from 17% to 80%. The study is based on a dynamic cohort in which the enrollment is continuous over time and there is an inevitable degree of losses to follow-up. We started to recruit subjects on January 1, 1987, and by December 31, 1991, 1,761 seronegative IVDUs (1,394 male, 367 female) had been enrolled (Fig. 2).

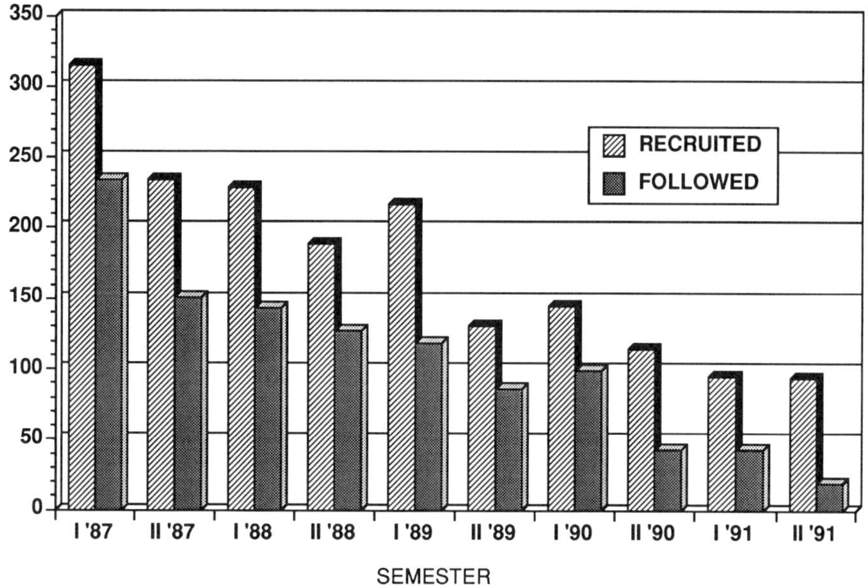

FIG. 2. Intravenous drug users recruited (*shaded*) and followed (*stippled*) in the NISDA study, by semester, 1987–1991.

The methods of enrollment and follow-up have been described in detail elsewhere (1). Briefly, IVDUs arriving at the treatment centers were asked their consent to participate in the study and then tested for HIV antibodies; the seronegative subjects were enrolled, examined, and interviewed by the attending physicians. Participants were then invited to follow-up visits, during which they were again tested and interviewed.

The occurrence of HIV infection was estimated in terms of incidence rate (the number of seroconversions divided by the number of person-years of follow-up) (2). The date of seroconversion was assumed to be midway between that of the visit at which the seroconversion was detected and the last visit at which the subject was negative for anti-HIV antibodies. Prevalence rates were calculated by dividing the number of individuals found to be HIV-positive by the number of subjects tested by the treatment center each year (almost 90% of all attending IVDUs).

In the follow-up analysis, incidence rate ratios (IRR) were estimated on the basis of the ratio between the incidence rates in exposed and unexposed subjects, the exposure variables being derived from the enrollment visit (3). In case-control analysis, exposure was classified on the basis of the experience of the entire follow-up as assessed at the last visit (e.g., for syringe sharing: never shared, do not share but used to share, rarely share, often share). Exposure information was acquired before the individual's HIV status was known. In this analysis, the seroconverters were the "cases" and the remaining seronegative subjects the "controls;" odds ratios (OR) were then calculated (4). Logistic regression analysis was used to control for confounding factors (5).

Incidence Rates of HIV Infection

A total of 1,063 subjects (60% of enrolled subjects) were followed for an average of 17.4 months. During follow-up, 63 seroconversions were observed. The seroconversion rate decreased from 6.3% in 1987 to 4.3% in 1991 (Table 1).

Since this study was based on a dynamic cohort, we were able to study the trends in risk behaviors over time among IVDUs at the moment of enrollment into the study. From January 1, 1987, to December 31, 1991, there were no changes in the frequency of IVDU at recruitment, whereas there was a progressive decline in the frequency of syringe sharing (from just under 80% to a little over 50%), possibly due to general anti-AIDS information and educational campaigns (Fig. 3). I would like to remind you that syringes are sold cheaply and without prescription in Italy. The frequency of syringe sharing dramatically decreased among followed subjects independently of the year of enrollment. This decrease was partly due to those who stopped injecting altogether and partly to those who continued injecting but reduced their frequency of syringe sharing.

The prevalence of HIV infection among IVDUs attending detoxification centers in different geographic areas was variable (range 17% to 80%). We studied the incidence rates among seronegative individuals in relation to the local baseline prevalence of infection. The areas were grouped in three strata of prevalence (less than 30%, 30% to 60%, and more than 60%). High incidence rates were found in areas where prevalence was high, and vice versa (6,7). This is the empirical demonstration of what would be expected, since

TABLE 1. *Incidence rate in a cohort of seronegative intravenous drug users 1987–1991*

Year	HIV+[a]	P-Y[b]	IR[c]	95% CI[d]
1987	13	207.2	6.3	3.3–10.7
1988	16	392.1	4.1	2.3–6.7
1989	13	427.2	3.0	1.6–5.2
1990	14	354.0	4.0	2.2–6.6
1991	7	163.6	4.3	1.7–8.9

[a]HIV-positive.
[b]Person-years.
[c]Incidence rate per 100 person-years.
[d]Ninety-five percent confidence interval.

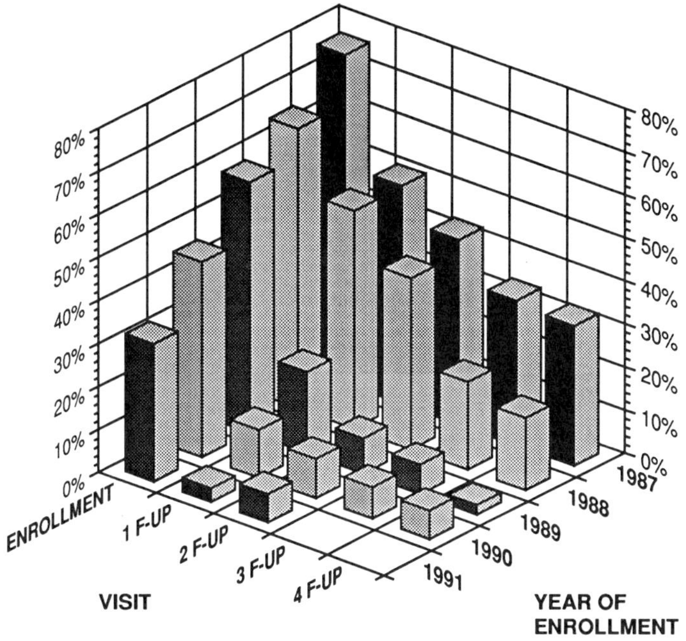

FIG. 3. Frequency of syringe sharing in IVDUs enrolled and followed in successive years.

prevalence reflects the diffusion of the virus in the local IVDU population and the probability that a used syringe or sexual partner is infected.

The incidence rate was 3.9 per 100 person-years (P-Y) in males and 4.7 in females, the rates being higher in younger subjects and in those with a shorter duration of i.v. drug use (Table 2). Incidence rates were higher in occasional users (IR = 8.4) and lower in users who injected at least once a day (IR = 3.4). The incidence of HIV infection in those reporting syringe sharing at enrollment was more than double that of those not sharing (8). To examine the role of heterosexual transmission, we compared the crude incidence rates of HIV infection of males and females according to the presence or absence of an IVDU or HIV-positive partner. In comparison with men, the relative risk of seroconversion of women not reporting sexual partners (RR = 0.8) was about half that of women reporting an IVDU (RR = 1.9) or known HIV-positive partner (RR = 1.6), although the estimates did not reach statistical significance.

Syringe Sharing: Cohort and Period Effects

Since our findings concerning the risks associated with young age and short IVDU contrast with those of cross-sectional studies (9-14) we decided

TABLE 2. *Incidence rate of HIV infection in intravenous drug users, 1987–1991*

	Conversions	P-Y	IR
Gender			
male	47	1204.98	3.9
female	16	339.18	4.7
Age			
<20	7	132.48	5.3
20–24	36	676.12	5.3
25–29	13	442.53	2.9
≥30	7	292.38	2.4
Years of i.v. drug use			
<2	20	287.99	6.9
2–5	21	480.95	4.4
6–10	11	377.90	2.9
>10	7	314.53	2.2
History of heroin use			
constant	33	963.21	3.4
periodic	15	317.70	4.7
occasional	13	155.04	8.4
History of syringe sharing			
yes	50	1065.11	4.7
no	13	479.05	2.7

to analyze this issue further. The increased risk of HIV infection for young subjects with a short duration of IVDU experience can probably be explained by their higher frequency of syringe sharing. It is a fact that IVDUs are more likely to share injecting equipment during the earlier periods of their i.v. drug use (when they are also younger) (15).

We considered the frequency of syringe sharing for different birth cohorts and different starting ages of i.v. drug use (Table 3). From the row totals we see that the frequency of syringe sharing was lower in the younger generations (from 67.8% to 52.9%). However, this finding alone does not necessarily mean that individuals who started injecting at a younger age have a lower frequency of syringe sharing than those starting at older ages, because it

TABLE 3. *Frequency (%) of syringe sharing at enrollment: cohort and period analysis, 1987–1991*

	Year of start of i.v. drug use							
Year of birth	72–74	75–77	78–80	81–83	84–86	87–89	90–91	Row totals
52–54	*69.5*	**83.3**	*85.7*	**33.3**	25	66	0	67.8
55–57	**69.5**	*74.2*	**62.5**	*70.5*	**50**	80	0	66.6
58–60	*70*	**68.5**	*72.7*	**65.5**	*62.1*	**33.3**	0	65.8
61–63	50	*87.5*	**71.6**	*67.2*	**45.4**	*34.8*	**14.2**	60.6
64–66	0	100	*69.3*	**68.8**	*57.6*	**58.1**	*33.3*	61.7
67–69	0	0	60	*71.7*	**67.9**	*49.1*	**12.5**	56.2
70–72	0	0	0	0	*56.2*	**61.9**	27.2	52.9
Column totals	68.9	76.6	70.7	67.5	58.2	51.8	20.6	

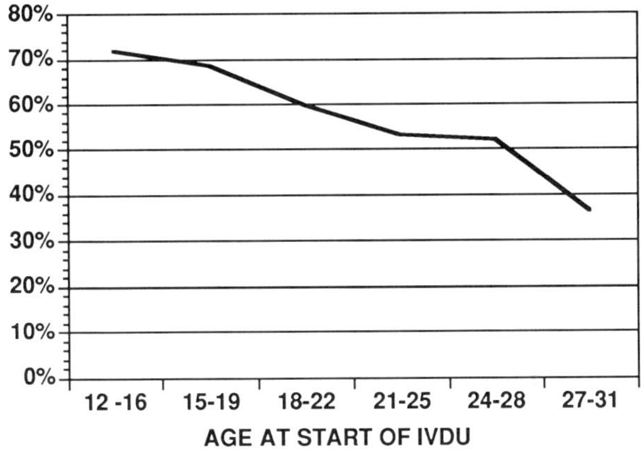

FIG. 4. Frequency of syringe sharing by age at start of intravenous drug use.

also reflects the time-period effect. As can be seen, the decrease in the frequency of syringe sharing is even greater when we consider the year of starting i.v. drug use regardless of age (from 68.9% in those starting in 1972 to 1974 to 20.6% in those starting in 1990 to 1991). To evaluate the effect of age at the start of i.v. drug use on the frequency of syringe sharing separately from the effects of time period and birth cohort, we used the data within Table 3. The diagonal lines define the cells representing the frequency of sharing among individuals who began injecting at the same age (although with some overlap) but in different time periods. If we calculate the average frequency of syringe sharing for each of the age groups (represented by the diagonal lines), we obtain the age group prevalence of syringe sharing, stratified for cohort and period effects. The results are shown in Fig. 4. The history of syringe sharing was 72% among individuals who started i.v. drug

TABLE 4. *Risk of HIV infection by frequency of syringe sharing and seropositive sexual partners*

	HIV-[a]	HIV+	OR[b]	95% CI
		Syringe sharing		
never shared	230	6	1	
quit	387	7	0.7	0.2–2.1
still sharing	238	33	5.3	2.4–11.9
		HIV-seropositive sexual partner		
never had	711	32	1	
quit	92	7	1.7	0.7–3.9
still has	52	7	3	1.3–6.8

[a]HIV-negative.
[b]Odds ratio.

TABLE 5. *Parenteral and sexual transmission*

	HIV+	HIV−	OR	95% CI
	Not syringe sharing			
Sex partner not HIV+	9	566	1	
Sex partner HIV+	1	24	2.7	0.3–23.4
	Syringe sharing			
Sex partner not HIV+	23	202	9.0	3.9–212.0
Sex partner HIV+	6	26	15.1	4.7–48.6

use before they were 17 years old, progressively declining to 36% in subjects who started i.v. drug use when they were almost 30 years old. These results demonstrate that young age is always a risk indicator for HIV infection, because it is strongly associated with a higher probability of sharing used, infected syringes.

Parenteral and Sexual Transmission

To study the role of parenteral and sexual transmission more accurately, we used a different method of analysis. A case-control analysis was nested inside the longitudinal study, allowing exposure to be categorized on the basis of the entire follow-up experience (16). Logistic regression was used to control for age, sex, geographic area, and prevalence (Table 4). The risk associated with syringe sharing was only present in subjects who continued sharing syringes (OR = 5.3), thus revealing the importance of using an appropriate time window for exposure.

A significant risk for HIV infection was also detected in the sexual partners of HIV-seropositive individuals. The odds ratio (3.0 in current partners) has been adjusted for syringe sharing and represents only sexual transmission. In another analysis, the risk was highest (OR = 15.1) in subjects who reported both syringe sharing and sexual contacts with HIV-positive individuals (Table 5).

MODELING TIME-DEPENDENT EXPOSURE

The characteristics of HIV infection and the behavior of IVDUs both give rise to methodological problems. The precise moment of infection is unknown because it is not possible to test each individual every day. Furthermore, as in most follow-up studies where participation is voluntary, the length of the intervals between visits varies. Another factor is that ELISA tests may remain negative for up to 6 months after the moment of infection (17). All we know is that detectable anti-HIV antibodies appeared between the last negative and the first positive test.

Analysis of the risk factors for the parenteral or sexual transmission of HIV has to take into account behavioral variables that change over time. During follow-up, it is possible that one participant who reported syringe sharing at the second visit says he did not share a single syringe between the second and the third visit, and then reports sharing at the fourth (Fig. 5). Similar time-dependent changes can be seen in relation to sexual exposure and nonexposure.

So, at the same time, we have a time-dependent exposure variable and different lengths of time between visits. As an exercise, we compared these different intervals using different definitions and statistical models. Since this is an example, we estimated the risk for HIV infection associated with syringe sharing using only two covariates, the year of birth and the year of beginning i.v. drug use.

Definition of Intervals

The goal of interval definition is to catch any changes in the exposure variable. We compared four interval definitions and ran three statistical models for each of them.

Firstly, we defined the intervals in such a way that they would coincide with any change in the exposure status of any subject during the entire follow-up. Forty-one "exact" intervals of this type were calculated (Table 6), which turned out to be of exactly 1 month until the 31st interval. Although

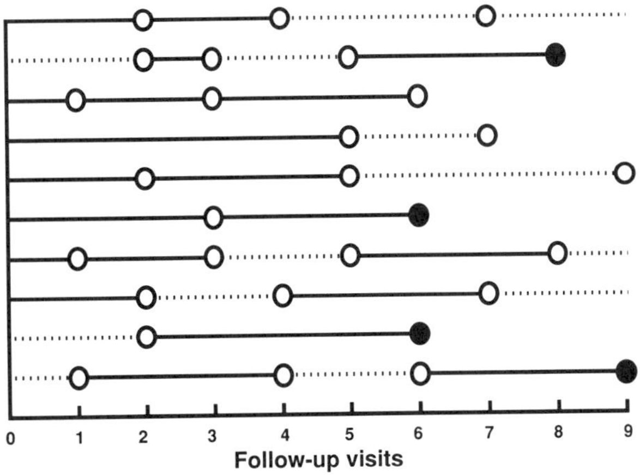

FIG. 5. Follow-up study with time-dependent exposure. Each line represents one individual, observed from time 0 (recruitment) through 9 (follow-up visits). The circles represent one visit (white when HIV test is negative and black in seroconversions). The line patterns indicate exposure status: continuous for syringe sharing, dotted for not sharing.

TABLE 6. *Interval stratification*

	Date of birth			
	1960–65 Date of start of i.v. drug use			
	≤1982 Sharing		>1982 Sharing	
Interval	No	Yes	No	Yes
1	124	98	167	89
2	124	97	167	89
3	123	97	165	88
4	119	96	151	76
5	119	85	151	76
.	.	.	.	.
.	.	.	.	.
.	.	.	.	.
41	4	2	3	1

Note: Layout of person-month intervals (sharing and not sharing syringes) stratified by birth cohort (born before 1960, between 1960 and 1965, and after 1965) and year of start of i.v. drug use (before and after 1982). The cells represent the person-time of individuals, born between 1960 and 1965 and IVDUs before and after 1982, who were and were not sharing syringes at each interval. The table is completed by two analogous tables, for individuals born before 1960 and those born after 1965, for a total of 450 cells.

this definition was the only one that exactly caught all of the changes in exposure over time, a 1-month interval has a limited overlap with the duration of the latency of infection. Furthermore, these calculations were very time consuming; this model involved 450 cells.

A second interval was arbitrarily fixed at 3 months. The number of cells was less (148 cells), but because not all of the changes in exposure were caught, we had to make an assumption about subjects who were both exposed and nonexposed during the same period. We decided to make an arbitrary but conservative choice, and considered the exposed subjects to be all those who were exposed during at least part of the time interval (although we understood that the bias would lead to an underestimation of the risk). On the other hand, a 3-month interval is a more reasonable approximation than that of 1 month in relation to the latent period of the infection.

As a further alternative definition of fixed intervals, we considered 6 months, which is a biologically plausible interval and greatly reduced the number of cells (80 cells).

Finally, we used the most natural intervals, those determined by the actual length of the time intervals between visits. The number of cells was very close to that of the 6-month definition (83 cells).

Alternative Statistical Models

The proportional hazards model (Cox regression analysis) is often used in the analysis of longitudinal studies (18):

$$\lambda(t;x) = \lambda_0(t)\exp\left(\sum_{i=1}^{k} \beta_i x_i\right) \qquad \text{or} \qquad \log \lambda(t;x) = \log \lambda_0(t) + \sum_{i=1}^{k} \beta_i x_i$$

In this model, $\lambda(t;x)$ is the instantaneous event rate at time t expressed as a function of the risk factors. Lambda zero is the underlying rate when the risk factors are set to zero. However, this form of the proportional hazards model considers continuous rather than grouped events, and is not appropriate to the data at hand when the events occur within an interval of time (between visits).

In order to analyze grouped events, the proportional hazards model takes the following from, where α_l is equal to the log of the integral of the underlying rate in the interval from time t to time $t+1$:

$$\log\left[-\log\left(1-p_l\right)\right] = \alpha_l + \Sigma \beta_i x_i$$

The left hand expression of this model is called the complementary log(-log) transform. This is the first of the three models we compared (19).

The second one is the logistic model, which lends itself to the analysis of grouped events when the exact date of onset is unknown, and it is widely used:

$$\text{logit}(p_l) = \log\left[p_l/(1-p_l)\right] = \alpha_l + \Sigma \beta_i x_i$$

The third and last of our comparative models was the log-linear model, which derives from the proportional hazards model when the underlying hazard rate is constant $[\lambda(t) = \lambda]$.

$$\lambda(t;x) = \lambda_0 \exp\left(\sum_{i=1}^{k} \beta_i x_i\right) \qquad \text{or} \qquad \log \lambda(t;x) = \sum_{i=0}^{k} \beta_i x_i$$

In this model, we defined the dependent variable as the observed rate (number of cases per person-time), following a Poisson distribution (20).

Comparison of Intervals and Models

For the 1-month interval, the three models produced almost identical estimates (Table 7). Estimates were a little lower and no longer equal when the 3-month interval was used. With an interval of 6 months, all of the models showed a decrease in risk estimates. In the follow-up interval, the log-linear model yielded an average estimate, while the other two models yielded an estimate which was even lower.

TABLE 7. *Comparison of models*

	Log-linear	Log-log	Logistic
Interval = 1 mo.; Cells = 450			
Deviance (44 df)	88.0	88.4	88.5
Coefficient	1.578	1.584	1.592
Relative risk	4.8	4.9	4.9
Interval = 3 mo.; Cells = 148			
Deviance (16 df)	59.9	63.4	63.5
Coefficient	1.528	1.562	1.580
Relative risk	4.6	4.8	4.9
Interval = 6 mo.; Cells = 80			
Deviance (10 df)	44.2	45.84	45.93
Coefficient	1.350	1.394	1.418
Relative risk	3.9	4.0	4.1
Interval = F-UP[a]; Cells = 83			
Deviance (11 df)	48.0	41.24	41.3
Coefficient	1.452	1.321	1.348
Relative risk	4.3	3.7	3.8

Note: The deviance refers to the variability explained by the model; the coefficient and the relative risk are estimates of HIV infection for individuals sharing syringes.
[a]Follow-up.

The difference between the log-linear model and the other two models is that the log-linear model assumes a Poisson distribution and uses person-time in the intervals. The log(-log) and the logistic models assume a binomial distribution, and so each cell counts as one individual, regardless of whether the subject remained for only a fraction of the interval. The models give virtually identical results if we use the variable person-time as binomial denominator in the log(-log) and logistic models.

In summary, it seems reasonable to use observed visits to define exposure intervals. Furthermore, the choice of a parsimonious model (with a moderate number of intervals) leads to a better fit, because it avoids the need for a number of cells greatly exceeding the number of cases. The three statistical models are equivalent, especially if the incidence rate is low (21). The Poisson log-linear model gives more consistent estimates because it uses person-time as the denominator.

Figure 6 shows the survival curves derived from the Poisson model. These curves show the probability of remaining seronegative up to the eighth follow-up visit, corresponding to 45 months of follow-up. The upper curve refers to nonsyringe sharing subjects born before 1960, who became IVDUs before 1982. The lower curve represents syringe sharing subjects born after 1965, who became IVDUs before 1982. This survival analysis shows that the incidence of HIV infection is higher in the earlier period of i.v. drug use, which is also associated with young age.

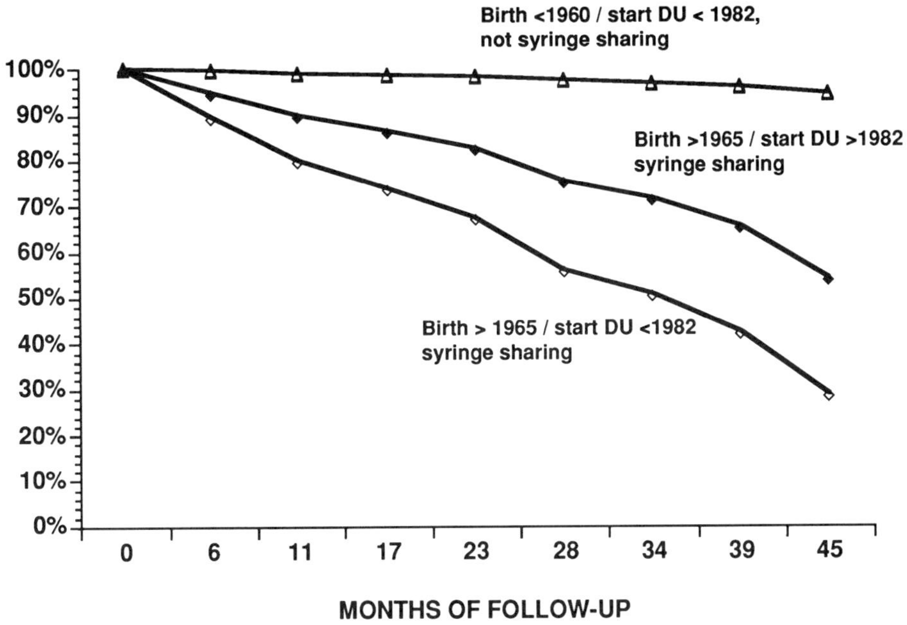

FIG. 6. Probability of remaining HIV-free according to syringe sharing, year of birth, and year of starting i.v. drug use, from the Poisson log-linear model.

CONCLUSIONS

The risk estimates of the NISDA study are higher than those reported by other studies of HIV infection in intravenous drug users (22-28) because of the differences between prospective and cross-sectional studies, as well as questions of misclassification and confounding. We studied incidence cases who were interviewed about their behavior immediately preceding or around the moment of seroconversion. This study design reduced the extent of exposure misclassification in comparison with that associated with cross-sectional studies; the time of seroconversion of prevalence cases is unknown, and consequently the behavioral data used to measure exposure do not refer to the behavior of individuals at the actual time of the infection. The case-control approach used in the analysis of this prospective study achieved a more refined classification of exposure levels by taking into account the fact that, in seronegative individuals, recent behaviors are more important in determining the risk of acquiring HIV infection than past habits. Parenteral and sexual transmission were studied simultaneously, controlling for other factors (such as the geographic prevalence of HIV) that affect the risk of both syringe sharing and sexual transmission. Finally, the restriction of sexual transmission to partners of known HIV-positive subjects allowed more accurate risk estimates than those provided by studies where exposure is assessed in more generic terms ("intravenous drug user partner").

PARTICIPANTS IN THE NISDA STUDY AND THEIR AFFILITATIONS

Angela Anfossi, Luca Gutierrez, Alessandro Garibaldi (USSL 73, Novi Ligure), Maurizio Amendola, Mariangela Autelitano, Danilo Ciaci, Alberto Osella (Istituto di Tecnologie Biomediche Avanzate, CNR, Milano), Claudio Arici, Giovanna Gavazzeni (Reparto Malattie Infettive, Ospedali Riuniti, Bergamo), Giorgio Bono, Silvia Molinari (Clinica Neurologica Mondino, Pavia), Anna Maria Camisani (USSL 51, Cremona), Maurizio Cefis (Centro Trasfusionale, Ospedale di Cassano d'Adda), Laura Ciaffi, Alberto Saracco (Clinica delle Malattie Infettive, Universita di Milano), Fabrizio Ciambelli, Alberto Schizzarotto (USSL 6, Gallarate), Edoardo Cozzolino, Rosa Pagani (USSL 59, Trezzo d'Adda), Virgilio Cruccu, Cristina Grondona (Ospedale Fatebenefratelli, Milano), Renato Durello (Ospedale di Bollate), Maurizio Fea (USSL 77, Pavia), Sergio Fonzi, Tiziano Miglierina, Italo Nessi (USSL 2, Cittiglio), Patrizio Frattini (USSL 1, Luino), Giovanni Guerra, Enrico Ximenes (USSL 56, Ospedale di Lodi), Silvano Lopez (Ospedale di Abbiategrasso), Guido Loretu, Vincenzo Marino (USSL 4, Arcisate), Giuliana Mamolo, Claudio Tosetto (USSL 3, Varese), Corrado Mattoni (USSL 59, Cassano D'Adda), Massimo Memoli, Antonio Prestini (CAD, Milano), Maria Merlo (USSL 9, Saronno), Piero Ronchi (NOT, Treviglio), Bernardino Salassa, Maria Luisa Soranzo (Ospedale Amedeo di Savoia, Torino), Vincenzo Stefano, Davide Vecellini (USSL 8, Busto Arsizio), Carlo Storer (USSL 57, Ospedale Predabissi, Vizzolo Predabissi), Dario Valsecchi (USSL 22, Sondrio), Claudio Velati (Ospedale di Bollate), Luisa Zampini (Ambulatorio Farmacodipendenze, Ospedale Sacco, Milano), Glorian Zapparoli (Zona 8, Milano).

ACKNOWLEDGMENTS

This research was supported in part by grants from the National Research Council of Italy (Progetto Finalizzato CNR "FATMA") and from the Ministry of Health (Instituto Superiore di Sanità—Progetto AIDS).

REFERENCES

1. Nicolosi A, Molinari S, Musicco M, et al. Positive modifications of injecting behavior among intravenous heroin users from Milan and Northern Italy, 1987–1989. *Br J Addict* 1991;86:91–102.
2. MacMahon B, Pugh TF. *Epidemiology: principles and methods*. Boston: Little, Brown & Co.; 1970.

3. Rothman KJ. *Modern epidemiology*. Boston: Little, Brown & Co.; 1986.
4. Miettinen OS. *Theoretical epidemiology: principles of occurrence research in medicine*. New York: John Wiley & Sons; 1985.
5. Schlesselman JJ. *Case-control studies: design, conduct, analysis*. New York: Oxford University Press; 1982:227–90.
6. Nicolosi A, Lazzarin A, for the NISDA Study. HIV seroconversion rates in intravenous drug abusers from Northern Italy [Letter]. *Lancet* 1989;ii:269.
7. Nicolosi A, Corrêa Leite ML, Musicco M, Molinari S, Saracco A, Lazzarin A. Prevalence and incidence trends of HIV infection in intravenous drug users attending treatment centers in Milan and Northern Italy, 1986–1990. *J Acquir Immune Defic Syndr* 1992;5:365–373.
8. Nicolosi A, Musicco M, Saracco A, et al. Incidence and risk factors of HIV infection: a prospective study of seronegative drug abusers from Milan and Northern Italy, 1987–1989. *Epidemiology* 1990;1:453–59.
9. Sasse H, Salmaso S, Conti S, and the First Drug User Multicenter Study Group. Risk behaviors for HIV-1 infection in Italian drug users: report from a multicenter study. *J Aquir Immune Defic Syndr* 1989;2:486–96.
10. Schoenbaum EE, Hartel D, Selwyn PA, et al. Risk factors for human immunodeficiency virus infection in intravenous drug users. *N Engl J Med* 1989;321:874–79.
11. Koblin BA, McCusker J, Lewis BF, et al. Racial/ethnic differences in HIV-1 seroprevalence and risky behaviors among intravenous drug users in a multisite study. *Am J Epidemiol* 1990;132:837–46.
12. Serraino D, Franceschi S, Vaccher E, et al. Risk factors for human immunodeficiency virus infection in 581 intravenous drug users, Northeast Italy, 1984–1988. *Int J Epidemiol* 1991;20:264–70.
13. Robles RR, Colòn HM, Sahai H, Matos TD, Marrero CA, Reyes JC. Behavioral risk factors and human immunodeficiency virus (HIV) prevalence among intravenous drug users in Puerto Rico. *Am J Epidemiol* 1992;135:531–40.
14. Papaevangelou G, Richardson C, Ancelle-Park, for the European Community Study Group on HIV in IDU. Factors associated with HIV seropositivity in European injecting drug users. Presented at the International Conference on AIDS, Amsterdam, The Netherlands, 1992 (abstract PuC 8170).
15. Turner CF, Miller HG, Moses LE. *AIDS: sexual behavior and intravenous drug use*. Washington, DC: National Academy Press; 1989.
16. Nicolosi A, Corrêa Leite ML, Musicco M, Molinari S, Lazzarin A. Parenteral and sexual transmission of human immunodeficiency virus in intravenous drug users: a study of seroconversion. *Am J Epidemiol* 1992;135:225–233.
17. Horsburg GR Jr, Citin YO, Jason J, Holmberg SD, et al. Duration of immunodeficiency virus infection before detection of antibody. *Lancet* 1989;ii:637–640.
18. Cox DR. Regression models and life tables. *J R Stat Soc B* 1972;34:187–220.
19. Abbott RD. Logistic regression in survival analysis. *Am J Epidemiol* 1985;121:405–71.
20. Frome EL, Checkoway H. Use of Poisson regression models in estimating incidence rates and ratios. *Am J Epidemiol* 1985;121:309–23.
21. Green MS, Symons MJ. A comparison of the logistic risk function and the proportional hazards model in prospective epidemiologic studies. *J Chron Dis* 1983;36:715–24.
22. Chaisson RE, Moss AR, Onishi R, et al. Human immunodeficiency virus infection in heterosexual intravenous drug users in San Francisco. *Am J Public Health* 1987;77:169–72.
23. van den Hoek JA, Coutinho RA, van Haastrecht HJA, et al. Prevalence and risk factors of HIV infections among drug users and drug-using prostitutes in Amsterdam. *AIDS* 1988;2:55–60.
24. Rezza G, Titti F, Tempesta E, et al. Needle sharing and other behaviours related to HIV spread among intravenous drug users. *AIDS* 1989;3:243–48.
25. Vlahov D, Muñoz A, Anthony JC, et al. Association of drug injection patterns with antibody to human immunodeficiency virus type 1 among intravenous drug users in Baltimore, Maryland. *Am J Epidemiol* 1990;132:847–56.
26. Friedland G. Parenteral drug users. In: Kaslow RA, Francis DP, eds. *The epidemiology of AIDS*. New York: Oxford University Press; 1989:153–78.
27. Des Jarlais DC, Friedman SR, Stoneburner RL. HIV infection and intravenous drug

use: critical issues in transmission dynamics, infection outcomes, and prevention. *Rev Infect Dis* 1988;10:151–58.
28. Battjes RJ, Pickens RW, Amsel Z, et al. Heterosexual transmission of human immunodeficiency virus among intravenous drug users. *J Infect Dis* 1990;162:1007–11.

DISCUSSION

Dr. Padian: On the one hand, it seems that there is a higher risk for seroconversion among younger people and recent users; on the other (if I understand correctly), it seems that the younger the subject, and the more recently he has begun using drugs, the less likely he is to share.

Dr. Nicolosi: If you take each variable separately, there is an association: the younger you are, the more likely you are to share; the longer you have been injecting, the less likely you are to share. But of course, these variables become mixed over time. If you only take the generation effect, the members of the younger generation share less because there is also a period effect. And, when we control for period and birth cohort, you see that syringe sharing decreases with advancing age at start of intravenous drug use.

Dr. Piot: Was there any intervention built into your study? If so, what was it, and how was it applied throughout the different centers?

Dr. Nicolosi: The intervention was carried out mainly because of ethical reasons. We were HIV testing and counseling for the study, and we informed the subjects about risk behaviors and recommended that they shouldn't share syringes, should use condoms, and so on. But intervention was not the point of the study; it was given to everybody, and there was no built-in comparison.

Dr. van den Hoek: Can you explain what methadone programs there are in Italy?

Dr. Nicolosi: In Italy, there is a detoxication program rather than just a methadone program. When people go to drug-dependence treatment centers, the physician chooses the most appropriate treatment for the individual (e.g., pharmacological without methadone, methadone, opioid-antagonists, psychological counseling, or mixed treatments). Methadone is not the primary treatment; in the same treatment center, there are people who use methadone and people who use other or combined treatments. We have made an analysis which showed that methadone patients are older, have a longer history of drug use, and share syringes less frequently.

Dr. van den Hoek: What I mean is, were the studied people in the methadone program also involved in the follow-up, or was it possible to participate in the follow-up study without following a methadone program?

Dr. Nicolosi: All of the people in the follow-up continued attending the center because, although the situation is now better, for a long time there was a waiting list to enter a detoxication center. Once somebody was accepted, he didn't like to drop out because he would have to go back on the waiting list.

Dr. van den Hoek: So people who drop out of the methadone program also dropped out of your study?

Dr. Nicolosi: That is correct.

Dr. Biggar: To go back to Anneke's data, that roughly 30% of the people who seroconverted apparently had no borrowing history (and the fact that it has been suggested that this is more common in females); if you stratified your data and only looked at males, would you enhance your power to detect something with respect to borrowing? I assume that the relative risk among males is much higher.

Dr. Nicolosi: We stratified males and females according to the status of their partners, and we saw that there was a higher incidence in men than in women among persons who did not report sexual contacts with seropositive partners or other IDUs, whereas there was a higher incidence in women than in men among persons who did report sexual contacts with seropositive partners or other IDUs. This leads us to suppose that HIV transmission is mostly parenteral among men.

Dr. Biggar: But if you just restricted your models to men, would you not find a higher relative risk with syringe sharing?

Dr. Nicolosi: Except for hypothesizing a different susceptibility to the virus for men and women, I cannot think of any reason why the risk of infection inherent in the act of using a syringe infected by an HIV-positive individual should vary according to gender. Relative risks for syringe sharing are virtually the same for men and women. In the whole pool, you can only see an increased risk for syringe sharing in men if you analyze parenteral and sexual transmission at the same time. But, if you only study sexual transmission, you see a higher risk for women than for men, probably because male-to-female is more efficient than female-to-male transmission.

Dr. Friedman: How do you define syringe sharing; what words do you use in your question?

Dr. Nicolosi: We ask, "Have you ever shared a syringe?", "Have you ever used a syringe borrowed from another person?" and, if the answer is yes, "How many times over the last 6 months (or over the last 4 weeks) have you shared a syringe?" We then elicit the percentage of times, from less than 10% to 100%.

Dr. Gail: I'd like to make a minor methodological point. You said that when you tried a logistic regression or a complementary log-log, but put person-years in instead of numbers of people, you got the same result as the Poisson regression. One nice thing about the Poisson regression is that under Poisson person-year–type assumptions, you can try various links and various ways of modeling the expected value, not only the multiplicative link, but also the logistic or the complementary log-log link; and when events are rare, all three links are basically the same. They are all basically log linear.

Dr. Nicolosi: That's absolutely right.

Dr. Halloran: What you say about the risk of being infected from sharing needles for females and males would only be true if they had the same partner pool. There are several components that go into the probability of being infected, and one of them is the probability that your partner is infected. So, if the women are sharing their needles with a different partner pool from that of the men, they could also have a different risk per share of being infected. The infectivity of the partner you are sharing with is important.

Dr. Musicco: The problem is that it is not very easy to know the real infectivity of the partner because, in this particular study, it was generally unknown whether the partner was infected.

Another problem with sex and syringe sharing is that you have the constant effect of syringe sharing independently of sex, and you have an interaction between sexual transmission and sex (which occurs more in women). When we look at the models, we never find a significant interaction (perhaps because of the small numbers involved), so we are not able to handle this. But I would like to ask whether using a different model (for example, the Poisson regression) would make it easier to handle this type of interaction?

Dr. Muñoz: When I saw the numbers, I thought they were too close. I suspect that you are fitting a different number of cells to the model you use, but that when the model fits, you only use the cell percentage covariant—or rather the sharing—in only one way. I suspect that you are collapsing a lot of categories at the level of estimation. It's like the algorithm saying, "I don't need this number of cells, I'm just going to put them together."

Dr. Tsiatis: I think it was Mitch Gail who said that, given the number of cells you're using, the three models are pretty equivalent; so I'm not at all surprised that the answers are the same. My comment is that, if you built in interaction terms, you would have exactly the same problem with all three models. I think the solution is larger numbers, not different models.

Dr. Nicolosi: I'd like to describe the rationale underlying this model comparison. We were concerned as to whether we were defining exposure in a meaningful way. In our AJE paper contrasting incidence and cross-sectional studies, we have suggested that the key point is the definition of exposure. If you use the past history of sharing as exposure status (as opposed to recent sharing history), this will lead to misclassification and to an underestimation of the true risk. At that time, most participants had not been followed for a long time and recent history of syringe sharing provided a reasonable measure of exposure. Now that longer follow-ups have accumulated, are we still correct in creating exposure categories for the entire follow-up based on the most recent interview? That was our concern, and so every time there was a change in exposure, we analyzed it and then went by degrees from the desirable model to what happens in practice. The fact that the models give almost the same results is quite reassuring, because it seems to show that we are doing things correctly.

Dr. Friedman: I'd just like to make a couple of general points. One is simply to inform people that, when you look at the relationship between city seroprevalence and seroincidence rates, it's very nice and linear in Italian studies, but, in our US studies, there is more of an increase than a leveling off. This may be due to technical reasons such as the number of cities, but it leveled off at something between 12% and 20%.

On the issue of sexual as against drug injection transmission, I don't think we have yet managed to develop the technique. It's not just a question of statistical models; I think it's still a question of the kind of data we have. We need to know whether we are able to see sexual transmission through the noise produced by drug injection variables (at least as I understand the Italian data). There are questions concerning the levels of interactivity; the fact that, when people are injecting, there seem to be gender differences in who goes first in sharing syringes (usually, it's the man who goes first). All of this requires very careful question wording, and it probably takes measurements beyond those which we can get from respondents.

There are also questions concerning the total pool of people with whom one takes risks, and exactly what is going on there. Maybe we can get some of this from partner data, where it exists; but we have to give it very, very careful attention.

And once again, there's the question of the unmeasured variables; sharing syringes is not the only way that injecting procedures can lead to shared viruses, but we don't have data on those variables. Obviously, the next generation of questionnaires will need to pick up on these things.

HIV Epidemiology: Models and Methods,
edited by Alfredo Nicolosi. Raven Press, Ltd.,
New York © 1994.

3

The ALIVE Study

HIV Seroconversion and Progression to AIDS Among Intravenous Drug Users in Baltimore

David Vlahov

Department of Epidemiology, The Johns Hopkins School of Hygiene and Public Health, Baltimore, Maryland, 21205

Intravenous drug users are at high risk for infection with the human immunodeficiency virus (HIV) in the United States, Europe, and parts of Asia (1–3). In response to the HIV epidemic, studies have been conducted to identify prevalence, incidence, risk factors, and natural history of infection among intravenous drug users (4–22). The purpose of this chapter is to review the work of the ALIVE Study being conducted in Baltimore, Maryland, USA. This paper will review methods and major findings from the baseline cross-sectional survey, the longitudinal follow-up of the seronegatives to seroconversion, the longitudinal follow-up of the HIV seropositives to a diagnosis of acquired immunodeficiency syndrome (AIDS), and, finally, data concerning the effectiveness of selected prevention strategies.

METHODS

The rationale, organization, and data collection methods for the study have been described in detail elsewhere (23,24). In brief, the study can be viewed as three parts: the first was the baseline cross-sectional survey; the second was the ongoing follow-up of HIV seropositives; the third was the ongoing follow-up of the HIV seronegatives.

For the first part, between February, 1988, and March, 1989, the Infectious Disease Program of the Epidemiology Department, The Johns Hopkins School of Hygiene and Public Health, enrolled intravenous drug users to undergo HIV testing and interviews to identify correlates of being HIV infected. Intravenous drug users were recruited by word-of-mouth from a variety of community agencies, including drug-abuse treatment centers, city health department clinics for sexually transmitted disease, local emergency rooms, state probation and parole offices, university hospital HIV and AIDS clinics, homeless shelters, and the street outreach AIDS prevention (SOAP) program of a local community education group (H.E.R.O.). Clinic staff members also distributed brochures at selected housing projects and locations where intravenous drug use was evident. Finally, study participants were encouraged to refer eligible friends to the study clinic. Eligibility requirements for enrollment in the study included an age of 18 years or older, a history of injecting illict drugs at any time in the previous 11 years, and AIDS-free at baseline.

Data collection at baseline was conducted on eligible and consenting intravenous drug users. After venipuncture to collect serum for HIV antibody testing and other assays (including HTLV-I/II, hepatitis B virus, hepatitis C virus), each participant was questioned face-to-face by a trained interviewer in a private room. The standardized baseline interview elicited demographic data; a medical history; injection history for the last 6 months of use, the first 3 months of use, and year-by-year since 1977; a 10 year history of sexual activity; knowledge and attitudes of HIV and AIDS (instrument from the National Center for Health Statistics, USA); as well as information on health insurance and medical services utilization (24). After data collection, participants were counseled regarding risk reduction and offered bleach (to disinfect needles), condoms, and referral into treatment for drug abuse. After being reimbursed 10 dollars for their time, participants were scheduled to return for HIV serologic test results in 2 to 3 weeks.

At the test results visit, separate HIV seropositive and HIV seronegative cohorts were established. The seropositive cohort was established for a detailed clinical immunologic follow-up study to identify prognostic indicators for development of AIDS. The goal was to enroll a cohort of about 800 intravenous drug users, of whom 80% were HIV seropositive and 20% were HIV seronegative. All HIV seropositive intravenous drug users were invited into this clinical immunologic cohort. Generally, after five seropositive individuals enrolled, the next seronegative subject to return for results of baseline serologic tests was invited into the clinical immunologic follow-up. Consenting individuals (630 seropositive and 160 seronegative) agreed to return at 6-month intervals for interviews, physical examinations, and venipuncture. Separate consents were obtained to secure release of medical information.

The HIV seronegative cohort was established by inviting all HIV seronegatives not selected for the clinical immunologic follow-up to return at 6 month intervals for interviews and repeated serologic testing to identify risk factors for seroconversion. Although no funding was available to maintain the seronegative cohort for 12 months after baseline, two-thirds of the original group returned voluntarily. The seronegative cohort, then, was defined as HIV-seronegative intravenous drug users who had returned for at least one follow-up visit.

Data collection for the follow-up visits of both the clinical immunologic cohort and the seronegative longitudinal cohort included a standardized interview schedule. The questionnaire elicited information on medical history, drug use, and sex practices in the prior 6 months. In addition, to assess validity of self-reports, a scale of socially desirable responding was administered (25).

Only the clinical immunologic cohort underwent a physical examination at each semiannual visit to obtain information on signs and symptoms of drug abuse and HIV-related disease; some volunteers underwent a detailed neuropsychologic and neurologic evaluation at 6-month intervals. Participants from both cohorts underwent venipuncture. The clinical immunologic cohort had serologic tests for HIV and syphilis, as well as measurement of T-cell subsets, routinely performed at each semiannual visit. The seronegative cohort had HIV tests performed at each visit; for a subgroup of volunteers, cells were obtained for polymerase chain reaction assays. For both cohorts, serum, plasma, and cells were cryopreserved in a biological repository for later assays.

LABORATORY STUDIES

Antibodies to HIV were detected by commercial enzyme-linked immunosorbent assay (ELISA; Genetic Systems, Seattle, WA) with confirmation of positive ELISA test by Western blot (DuPont, Wilmington, DE). Antibody to HLTV-I/II was performed using ELISA and Western blot (Cambridge Bioscience, Rockville, MD); antibodies to hepatitis B by ELISA or radioimmunoassay (RIA; Abbott, North Chicago, IL), hepatitis C by ELISA confirmed by radioimmunoblot assay (RIBA; Ortho Diagnostics, Raritan, NJ). Syphilis assays were performed using (RPR) with (FTA-ABS) confirmation (Smith-Kline, King of Prussia, PA). For measurement of T-cell subsets, specimens of heparinized whole blood were stained with monoclonal antibodies using the whole blood method of Hoffman, et al. (26) as modified by Giorgi, et al. (27); percentages of CD3+, CD4+, and CD8+ T-cells were determined by flow cytometry. Using these percentages with the complete blood count and differential, we determined the count of T-cell subsets. Hemoglobin levels and platelet count were also obtained from the complete blood count (Smith-Kline). Serum β_2 microglobulin and neopterin were measured by RIA (Pharmacia, Uppsala, Sweden; and Neopterin RIAcid, Henning, Berlin, Germany, respectively). The immunoglobulin A (IgA) assay used FIAX Sti Q (M.A. Bioproducts, Walkerville, MD) coated with immunosorbents to bind IgA, which was then immersed in fluorescein isothiocyanate-labeled, goat antihuman immunoglobulin-specific IgA, and the fluorescence of the bound antibodies was measured.

STATISTICAL ANALYSES

A full description of methods is beyond the scope of this paper. However, it is worth noting here that the ALIVE Study has used a broad range of designs and statistical techniques. For the cross-sectional data, descriptive statistics and exploratory data analysis techniques (28) appropriate to level of measurement have been performed, followed, for categorical data, by Mantel-Haenszel techniques and logistic regression (29). For continuous outcomes, linear regression techniques have been used (30). For the clinical immunologic cohort, we have used survival techniques, including Kaplan-Meier and proportional hazards techniques (31). For continuous outcomes, we have used longitudinal data analysis techniques (32). For the seronegative cohort, we have used person-time tecniques, including Poisson regression. In select circumstances we have used a nested case-control design using conditional logistic regression on matched data (32).

RESULTS

Description of the Initial Cross-Section

Of the 3,375 individuals who registered for screening at the study clinic, 378 (11.2%) did not qualify (aged under 18 years old or no injection drug use reported in the past 10 years). Of the 2,997 remaining, 76 (2.5%) were excluded for a variety of reasons (including subsequent denial of injection drug use, diagnosis of AIDS before baseline, duplicate enrollment under different names, and equivocal HIV-test results). Of the 2,921 eligible and consenting participants, stigmata of i.v. drug use were present in 94% of those recorded by the phlebotomist, using only inspection of the upper extremities. Although a variety of agencies had been enlisted to disseminate information about the study, 85.7% of the participants reported that they had first learned about the study by word-of-mouth from a friend or another participant.

Of the 2,921 participants, the median age was 34 years (range: 18 to 68 years), 90% were black, 81% were male, 72% had a legal income less than $5,000 per year, 55% had 12 years or less of education, 23% were currently employed, 36% had a history of homelessness, 75% had a history of arrest, 66% had a history of incarceration, and 51% had a history of treatment for drug abuse. The median duration of injection drug use was 12 years (range: 1 to 50 years). Of the 2,921 participants, 2,616 (90%) claimed their most recent injection was within the same calendar year as their baseline visit, and 2,252 (77%) reported their most recent injection was within 1 month prior to interview; 40% reported injecting at least daily, 70% reported sharing needles, and 32% reported use of shooting galleries in the last 6 months of drug use. Among males, 10% reported homosexual or bisexual activity in the past 10 years. Among men and women, 5% reported receptive anal intercourse. In this predominantly minority, lower socioeconomic status, urban, active drug injection population from Baltimore, Maryland, the prevalence of antibody to HIV in 1988 to 1989 was 24% (33).

Cross-Sectional Analyses

Factors associated with prevalent HIV infection at baseline in a multivariate analysis include being black [adjusted odds ratio (AOR) = 3.90], needle sharing (AOR = 1.59), use of shooting galleries (AOR = 2.21), and receptive anal intercourse among males (AOR = 11.53); gender, receptive anal intercourse among females, and number of different sex partners were not significantly associated with being HIV infected (34). In this same analysis, which used a 10 year retrospective interview on drug injection practices, data were consistent with an inference that the first several years of an injection career were associated with an elevated risk of HIV infection (34). A subsequent analysis examined history of sexually transmitted diseases; a history of syphilis was independently associated with being HIV seropositive at baseline, but only among male homosexual injection drug users (35). More recently, injection of cocaine was examined as a correlate of HIV infection and was identified as a statistically significant predictor among drug users outside of treatment, after adjusting for multiple potential confounders such as frequency of injection, use of shooting galleries, number of sex partners, or history of sexually transmitted diseases (36). The practice of frontloading was infrequent and, similar to sharing of cookers, was not associated with being HIV seropositive (37).

Using the AIDS Awareness Test from the National Center for Health Statistics, knowledge about AIDS in this cohort of injection drug users was higher than for a random sample of the US population surveyed at the same time (38). The primary sources of information about AIDS was from television and radio, with only a very small proportion reporting contact with street outreach AIDS education teams; although this latter finding could have been a function of selection into this study, the major finding was that mass media reaches this population (39). Although television executives were reluctant to consider presentation of explicit prevention messages directed at injection drug users (39), use of mass media should be explored further. For example, we assessed knowledge about antiretroviral therapies in this population and found considerable knowledge deficits (40); this less sensitive topic could be addressed through mass media approaches.

Despite high levels of knowledge about HIV transmission and prevention in this population, we noted a knowledge-behavior discrepancy in that 98% knew that condoms could prevent HIV transmission, yet 66% reported at baseline that they never used condoms; likewise, 98% knew HIV could be transmitted through shared needles, yet 70% reported recent sharing of needles. One factor that was associated with this discrepancy was perception of risk; 60% of high-risk injection drug users failed to perceive themselves to be at high risk (38). Thus, knowledge of HIV itself is necessary but not sufficient to effect risk reduction; altering perception of individual risk appears to be important to consider.

Behavior change is difficult to gauge accurately in cross-sectional or prospective studies because of the potential for socially desirable responding. At baseline, 40% of injection drug users with a history of shooting gallery use reported cessation of this activity before the initial interview (38); and although about 25% of injection drug users reported a history of blood or plasma donation, the proportion had decreased in recent years (41). We attempted to address the issue of behavior change, minimizing the potential for socially desirable responding, by analyzing data from the baseline interview on six sequential cohorts initiated into injection drug use between 1982 and 1987. The intriguing feature of this approach was that it asked about periods remote from the baseline in 1988 (thus, less subject to socially desirable responding) but focused on the period of initiation into injection drug use (because vividly recalled, validity of reports should be constant across time). The proportion of drug users who reported more than one needle-sharing partner in the first 3 months of injection drug use declined from 42% in 1982 to 25% in 1987, which was a statistically significant trend (42). More recently, data collected prospectively since baseline has suggested a greater decline in risk behaviors among persons who were told their HIV-test result was seropositive, but that change was limited to soon after learning test results (43).

Validity of self-reports among injection drug users is a topic that has been of long-standing concern among researchers (44,45). For example, traditional approaches using corroboration with official records or urine tests are inadequate to validate route of drug administration or the practice of needle sharing. We validated route of administration by inspection for track marks. For needle sharing, we estimated construct validity using biological markers, hypothesizing higher frequency risk histories in HIV seropositives than seronegatives, and more remote higher risk histories among HIV seropositives with lower CD4+ cell counts (a target organ of HIV infection). Data were consistent with these hypothesized associations, which increased our confidence that validity of self-reports in this population was reasonable (24). A separate approach was to apply Paulhus' two-component model scale of socially desirable responding (i.e., self-deception and impression management) to assess self-reports in this population (25). Although we found variable levels of socially desirable responding among subgroups of injection drug users, these findings did not confound estimates of risk for being HIV infected; these data indicate that while "noise" is present in self-reports, estimates of HIV risk are probably of reasonable validity (46). In addition, because terminology for drug injection practices was highly variable in pilot studies, we used photographs of select practices to elicit respondents' own terms and then used respondents' own terms throughout the interview (47).

Selection bias among studies of injection drug users is another methodologic issue that has been of long-standing concern among researchers (44,45). In particular, many studies of injection drug users are conducted on treatment-based samples; however, only 10% to 15% of drug users are in treatment for drug abuse at any given time. In our study population, we noted that characteristics of injection drug users varied considerably by history of arrest or treatment for drug abuse (48). However, when we examined the extent to which current enrollment in a drug-treatment program (yes/no) affected estimates of other factors being associated with HIV infection at baseline, differences were modest. These analyses suggested that treatment-based samples, with some qualifications, provide a reasonable means to study HIV infection among injection drug users (49).

Several infections other than HIV are common among injection drug users. At baseline, over 60% of injection drug users reported a history of a sexually transmitted disease; a history of diagnosis or treatment for syphilis was reported by 17% of HIV seropositives and 11% of seronegatives (35). Markers for hepatitis B virus infection (HBsAg, HBsAb, HBcAB) were present in 92% of HIV seropositives and 78% of HIV seronegatives. Antibodies to hepatitis C virus were present in 84% of HIV seropositives and 86% of HIV seronegatives tested (50). Among nearly 2,000 injection drug users, 8.5% were seropositive for antibody to HTLV-I/II, nearly 12% for HIV seropositives and 7% for HIV seronegatives (51). More recently, in collaboration with the city health department, we have performed PPD-tuberculin skin testing on 395 participants, of whom 257 returned for skin-test reading. The rate of PPD positivity was 22% among HIV seropositives and 29.5% among HIV seronegatives; anergy was significantly more common among the HIV seropositives (52).

Prospective

HIV Seropositive Clinical Immunologic Subcohort

Analyses were performed to characterize progression to immunosuppression (CD4+ cell decline) and to AIDS. In the first analysis, lymphocytes and complete blood counts were available on 621 HIV seropositives, 152 seronegatives, and 86 HIV seroconverters through July, 1991 (53). Proportions (%) and absolute numbers (mm^{-3}) of CD3+, CD4+, and CD8+ lymphocytes were determined by flow cytometry and complete blood count (CBC) with differential. Median numbers per mm^3 of CD4+ and CD8+ lymphocytes were 1,061 and 627 for seronegatives, and 508 and 894 for seropositives; for seroconverters, corresponding levels were 734 and 889 at the first visit (median = 4.5 months) after estimated time of seroconversion. For HIV seropositives, the median rate of decline in absolute numbers (and %) of CD4+ lymphocytes were 8 cells (0%) per 6 months (median follow-up = 18 months). For seroconverters, these figures were 49 cells (1.9%) per 6 months post-seroconversion (median follow-up = 12 months). These results were not affected by excluding the few individuals who received AZT subsequent to baseline when none were on AZT or pentamidine. Results indicated no difference in T-cell levels or number of clinical symptoms between those who remained and those who dropped out of follow-up, suggesting little or no bias related to drop out. Forty-eight cases of AIDS were identified primarily in those with low initial CD4+ cell levels. Rate of change for CD4+ did not vary by injection status (active/inactive) or frequency of injection at baseline. This rate of CD4+ cell decline was more gradual than previously reported for other groups and did not appear to be due to treatment or methodologic bias. Confidence in the observed results was strengthened by the following observations: (i) as expected, CD4+ lymphocytes declined substantially immediately after seroconversion, (ii) initial CD4+ levels were lower for seropositives than seronegatives, and (iii) progression to AIDS was observed among those with low CD4+ levels at baseline. More recently, this analysis was updated, with essentially the same results (54).

To identify prognostic indicators for the development of AIDS (55), we conducted medical record searches on 554 of the 630 persons HIV seroprevalent at baseline who consented to release medical records. Among the 554, 13 non-AIDS deaths and 48 (9%) cases of AIDS (meeting the 1987 Centers for Disease Control definition of AIDS) were identified through December, 1990. Using CD4+ numbers less than 200 per mm^3 as the reference, the relative hazards in a proportional hazards model for CD4+ numbers between 200 and 500 per mm^3 and CD4+ numbers greater than 500 per mm^3 were 0.32 (95%CI = 0.14, 0.71) and 0.09 (95%CI = 0.04, 0.24), respectively. After controlling for CD4+ level, addition of variables one at a time indicated that serum neopterin above 11.7 nmol/L and presence of more than one clinical symptom of ARC at baseline were each significantly associated with progression to AIDS within 2 years; all three variables remained significantly associated with progression to AIDS in a multivariate model. Of note, age, current drug use (yes/no) at baseline, platelets, serum IgA level, and serum $\beta 2$ microglobulin did not significantly add prognostic information to the model. In a subsequent analysis, results were similar, noting that oral thrush at baseline, rather than number of symptoms, was prognostically important; progression to AIDS did not vary by gender (56). We analyzed levels of serum neopterin, serum β2 microglobulin, and serum IgA levels by CD4+ cell levels and found all three markers increased as CD4+ cell levels decreased, but that levels were not significantly associated with demographic or drug-use variables (57).

Estimation of the incubation period from HIV seroconversion to AIDS for injection drug users was performed using multiple imputation methods described by Muñoz, et al. (58), combining data from two cohorts: the ALIVE Study and the Montefiore injection drug-user cohort (Dr. Gerald Friedland, principal investigator). The median incubation period was 10.7 years, which is consistent with estimates derived from other cohorts and other methods (59).

More recently, we have combined data from the ALIVE Study with data from the Baltimore component of the Multicenter AIDS Cohort Study of homosexual men (54,56,60). Those analyses are particularly important, because they compare two groups being studied at the same time, in the same city, using the same laboratories.

HIV Seronegative Cohort Follow-up

We followed injection drug users who were initially HIV seronegative with semiannual serologic screening and interviews about drug use and sex practices between visits. We used person-time techniques to calculate rates of seroconversion per semiannual visit in calendar time (person-semesters; Table 1). These data indicate (after an initial start-up period) an HIV seroconversion rate of almost 4% per year, which has remained essentially unchanged throughout the study period. Using Poisson regression, we identified a higher rate for women than men (relative risk = 1.6; 95%CI = 1.01, 2.56). Although the rate of new infections among actively injecting users showed a slight decline over time, the trend was not statistically significant.

The higher rate of HIV seroconversion in women than men was analyzed in further detail using a matched case-control design (62). Gender related differences in risk factors were identified; sexual practices, but no drug in-

TABLE 1. *Seroconversion rates of HIV seronegative cohort of injection drug users*

Calendar semester	Jan–Jun '88	July–Dec '88	Jan–Jun '89	Jul–Dec '89	Jan–Jun '90
Seroconverters (no.)	2	25	30	28	18
Person-semesters	294	1094	1331	1089	946
Rate[a]	0.7%	2.3%	2.3%	2.6%	1.9%

From Nelson KE, et al. (61).
[a]Rate per person-semester.

jection variables, were significantly associated with HIV seroconversion in women drug users.

To estimate the frequency of latent HIV infection among seronegative injection drug users, we performed polymerase chain reaction (PCR) technique on 2,159 blood specimens (63). Of these specimens, 98.8% were both PCR and serologically negative. Seven (0.3%) were seronegative and PCR positive with at least two primer pairs; within 6 months, all five who returned for follow-up evaluation seroconverted. Nineteen specimens (0.9%) were equivocal by PCR analysis (i.e., showing only one primer pair amplification): one seroconverted at the same visit, 15 remained seronegative at follow-up, and three did not return. Among 62 seropositive participants, 87.1% were PCR positive, 1.6% was equivocal, and 11.3% were PCR negative. The concordance between PCR and serological results was 98.6%. This analysis indicates that latent HIV infection detected by PCR among seronegative persons who inject illicit drugs is uncommon; standard serologic screening is highly sensitive.

Evaluation of Interventions to Prevent Transmission of HIV and Other Infections Among Injection Drug Users

While many infectious and noninfectious diseases were noted to be more common in HIV-seropositive than seronegative intravenous drug users, we noted a protective association for a history of diabetes; the HIV rate was 10% among diabetic and 24% among nondiabetic drug users (64). On careful, stratified analysis of this association, we noted that diabetes was "protective" against HIV infection in intravenous drug users because of the safer injection practices afforded by their ready access to sterile injection equipment and immunity from prosecution for violation of paraphernalia laws. With sparse data on effectiveness of needle exchange programs, this analysis provides indirect evidence to suggest that availability of sterile needles might have a beneficial impact on preventing parenteral transmission of HIV infection.

Another approach to preventing transmission of HIV infection among injection drug users has been the use of bleach to disinfect needles between injections; however, data on field effectiveness are sparse. Using data on HIV seroconverters and persistently seronegative injection drug users as controls, we conducted a matched case-control study using conditional logistic regression (65). After restricting the sample to black heterosexuals who reported sharing needles, matching criteria were date of study entry, date of follow-up, gender, and use of cocaine. The adjusted odds ratio for use of disinfectants "less than all the time" (compared to those who denied use of disinfectants) was 0.91, and that for disinfectant use "all the time" was 0.71. These preliminary data from 22 seroconverters and 95 matched controls suggests a modest protective effect for use of needle disinfectants under field conditions.

More recently, an analysis was performed to examine the effects of skin cleaning prior to injection on the occurrence of self-reported abscesses at the injection site and endocarditis (65). The occurrence of these infections was lower among those reporting skin cleaning, and the associations persisted after accounting for several potential confounders.

Neuropsychological Evaluation of Injection Drug Users

Drs. Justin McArthur, Ola Selnes, and Walter Royal have been studying a subgroup of the ALIVE cohort to assess neurological manifestations of HIV infection. In cross-sectional and limited longitudinal analyses, neither HIV infection among initially asymptomatic individuals nor chronic use of drugs was associated with neurologic findings or neuropsychological test scores, after accounting for age and education (66,67).

CONCLUSION

The ALIVE Study was started with the objectives of identifying correlates for being HIV seropositive, estimating rates and risk factors for HIV seroconversion, and identifying factors associated with progression to both immunosuppression and AIDS among injecting drug users. Multiple reports have been presented and published in addressing these objectives. However, findings have been disseminated in a broad range of journals. The purpose here was to summarize findings in one place and to provide an overview of results to date.

As has been presented, many questions about HIV infection, specifically among intravenous drug users, have been addressed. Perhaps the most unexpected finding has been the gradual rate of decline in CD4+ cell levels. The study continues to follow participants, and with time this issue should become more clear. Future directions include more detailed analyses on the occurrence of HIV-related–non-AIDS diagnoses, possible cardiac and gynecologic manifestations of HIV infection, effects of antiretrovirals, studies of mortality, and continued analyses of the cohort of injection drug users and homosexual men being followed in Baltimore. The study of the natural history of HIV infection in this population also permits a unique opportunity to study longitudinal aspects of infection drug use, including determinants of entry into and withdrawal from treatment for drug abuse, as well as cessation from drug use without formal assistance of treatment programs. Earlier analyses of this cohort examined predictors for entry into injection drug use (68).

The identification and follow-up of a high-risk HIV-seronegative cohort is a valuable resource in planning for candidate HIV vaccines. Intravenous drug users can be recruited into vaccine studies and do return for follow-up visits (69,70). The data to date suggest that the natural history of HIV infection appears to be similar between injection drug users and other risk groups studied in developed countries. With one of the highest rates of new HIV infection, this population may be important to consider as a group to include in HIV vaccine studies.

Summarizing results to date from one ongoing longitudinal study runs the risk of incorrectly communicating that only one study is addressing the major research questions. Nothing could be further from the truth. Only a partial listing of important research teams were provided in the introduction, and all have been of vital importance to addressing scientific issues and stimulating further questions. Rather, the purpose here has been to gather our work to facilitate further dialogue so that all groups together can move closer toward an end to this epidemic.

ACKNOWLEDGMENTS

I would like to acknowledge the National Institute on Drug Abuse (USA) for supporting the studies; Drs. Kenrad E. Nelson, Alvaro Muñoz, Liza Solomon, James C. Anthony, Joseph B. Margolick, David D. Celentano, Wallace Mandell, Richard E. Chaisson, Mark D. Smith, Noya Galai, Justin McArthur, Ola Selnes, and Walter Royal for their superb investigative skills; B. Frank Polk for advice and leadership; and the staff and participants of the ALIVE Study for their work advancing knowledge about drug abuse and AIDS.

REFERENCES

1. Coutinho RA. Epidemiology and prevention among intravenous drug users. *J Acquir Immune Defic Syndr* 1990;3:413–416.
2. Des Jarlais DC, Friedman SR. Editorial Review. HIV infection among intravenous drug users: epidemiology and risk reduction. *AIDS* 1987;1:67–76.
3. Hahn RA, Onorato IM, Jones TS, Dougherty J. Prevalence of HIV infection among intravenous drug users in the United States. *JAMA* 1989;261:2677–2684.
4. Chaisson RE, Moss AR, Onishi R, Osmond D, Carlson JR. Human immunodeficiency virus infection in heterosexual intravenous drug users in San Francisco. *Am J Public Health* 1987;77:169–172.
5. Des Jarlais DC, Friedman SR, Marmor M, et al. Development of AIDS, HIV seroconversion and co-factors for T-cell loss in a cohort of intravenous drug users. *AIDS* 1987;1:105–111.
6. Robertson JR, Skidmore CA, Roberts JJK. HIV infection in intravenous drug users: a follow-up study indicating changes in risk-taking behavior. *Br J Addict* 1988;83:387–391.
7. Goedert JJ, Biggar R, Weiss S, Eyster M, Melbye M, Wilson S, Ginzberg H. Three year incidence of AIDS among HTLV-III infected risk group members: a comparison of the cohorts. *Science* 1985;28:992–995.

8. Chitwood DD, McCoy CB, Inciardi JA, McBride DC, Comerford M, Tropido E, McCoy V, Page B, Griffin J, Fletcher MA, Ashman MA. HIV seropositivity of needles from shooting galleries in South Florida. *Am J Public Health* 1990;80:150–152.
9. Friedland GH, Harris C, Butkus-Small C, Shine D, Moll B, Darrow W, Klein RS. Intravenous drug abusers and the acquired immunodeficiency syndrome (AIDS): Demographic, drug use and needle sharing patterns. *Arch Intern Med* 1985;145:1413–1417.
10. van den Hoek JAR, Coutinho RA, van Haastretcht HJA. Prevalence and risk factors of HIV infection among drug users and drug-using prostitutes in Amsterdam. *AIDS* 1988;2:55–60.
11. Page JB. Shooting scenarios and risk of HIV-1 infection. *Behav Sci* 1990;33:478–490.
12. McCusker J, Koblin B, Lewis BF, Sullivan J. Demographic characteristics, risk behaviors, and HIV seroprevalence among intravenous drug users by site of contact: results from a community-wide HIV surveillance project. *Am J Public Health* 1990;80:1062–1067.
13. Brettle RP, Bisset K, Burns S, Davidson SJ, Gray JMN, Inglis JM, Lees JS, Mok J. Human immunodeficiency virus and drug misuse: the Edinburgh experience. *BMJ* 1987;295:421–424.
14. Rezza G, Lazzarin A, Angarano G, et al. The natural history of HIV infection in intravenous drug users: risk of disease progression in a cohort of seroconverters. *AIDS* 1989;3:87–90.
15. Stimson GV. Syringe exchange programs for injecting drug users. *AIDS* 1989;3:253–260.
16. Haverkos HW, Lange WR. Serious infections other than human immunodeficiency virus among intravenous drug users. *J Infect Dis* 1990;161:894–902.
17. Selwyn P, Hartel D, Wasserman W, Drucker E. Impact of the AIDS epidemic on morbidity and mortality among intravenous drug users in a New York City methadone maintenance program. *Am J Public Health* 1989;79:1358–1362.
18. Watters JM. Observations on the importance of social context in HIV transmission among IVDUs. *J Drug Issues* 1989;19:9–26.
19. Galli M, Lazzarin A, Saracco A. Clinical and immunological aspects of HIV infection in drug addicts. *Clin Immunol Immunopathol* 1989;50:S166–S176.
20. Nicolosi A, Mussico M, Saracco A, et al. Incidence and risk factors of HIV infection: a prospective study of seronegative drug users from Milan and Northern Italy. *Epidemiology* 1990;1:453–459.
21. Battjes RJ, Pickins RW, Amsel Z, Brown BS. Heterosexual transmission of human immunodeficiency virus among intravenous drug users. *J Infect Dis* 1990;162:1007–1011.
22. Zaccarelli, Rezza G, Girardi E, et al. Monitoring HIV trends in injecting drug users: an Italian experience. *AIDS* 1990;4:1007–1010.
23. Vlahov D, Anthony JC, Mūnoz A, Margolick JB, Nelson KE, Polk BF. The ALIVE study: a longitudinal study of HIV infection among intravenous drug users. *J Drug Issues* 1991;21(4):755–771.
24. Anthony JC, Vlahov D, Celentano DD, Menon AS, Margolick JB, Cohn S, Nelson KE, Polk BF. Self-reported interview data for a study of HIV-1 infection among intravenous drug users: description of methods and preliminary evidence of validity. *J Drug Issues* 1991;21(4):739–757.
25. Paulhus DL. Two-component models of socially desirable responding. *J Pers Soc Psychol* 1984;46:598–609.
26. Hoffman RA, Kung PC, Hansen WP, Goldstein, G. Simple and rapid measurement of human T-lymphocytes and their subclasses in peripheral blood. *Proc Natl Acad Sci USA* 1980;77:4914–4917.
27. Giorgi JV, Cheng HL, Margolick JB. Quality control in the flow cytometric measurement of T-lymphocyte subsets: the Multicenter AIDS Cohort Experience. *Clin Immunol Immunopathol* 1990;55:173–186.
28. Tukey J. *Exploratory data analysis*. Reading, MA: Addison-Wesley; 1977.
29. Breslow NE, Day NE. Statistical methods in cancer research: Vol. I: The design and analysis of case-control studies. International Agency on Research on Cancer. Lyon, France, 1982.
30. Rosner B. *Fundamentals of biostatistics*. 2nd ed. Boston: Duxbury Press; 1988.
31. Miller RG, Gong G, Muñoz A. *Survival analysis*. New York: John Wiley & Sons; 1981.
32. Breslow NE, Day NE. Statistical methods in cancer research: Vol. II: The design and

analysis of cohort studies. International Agency for Research on Cancer. Lyon, France, 1987.
33. Vlahov D, Anthony JC, Muñoz A, Margolick J, Nelson KE, Celentano DD, Solomon L, Polk BF. The ALIVE study: a longitudinal study of HIV-1 infection in intravenous drug users: description of methods. *J Drug Issues* 1991;21:759–776.
34. Vlahov D, Muñoz A, Cohn S, Celentano DD, Anthony JC, Nelson KE. Association of drug injection patterns with antibody to human immunodeficiency virus type 1 (HIV-1) among intravenous drug users in Baltimore. *Am J Epidemiol* 1990;132:847–856.
35. Nelson KE, Vlahov D, Cohn S, Odamabaku M, Hook E. Sexually transmitted disease (STDs) in a cohort of intravenous drug users: association with HIV serostatus. *J Infect Dis* 1991;164:457–463.
36. Anthony JC, Vlahov D, Cohn S, Nelson KE. New evidence on cocaine use and risk of HIV infection. *Am J Epidemiol* 1991;134:1175–1189.
37. Samuels JF, Vlahov D, Anthony JC, Solomon L, Celentano DD. The practice of frontloading among intravenous drug users: association with HIV antibody. *AIDS* 1991;5:343.
38. Celentano DD, Vlahov D, Menon AS, Polk BF. HIV knowledge and attitudes among intravenous drug users: comparisons to the U.S. population and by drug use behaviors. *J Drug Issues* 1991;21(3):647–661.
39. Jason J, Solomon L, Celentano DD, Vlahov D. HIV-infection prevention messages for injecting drug users: sources of information and use of mass media, Baltimore, 1989. MMWR Morb Mortality Wkly Rep 1991:40(28):465–469.
40. Smith MD, Celentano DD, Solomon L, Astemborski J, Vlahov D. Knowledge of therapeutics for human immunodeficiency virus infection among intravenous drug users. *J Infect Dis* 1992;166:685–686.
41. Nelson KE, Vlahov D, Margolick JB, Bernal M. Blood and plasma donations among active intravenous drug users in Baltimore. *JAMA* 1990;263:2194–2197.
42. Vlahov D, Muñoz A, Celentano DD, Cohn S, Anthony JC, Chilcoat H, Nelson KE. HIV seroconversion and disinfection of injection equipment among intravenous drug users, Baltimore, Maryland. *Epidemiology* 1991;2:442–444.
43. Celentano DD, Muñoz A, Cohn S, Vlahov D. Drug-related behavior change for HIV transmission among injection drug users. Presented at the VIII International Conference on AIDS. Amsterdam, The Netherlands, July 19–24, 1992.
44. Vlahov D, Polk BF. Perspectives on infection with HIV-1 among intravenous drug users. *Psychopharmacol Bull* 1988;24(3):325–329.
45. Samuels J, Vlahov D, Anthony JC, Chaisson RE. Measurement of risk behaviors among intravenous drug users. *Br J Addict* 1992;87:417–428.
46. Latkin CA, Vlahov D, Anthony JC. Socially desirable responding and self-reported HIV infection risk behaviors among intravenous drug users. *Br J Addict* 1993;88:517–526.
47. Smith AM, Vlahov D, Menon AS, Anthony JC. Variation in terminology for drug injection practices among intravenous drug users in Baltimore. *Int J Addict* 1992;27(14):435–453.
48. Alcabes P, Vlahov D, Anthony JC. Characteristics of intravenous drug users by history of arrest and treatment for drug abuse. *J Nerv Ment Dis* 1992;180:48–54.
49. Alcabes P, Vlahov D, Anthony JC. Correlates of human immunodeficiency virus infection in intravenous drug users: are treatment program samples misleading? *Br J Addict* 1992;87:47–54.
50. Donahue JG, Nelson KE, Muñoz A, Vlahov D, Rennie LL, Taylor EL, Saah AJ, Cohn S, Odaka NJ, Farzadegan H. Antibody to hepatitis-C virus among cardiac surgery patients, homosexual men, and intravenous drug users in Baltimore, Maryland. *Am J Epidemiol* 1991;134:1206–1211.
51. Proietti F, Vlahov D, Alexander S, Taylor E, Cohn S, Kirby A, Blattner W, Saah A. Correlates of HTLV-II/HIV-1 seroprevalence and incidence of HTLV-II infection among intravenous drug users. Presented at the VIII International Conference on AIDS, Amsterdam, The Netherlands, 1992.
52. Graham NMH, Nelson KE, Solomon L, Bonds M, Rizzo RT, Scavotto J, Astemborski J, Vlahov D. Prevalence of tuberculin positivity and skin test anergy in HIV-1 seropositive and seronegative intravenous drug users. *JAMA* 1992;267:369–373.

53. Margolick JB, Muñoz A, Vlahov D, Solomon L, Astemborski J, Cohn S, Nelson KE. Longitudinal changes in T-lymphocyte subsets in a cohort of intravenous drug users with prevalent or incident HIV-1 infection. *JAMA* 1992;267:1631–1636.
54. Margolick JB, Muñoz A, Vlahov D, Solomon L, Astemborski J, He Y, Saah A. Rates of decline in CD4 lymphocytes in homosexual men and IV drug users studied in a single laboratory. Presented at the VIII International Conference on AIDS, Amsterdam, The Netherlands, 1992.
55. Muñoz A, Vlahov D, Solomon L, Margolick JB, Bareta J, Cohn S, Astemborski J, Nelson KE. Prognostic indicators for development of AIDS among intravenous drug users. *J Acquir Immune Defic Syndr* 1992;5:694–700.
56. Vlahov D, Muñoz A, Saah AJ, Solomon L, Palenicek J, Margolick JB, Astemborski J, Bareta J, Nelson KE. Prognostic indicators for development of AIDS in two cohorts. Presented at the VIII International Conference on AIDS. Amsterdam, The Netherlands, July 19–24, 1992.
57. Chaisson RE, Taylor E, Margolick JB, Muñoz A, Solomon L, Cohn S, Nelson KE, Vlahov D. Immune serum markers and CD4 cell counts in HIV-infected intravenous drug users. *J Acquir Immune Defic Syndr* 1992;5:456–460.
58. Muñoz A, Wang MC, Bass S, Taylor JMG, Kingsley LA, Chmiel JS, Polk BF. Acquired immunodeficiency syndrome (AIDS)-free time after human immunodeficiency virus type-1 (HIV-1) seroconversion in homosexual men. *Am J Epidemiol* 1989;130:530–539.
59. Alcabes P, Muñoz A, Vlahov D, Friedland G. Estimation of time from seroconversion to AIDS in HIV-infected intravenous drug users in the U.S. Presented at the VIII International Conference on AIDS, Amsterdam, The Netherlands, 1992.
60. Palenicek J, Nelson K, Cohn S, Rubb S, Muñoz A, Vlahov D, Saah A. Comparison of clinical manifestations of HIV-1 disease between IVDUs and homosexual men (HM). Presented at the VIII International Conference on AIDS, Amsterdam, The Netherlands, 1992.
61. Nelson KE, Muñoz A, Vlahov D, Cohn S, Solomon L. HIV-1 seroconversion in a cohort of intravenous drug users. In: Rossi GB, et al., eds. *Science challenging AIDS: proceedings of the VII International Conference on AIDS, Florence.* Basel, Switzerland: Karger; 1992.
62. Solomon L, Astemborski J, Warren D, Muñoz A, Cohn S, Vlahov D, Nelson KE. Differences in risk factors for HIV-1 seroconversion among male and female intravenous drug users. *Am J Epidemiol* 1993;137:892–898.
63. Farzadegan H, Vlahov D, Solomon L, Muñoz A, Astemborski J, Taylor E, Burnley A, Nelson KE. Detection of HIV-1 infection by polymerase chain reaction (PCR) in a cohort of seronegative intravenous drug users [*submitted*].
64. Nelson KE, Vlahov D, Cohn S, Lindsay A, Solomon L, Anthony JC. Human immunodeficiency virus infection in diabetic intravenous drug users. *JAMA* 1991;266:2259–2261.
65. Vlahov D, Sullivan M, Astemborski J, Nelson KE. Bacterial infections and skin cleaning prior to injection among intravenous drug users. *Public Health Rep* 1992 [*in press*].
66. Royal W, III, Updike M, Selnes OA, Proctor TV, Nance-Sproson L, Solomon L, Vlahov D, Cornblath DR, McArthur JC. HIV-1 infection and nervous system abnormalities among a cohort of intravenous drug users. *Neurology* 1991;41:1905–1910.
67. Concha M, Graham N, Muñoz A, Vlahov D, Royal W, Updike M, Nance-Sproson T, Selnes OA, McArthur J. Effect of chronic substance abuse on the neuropsychological test performance in intravenous drug users infected with HIV-1. *Am J Epidemiol* 1992;136:1338–1348.
68. Selnes OA, McArthur JC, Royal W, Updike ML, Nance-Sproson T, Concha M, Gordon B, Solomon L, Vlahov D. HIV-1 infection and intravenous drug use: longitudinal neuropsychological evaluation of asypmtomatic subjects. *Neurology* 1992 [*in press*].
69. Tomas JM, Vlahov D, Anthony JC. Association between intravenous drug use and early misbehavior. *Drug Alcohol Depend* 1990;25:79–89.
70. Steinhoff MC, Auerbach BS, Nelson KE, Vlahov D, Becker RL, Graham NMH, Schwartz DH, Lucas AH, Chaisson RE. Antibody responses to Haemophilus Influenzae type B vaccines in men with human immunodeficiency virus infection. *N Engl J Med* 1991;325;1837–1842.

DISCUSSION

Dr. Rezza: Is it that you don't find any age effect when you do a multivariate analysis, or is it that you don't find any univariate effect?

Dr. Vlahov: We don't find it in either situation, but I think there's a reason why we don't find it and you do (just as Jim Goedert found it in the hemophiliac cohort). What we have here is a prevalent cohort from the start, and we are addressing the clinical question of prognostic indicators. You are working with seroconverters, which is something different.

Dr. Rezza: But if we put age and CD4 levels into the same multivariate model, the effect of age disappears, which means that CD4 is very closely associated with HIV progression. I think that's why you don't find any age effect.

My second question is about the decline in CD4 levels. I'm struck by the fact that there is a stabilization in your cohort. After reading your articles, we did the same thing in a seroconverter cohort which we followed for 3 years, but we found a continuous decrease in the number of CD4 cells. Do you think that this stabilization occurs after a certain period of time (5 or 7 years, for example), or is there another explanation for it?

Dr. Vlahov: I think there are a number of possible explanations. Our data give us a window of 12 to 18 months, and so we are in the continuum of HIV infection. The question is whether we are selecting the cohort (as a population) in terms of the maturity of their infection. We have shown that there is a steep rate of decline after seroconversion, and I think that that's consistent with your data, as well as the data from the MACS.

The data from the seroprevalent cohort are consistent with stabilization, and, although I don't want to go into too much detail about all of the possible explanations, it does seem that there is a plateau phase somewhere in the middle. However, the duration of this plateau is difficult to determine unless we have more follow-up.

Dr. Detels: I think that one of the problems in looking at CD4 cells is that we tend to look at averages, or slopes. If nobody has an increasing number of CD4 cells (which is essentially the case with HIV-positive men), but a few have a declining number and the majority a largely stable number, it's inevitable that the average goes down. We have to look at distributions if we want to find that stable component.

I also think that the rate of fall-off from the plateau shows that it is not a constant interval. I suspect it is different in different individuals, and that it is very much influenced by repeated exposures to HIV or other factors. It's a methodological issue, I think.

Dr. Tsiatis: Did you estimate the decline by averaging each of the slopes?

Dr. Vlahov: It was by population, not person-by-person (at least in that particular analysis).

Dr. Tsiatis: But it would take care of some of the follow-up problem if you did it person-by-person.

My other comment is that, if you looked at the slopes of individuals, you could correlate them with their CD4 levels at the beginning of the study. Presumably, the people with higher CD4 levels are at an earlier stage of infection, but you would be able to see whether there really is a relationship. Have you done any analyses like that?

Dr. Vlahov: Yes. And I think I made a mistake when I answered your first question, because we did look at the individuals.

Dr. Muñoz: It's a very interesting picture when you do the slopes from the initial level, especially when you make a head-to-head comparison with the cohort of homosexual men (who are older in terms of the maturity of infection). There is a strong regression to the mean in intravenous drug users, but this is much less in the cohort of homosexual men. It's as if biology were taking over the silliness of a regression to the mean.

Dr. Halloran: Coming back to the question of the sudden fall-off, Longini used the Markov model in a series of papers to identify seven different stages of CD4 cell decline. In estimating the rate of transition from one stage to the next (and he put in several different cofactors, including treatment), he also showed a very rapid fall-off, which seems to be consistent with your data.

Dr. Moss: Our studies have shown that just the use of drugs alone leads to an elevation in β-2 levels of about 0.6. Perhaps that's why β-2 levels don't work so well as a predictor in drug users.

Dr. Gail: Have you been able to get any information on cumulative incidence in seroconverters?

Dr. Vlahov: The number of endpoints is very small at this moment, so we haven't had that chance yet. But we have combined data with the Montefiore cohort, a seroprevalent cohort that has been followed for a number of years. They have a number of endpoints, and we have combined our seroconverters with theirs by using the imputation method described by Muñoz in 1989 in the American Journal of Epidemiology. If I remember correctly, the median incubation period is 10.7 years from infection to AIDS.

Dr. Gail: Apart from imputation, how many endpoints do you have in the combined seroconverting cohorts?

Dr. Vlahov: Twenty-two.

Dr. van den Hoek: How many AIDS cases did you have among drug users in Baltimore when you started your cohort study?

Dr. Vlahov: Around 1988, there were about a thousand cases of AIDS in Baltimore City, and about 300 among intravenous drug users.

Dr. van den Hoek: You are following a cohort of seropositive drug users who were already seropositive at intake; that means you are dealing with survivors, doesn't it?

Dr. Vlahov: Yes, I think that in any seroprevalent cohort, you have to worry about the survival phenomenon. The question of incubation will be clarified by following seroconverters over time, but I still think that survivors can provide relevant information for addressing the clinical question of prognostic indicators for the development of AIDS.

Dr. van den Hoek: What is your long-range mortality rate?

Dr. Vlahov: We have had 130 deaths since the beginning of the study: 28 from AIDS and about half of the rest from narcotic overdoses. It's interesting that, in our cohort, if we calculate relative risks for persistently seronegative cases versus seroconverters versus prevalent seropositives, the relative risk for mortality is five among the prevalent seropositives, and two among the seroconverters. So, with about 4 years of follow-up (and an average follow-up of about 2 years for seroconverters), there is excess mortality among seroconverters over a very short follow-up time. This is related to narcotic overdose, and makes me wonder what impact this may have; it's possible we should consider it in terms of suicide.

Dr. van den Hoek: Yes, in our cohort, we have 17 deaths and only 24 AIDS cases.

Dr. Halloran: Coming back to the question about exposure to infection and transmission probability, all of these intervention studies have something to do with affecting transmission. Could you comment on what you believe bleach is doing in terms of reducing the probability of transmission?

Dr. Vlahov: HIV is exquisitely susceptible to the effects of a wide variety of disinfectants in a laboratory situation, but it's very different once you get out into the field. One of the things we have to worry about with bleach in the field is the same as one of the things we have to worry about with surgical instruments in a hospital: you have to be able to reduce the bio-burden surrounding this virus. Bleach binds with the proteinaceous material and then inactivates rapidly. We have not asked intravenous drug users to reduce the bio-burden by cleaning with soap and water before disinfecting (as we do with surgical instruments), because if people accidentally inject bleach it binds with the protein, leading to well-known negative effects; if they do it with a detergent, there can be considerable harm.

A second problem is whether drug users would do it all the time. And a third is contact time. Laboratory studies have shown that a minimum of a minute is required in laboratory situations; would drug users be prepared to wait a full minute when they're in withdrawal and have the drug in front of them? A lot of work is being done on this now. For example, we have a study in which we are videotaping i.v. drug users going through some of their procedures in order to be able to observe timings, rather than rely on asking them to report how long they spend on various steps, and in what phase they actually clean their injection equipment.

Dr. Halloran: The essential point concerning transmission is whether bleach completely blocks or just reduces the transmission probability. It seems to me that it does reduce the probability of transmission, but probably not to zero. So it's the kind of intervention that doesn't remove the risk of infection, even under optimal conditions.

Dr. Vlahov: I would agree with that.

Dr. Friedman: You say that it takes about a minute to inactivate the virus; Clyde McCoy and his people in Miami are saying that it's 30 seconds, and, of course, that's an absolutely critical difference.

Dr. Vlahov: I wasn't aware of McCoy's data; I was referring to the three published studies in the literature (Lionel Resnick, Linda Martin, and an article in Lancet in 1984 from a French group).

Dr. Friedman: So you're talking about inactivating the free virus. A much harder question is inactivating the infected cells, and I don't think we have the necessary lab work to know that.

One comment about your bleach study and the 0.77 estimate. As I remember your methodology, this figure is dependent on follow-up behavioral self-reports about bleach use among seroconverters. Once again, I really think we have a potential problem in relation to the validity of follow-up data in comparison with intake data.

Dr. Vlahov: Although the interviews are done when the blood is drawn, this is prior to the results being available to the individual; neither the individual nor the interviewer is aware of who has seroconverted and who hasn't.

Dr. Friedman: Maybe not, but it's not the first time that they have talked to your study, and the effect may be even stronger if the interview is conducted by the same person. One of the things that we have been worrying about is that, when we try to study behavioral change by using behavioral change indicators as dependent variables, the data always look very good. But the problem is the quality of the follow-up data. We've got to find ways of doing studies on follow-up data (like the one you did using intake data) in order to see whether they are equally good predictors of the various kinds of biological markers we can be reasonably confident about. And, furthermore, that there are no serious interaction effects.

Dr. Moss: As far as I know, nobody has shown that self-reported bleach use is associated with protection; and everybody seems to agree that the variable associated with risk is the number of sexual partners. When you get right down to it, I think it's possible that drug-user studies are really sexual transmission studies, and that bleach is not very relevant.

Dr. Friedman: In our seroconversion studies for the NADR data, we are finding no sexual risk variables except among women, in whom having had sex with another woman in the previous 6 months is a risk factor. We are interpreting this in network rather than in biological terms (who is it that they have been having sex or sharing needles with?) and then making predictions in the same way as for gay men who inject drugs, who are more likely to be infected in some cities than nongay i.v. users. But we are finding that a number of behavioral predictors relating to drug use are relevant, even within cohorts, or categories of cities, stratified by seroprevalence levels. Although there is a lot more we have to learn, drug-use variables are still involved, and to argue that it's all sexual. . . .

Dr. Nicolosi: With reference to sexual and parenteral transmission among i.v. drug users, a CDC study in Thailand, presented at the recent International AIDS Conference, reported about two different HIV variants, one mainly transmitted by sexual contacts, the other mainly transmitted by intravenous drug use. From the abstract, it would appear that this study points out another variable which needs to be taken into account, which may make further studies easier or more difficult.

Dr. Padian: I would like to point out that, when they talk about the difference between sexual and drug-use transmission, a lot of people say that the opposite is true. When you look at the developed world, most sexual transmission comes from the partners of i.v. drug users. It may be true that what is associated with drug use is frequently related to sexual transmission, but it is also true that transmissions attributed to sexual behavior, particularly between partners of i.v. drug users, may be related to drug-using behavior.

Dr. Vlahov: I should point out that the data I was referring to concerning the number of sex partners referred to female drug users; among male drug users, there were both injection and sexual variables.

Dr. Biggar: Concerning the population pool, you began by saying that there were 32,000 i.v. drug users in Baltimore. This estimate seems to be quite extraordinary if 25% are positive. That's 8,000 people just in the drug-abuse community, and if this community represents 30% of the inhabitants, that means 24% HIV positives in Baltimore. Do you have any other way (for example, back-calculation of AIDS cases) to verify these numbers, because they bear on how representative your studies are?

Dr. Vlahov: The person who has done the studies in Baltimore is David Nurco, who has used capture-recapture techniques to estimate the number of drug users. When I called to ask him how he feels about the results he gets, he admits that we really don't know the number of drug users, or how to establish it properly. I only offer that number in order to provide a very general framework, but it should not be used as a fundamental basis for discussion.

Dr. Friedman: It's true that small area differences exist in many city seroprevalence levels.

Dr. Gail: Do you have any information as to the kinds of treatment (for example AZT) that are being received by the subjects in your follow-up study on the development of AIDS, and how these compare with other kinds of cover?

Dr. Vlahov: At the beginning of our study in 1988, virtually nobody was on treatment, and, when we look at the first 12 months, the number was still trivial, although we strongly encouraged our people by referring them to a hospital two blocks away to try to get treatment.

Now, about one-third of those eligible for treatment are actually receiving it. We did an analysis to consider the predictors for getting into treatment, because the CDC recommended that high-risk people should be tested, that those who are positive should have CD4 tests done periodically, and that those with a level of 500 and below should be got into treatment. Our population is in any case tested and submitted to CD4 analysis, and we find that, even with such a small proportion of eligible subjects taken into treatment, the biggest single predictive variable is the presence of symptoms. It's only once people get sick that they take themselves into hospital; we're at that point. Whether this is something to do with access to health care, or whether it reflects the suspicion that drug users have in relation to hospitals and hospital environments, is now being studied in Phase II.

We have also analyzed the knowledge that people had of AIDS therapeutics, which will be published in the September issue of the Journal of Infectious Diseases. But the bottom line is that, although drug users are highly knowledgeable about the transmission and prevention of HIV, their knowledge of AIDS therapeutics is very limited, even with the education given to this cohort.

Dr. Detels: I'd like to go back to the bleach issue. I found out the hard way, when I made an analysis of condom use, that you have to ask the question the right way. Did you ask the question, "Do you use bleach after sharing with every partner?" or did you ask, "Do you use bleach after every instance of sharing a needle?"

Dr. Vlahov: The way we approached the question was a little more open-ended. We took people who reported using needles that they were not absolutely sure that only they had used, and we asked them what they did with the needle between uses. We then recorded the solutions they used and the procedures they went through. Afterwards, we asked what they typically did, and then we asked what proportion of the time spent in injecting they spent on cleaning: all of the time, more than half, less than half, little or none. Given that we had a small number of seroconverters in that analysis, we dichotomized the response into all the time and not all the time.

Dr. Detels: The other question I had was whether you looked for time-trend changes. In the MACS, one of the things that we found when we were looking for sexual activities was that the personal cost of admitting to being anal receptive was not very high when we began, but that, as the study progressed, it became much more difficult for subjects to admit that they were doing something ultimately very stupid, and we started getting a lot of "immaculate" infections.

Dr. Vlahov: I think that's a problem which is common across cohorts, where you have an ethical obligation to give counseling and education, and then have to rely on self-reports later on.

HIV Epidemiology: Models and Methods,
edited by Alfredo Nicolosi. Raven Press, Ltd.,
New York © 1994.

4

Cause-Specific Mortality Among Intravenous Drug Users in Milan 1981–1991

*Massimo Galli and †Massimo Musicco
for the COMCAT Study Group

**Institute of Infectious Diseases, University of Milan, Italy; Ospedale L. Sacco, 20157 Milan, Italy; †Department of Epidemiology and Medical Informatics, Institute of Advanced Biomedical Technologies, National Research Council, 20131 Milan, Italy*

Intravenous drug abuse is a considerable social and health problem in developed countries. Intravenous drug users (IVDUs) are known to be at increased risk from several infectious diseases (1–3); moreover, since before the AIDS era, they have been considered to be at higher risk to die of drug overdose, infectious disease, alcoholism, and violence than the general population of the same age and gender (4–7). Recent studies have reported a further mortality increase as a consequence of the appearance of HIV-1. Stoneburner et al. (8) have shown a marked increase in the number of narcotic-related deaths in New York City between 1978 and 1986, prevalently due to AIDS and other infectious diseases (mainly pneumonia). Selwyn et al. (9) have suggested that the impact of the HIV-1 epidemic on the mortality of IVDUs is limited to AIDS and AIDS-related causes of death. These authors documented a dramatic increase in mortality from AIDS in New York City between 1982 and 1987 and no substantial variation in death rates from other causes. However, this result does not seem generalizable. In Italy, for example, a marked increase in death from overdose parallels that from AIDS, and overdose has been reported as the main cause of death in the period from 1980 to 1988 in a cohort of IVDUs recruited in Rome (10).

The aim of this study was to analyze cause-specific death rates in a cohort of IVDUs living in the Metropolitan Area of Milan (MMA).

SUBJECTS AND METHODS

Between November, 1980, and December, 1988, we recruited all of the IVDUs resident in the municipalities of the MMA who were attending Milan's four public treatment centers for drug abuse. These centers were located in four main city hospitals and remained the only public centers until 1986.

The most frequent request made to the centers was for detoxication, mainly through methadone therapy. Social and psychological support, and other pharmacological treatments, were also frequently asked for, generally as a second request. Subjects received on-site primary medical care services. Between 1980 and 1988, methadone was administered in different schedules and for different periods to 72% of the subjects included in the cohort. Its use peaked in 1984, when 94% of the IVDUs attending the centers were on methadone therapy, and began to decrease in 1985. In 1990, only 16% of IVDUs attending the centers were on methadone maintenance.

Starting in 1981, the vital status of the subjects enrolled was ascertained at the registry offices of the municipalities of residence once a year. When a subject changed his or her residence to a municipality outside the MMA, he or she was considered alive until the time of the change and then lost to follow-up. When we had information of the death of a member of the cohort, we carried out an in-depth investigation in order to ascertain the cause of death by consulting the death certificates, the clinical records of the centers, and, when available, hospital case records and the autopsy reports from Milan's city morgue.

For the purposes of analysis, the causes of death were divided into six groups: overdose, AIDS, violent death (homicide, suicide, and accident), infectious diseases, other causes (liver cirrhosis, tumors, cardiovascular diseases), and undetermined. The cause of death was considered undetermined when the available documents were insufficient to support a causal judgment (e.g., cardiocirculatory arrest as the only cause of death reported on the death certificate, without any supplementary information from hospital or necropsy records).

Death rates were evaluated by the person-years method, and confidence intervals were calculated by the test-based method (11).

RESULTS

From November 1, 1980, to June 30, 1988, we recruited 2,432 IVDUs who were resident in the MMA (Table 1). More than 75% of them were enrolled before 1986. Their mean age at enrollment was 24.5 years (range 14 to 57); 1,905 were males (78.3%, mean age 24.5 years, range 14 to 46), and 527 were

TABLE 1. *IVDUs recruited in the cohort by calendar year (after exclusion of subjects residing outside the Milan metropolitan area or not traced at registry offices)*

Year	Percentage	Number
1980	11.7	285
1981	18.0	437
1982	12.8	312
1983	12.3	299
1984	11.0	267
1985	11.4	276
1986	9.4	229
1987	6.7	164
1988	6.7	163
Total	100.0%	2432

TABLE 2. *Mortality rates by cause in a cohort of intravenous drug users in Milan, 1981–1991*

Cause	D[a] (%)	MR[b]	95% CI[c]
Overdose	151 (36.6)	9.2	7.8–10.8
AIDS	144 (34.9)	8.8	7.4–10.3
Undetermined	44 (10.6)	2.7	1.9–3.6
Violence	35 (8.5)	2.1	1.2–3.1
Accident[d]	19 (4.6)	1.2	0.7–1.8
Suicide	10 (2.4)	0.6	0.3–1.1
Homicide	6 (1.5)	0.4	0.1–0.8
Other	28 (6.8)	1.7	1.0–2.8
Liver cirrhosis	18 (4.4)	1.1	0.6–1.7
Tumor	6 (1.5)	0.4	0.1–0.8
Myocardial infarction	3 (0.7)	0.2	0–0.5
Nephritis	1 (0.2)	0.1	0–0.3
Infectious diseases	11 (2.7)	0.7	0.4–1.3
Pneumonia/septic shock	6 (1.5)	0.4	0.1–0.8
Tuberculosis	2 (0.5)	0.1	0–0.4
Endocarditis	1 (0.2)	0.1	0–0.3
Fulminant hepatitis	1 (0.2)	0.1	0–0.3
Tetanus	1 (0.2)	0.1	0–0.3
Total	413 (100)	25.2	22.8–27.7

[a]D, number of deaths.
[b]MR, mortality rate per 1,000 person-years.
[c]Ninety-five percent confidence interval.
[d]17 car accidents, 2 burns.

TABLE 3. *Cause- and gender-specific mortality rates in a cohort of intravenous drug users in Milan, 1981–1991*

	Males (13,063 p-y[a])			Females (3,352 p-y)		
Cause	Deaths	MR	95% CI	Deaths	MR	95% CI
Overdose	121	9.3	7.7–11.1	30	9.0	6.0–12.8
AIDS	117	9.0	7.4–10.7	27	8.0	5.3–11.7
Violence	28	2.1	1.4–3.1	7	2.1	0.8–4.3
Infect. dis.[b]	7	0.5	0.2–1.1	4	1.2	0.3–3.1
Other	24	1.8	1.2–2.7	4	1.2	0.3–3.1
Undet.[c]	40	3.1	2.2–4.2	4	1.2	0.3–3.1
Total	337	25.8	23.1–28.7	76	22.7	17.9–28.4

[a]P-y, person-year.
[b]Infectious diseases.
[c]Undetermined.

females (21.3%, mean age 24.4 years, range 16–57). Until June, 1991, this cohort had contributed for 16,415 person-years (p-y) of observation.

By June, 1991, we had observed 413 deaths (16.9% of the enrolled subjects), a mortality rate of 25.2 per 1,000 p-y (95%CI = 22.8–27.7). The leading cause of death was overdose, followed by AIDS (Table 2).

Males and females had a similar overall mortality rate, but mortality for undetermined causes (which accounted for less than 11% of all deaths) was significantly higher in men (Table 3).

Death rates by cause and calendar year are given in Table 4. About 50% (205/413) of the deaths were observed in the last 3 years of follow-up. Death rates were stable from 1981 to 1986, ranging from 10.6 per 1,000 p-y in 1983 to 15.6 in 1986. From 1987 on, mortality progressively increased from 25.6 per 1,000 p-y to 63.8 in the first semester of 1991. Overdose and AIDS accounted for all of this increase. The first deaths for AIDS were observed in 1984; mortality from this cause increased from 1.4 per 1,000 p-y in 1984 to 36.8 in 1991, by which time it had become the leading cause of death. Deaths from overdose were present from 1981. They remained stable from 1982 to 1986 (ranging between 4.4 and 7.0 per 1,000 p-y) but markedly increased from 1987, in parallel with those for AIDS (Fig. 1). Until 1987, overdose was the leading cause of death; after that year, its weight on mortality was similar to that of AIDS. Globally, of the 205 deaths observed from 1989, 47.3% were due to AIDS and 33.6% to overdose. No obvious temporal trend was observed in mortality from violent causes. Infectious diseases accounted for a minority of deaths, with no increase or decrease over time. Death rates for undetermined and other causes remained substantially constant, although they were 50% (4/8 of all causes) in 1981 and only 7.7% (4/52) in 1991.

TABLE 4. *Number of deaths and cause-specific mortality rates by calendar year among a cohort of intravenous drug users in Milan, 1981–1991*

Year (p-y)		Drug overdose	AIDS	Violence	Infectious disease	Other	Undetermined	Total
1981	D	1	0	2	1	1	3	8
(519.3)	MR	1.9	0	3.9	1.9	1.9	5.8	15.4
	CI	0–11	0–7.5	0.4–14.2	0–11	0–11	1.1–17.1	6.6–30.5
1982	D	6	0	3	0	0	2	11
(856.9)	MR	7.0	0	3.5	0	0	2.3	12.8
	CI	2.5–15.3	1.1–4.6	0.7–10.4	0–4.6	0–4.6	0.2–8.6	6.4–23.0
1983	D	5	0	2	0	0	5	12
(1138.2)	MR	4.4	0	1.8	0	0	4.4	10.6
	CI	1.4–10.3	0–3.4	0.2–6.5	0–3.4	0–3.4	1.4–10.3	5.4–18.5
1984	D	7	2	3	2	1	4	19
(1409.7)	MR	5.0	1.4	2.1	1.4	0.7	2.8	13.5
	CI	2–10.3	0.1–5.2	0.4–6.3	0.1–5.2	0–4.1	0.7–7.3	8.1–21.1
1985	D	8	2	2	1	3	4	20
(1637.9)	MR	4.9	1.2	1.2	0.6	1.8	2.4	12.2
	CI	2.1–9.7	0.1–4.5	0.1–4.5	0–3.5	0.3–5.4	0.6–6.3	7.4–18.9
1986	D	11	8	4	0	4	2	29
(1858.0)	MR	5.9	4.3	2.2	0	2.2	1.1	15.6
	CI	2.9–10.6	1.8–8.5	0.6–5.6	0–2.1	0.6–5.6	0.1–4	10.4–22.4
1987	D	17	18	7	2	3	4	51
(1993.2)	MR	8.5	9.0	3.5	1.0	1.5	2.0	25.6
	CI	5–13.7	5.3–14.3	1.4–7.3	0.1–3.7	0.3–4.5	0.5–5.2	19.0–33.7
1988	D	26	17	6	0	4	3	56
(2063.4)	MR	12.6	8.2	2.9	0	1.9	1.5	27.1
	CI	8.2–18.5	4.8–13.2	1.0–6.4	0–1.9	0.5–5.0	0.3–4.3	20.5–35.3
1989	D	25	27	4	2	5	6	69
(2054.3)	MR	12.2	13.1	1.9	1.0	2.4	2.9	33.6
	CI	7.9–18.0	8.7–19.1	0.5–5.0	0.1–3.6	0.8–5.7	1.1–6.4	26.1–42.5
1990	D	28	40	1	2	4	10	84
(1944.2)	MR	14.4	20.6	0.5	1.0	2.1	5.1	43.7
	CI	9.6–20.8	14.7–28.0	0–2.9	0.9–3.8	0.5–5.3	2.4–9.5	34.5–53.5
1991	D	16	30	1	1	3	1	52
(815.9)	MR	19.6	36.8	1.2	1.2	3.7	12.2	63.8
	CI	11.2–31.9	24.8–52.5	0–7.0	0–7.0	0.7–10.9	0–7.0	47.7–83.6

Note: In November and December, 1980, only one death was registered due to drug overdose.

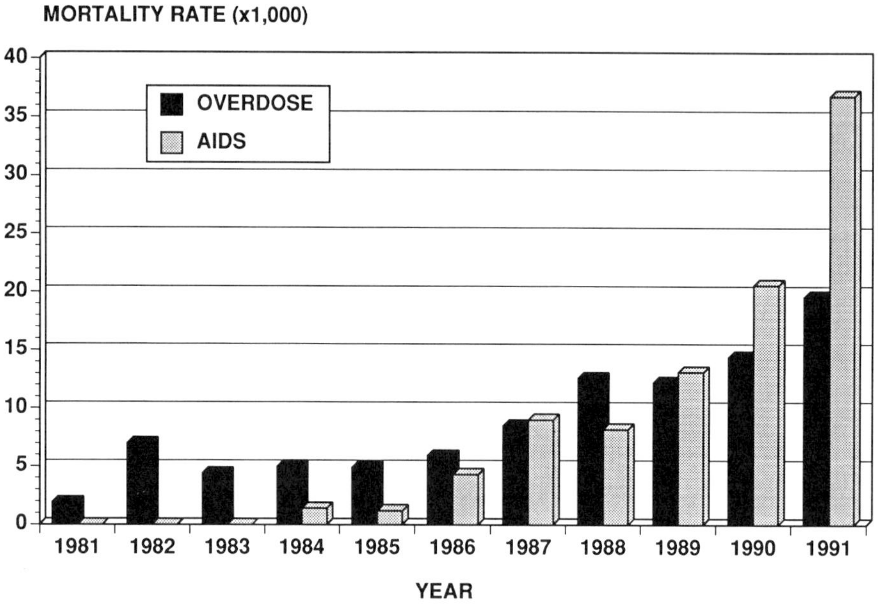

FIG. 1. Deaths from overdose and AIDS in a cohort of intravenous drug users in Milan, 1981–1991.

CONCLUSION

In the period from 1980 to 1989, overall mortality among the general population of Milan aged 25 to 29 years was 0.71 per 1,000 p-y (1.05 for men and 0.38 for women; Table 5). The mortality rate was lower during the early 1980s but progressively increased, reaching 1.78 per 1,000 p-y in men and 0.54 per 1,000 p-y in women in 1989. This increase in mortality has been related to the increase of deaths from overdose and AIDS in young adults, and a further increase is predictable. Over the same 1980 to 1989 period, our cohort accounted for 13,655 p-y; the observed number of deaths was 276 (against the 13.5 expected), giving a standardized mortality rate (SMR) of 21.8. In 1989, the SMR was 19.5 for male IVDUs and 54.2 for female IVDUs (Fig. 2).

The results of our study reveal a marked increase in mortality from 1987 as a consequence of increased mortality from AIDS and overdose. A study performed in New York City by Selwyn et al. (9) showed a similar trend (but with important differences in terms of the causes of death): The mortality rate increased from 12.9 per 1,000 p-y in 1984 to 44.0 in 1987. The death rate due to AIDS increased from 3.6 to 14.7 per 1,000 p-y, and that for bacterial pneumonias and sepsis went from 3.6 to 13.6; the mortality from overdose and other causes remained stable. By reviewing the 7,884 deaths occurring among New York City residents between 1978 and 1986 that were registered

TABLE 5. *Mortality from 1980 to 1991 in IVDU and in general population of the same age and gender in the city of Milan*

	Overall MR[a]				Deaths		
	City of Milan		IVDUs				
Year	Men	Women	Men	Women	Obs.[b]	Exp.[c]	SMR[d]
1980	0.787	0.338	15.8	0	1	0.05	20.0
1981	1.032	0.396	16.3	11.3	8	0.5	16.0
1982	0.953	0.281	12.6	14.0	11	0.72	15.3
1983	0.919	0.338	11.8	4.8	12	0.93	12.9
1984	0.819	0.278	15.9	3.6	19	1.04	18.3
1985	0.828	0.404	10.0	21.0	20	1.22	16.4
1986	1.031	0.377	16.3	13.1	29	1.67	17.4
1987	1.082	0.377	24.1	31.0	51	1.86	27.4
1988	1.345	0.481	27.2	27.0	56	2.39	23.4
1989	1.785	0.544	34.8	29.3	69	3.12	22.1
1990			46.7	33.0	85		
1991[e]			69.2	38.8	51		

[a]Mortality rate per 1,000 person-years.
[b]Observed number.
[c]Expected number based on mortality rates of Milan.
[d]Standardized mortality rates for age and gender.
[e]Deaths observed from January to June.

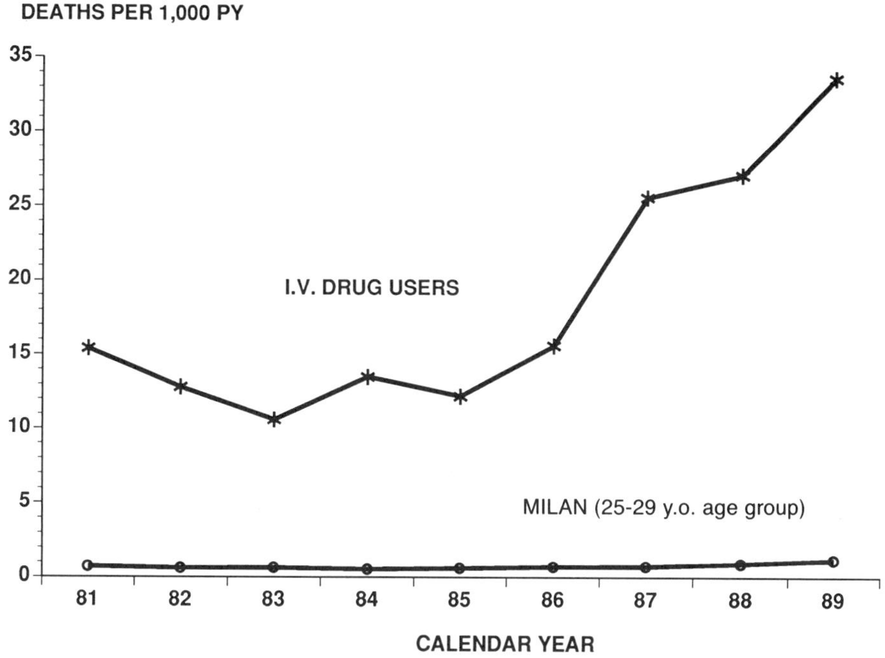

FIG. 2. Comparison of mortality (per 1,000 person-years) between the Milan population of 25 to 29 year-olds and a cohort of intravenous drug users in Milan, 1981–1989.

as being narcotic related, Stoneburner et al. (8) observed a relatively stable number per year, but a decreasing percentage of deaths from overdose. Drug-related deaths represented 61.6% of the deaths not attributable to AIDS in 1978, but only 22.6% in 1986. Increased morbidity for HIV-1 infection, without any rise in non-AIDS mortality, was observed in Amsterdam from 1986 to 1989 (12). D. Des Jarlais (*personal communication,* 1992) reported an overall mortality of 30.0 per 1,000 p-y in the period from 1984 to 1991; the mortality rate was 7.6 per 1,000 p-y for AIDS, 2.5 per 1,000 p-y for infectious diseases, and 4.3 per 1,000 p-y for overdose. During the same years, the mortality rate in our cohort was 27.6 per 1,000 p-y, 10.5 for AIDS, and 9.9 for overdose (Fig. 3). The death rate for infectious diseases other than AIDS and post-hepatitis liver cirrhosis was 0.7 per 1,000 p-y.

Recent data on IVDU mortality in other US cities are limited and have been collected using different methods. Klatt, Mills, and Noguchi (13) reviewed 274 IVDU autopsies performed in Los Angeles from 1981 through June, 1989, which revealed drug overdose as the cause of death in 11% and AIDS in 26% of cases; infectious diseases as a whole were responsible for 50% of deaths, and chronic alcoholism for 19%. In 1987, Joe and Simpson (14) reported the results of a 6-year follow-up of 555 IVDUs recruited from 18 agencies located across the US. Carried out before the AIDS epidemic in IVDUs, this study observed a mortality rate from all causes of 13.8 per 1,000 p-y, mainly attributable to drugs (48%) and violence (29%). This reflects the epidemiological patterns of IVDU mortality observed before the AIDS epidemic in Washington, DC, Atlanta, and other US cities (14,18,19).

Little information is available on IVDU mortality in Europe. Two studies, referring to the Greater London (20) and Paris areas (21), were performed before the AIDS epidemic; more recent data are those from the Amsterdam (12) and Rome studies (10). Although designed in a partially different way, the Rome study does allow us to compare the IVDU mortality rates recorded in the two largest Italian cities. In Rome, overdose was the main cause of IVDU deaths until 1988. The lower proportion of deaths due to AIDS in Rome than in Milan probably reflects a temporal gap in the spread of HIV among the IVDUs of the two cities; in fact, the earliest documented HIV-1 infections, the greater spread of HIV-1 among IVDUs, and the highest incidence of AIDS in Italy were all recorded in Milan (22–25). By the same token, the higher AIDS mortality observed in New York than in Milan is also the consequence of the earlier spread of HIV infection in the US.

In New York City, a recent increase in mortality for pneumonia among young adults has been described and related to the HIV epidemic (26). Selwyn et al. (27) describe an increased risk for bacterial pneumonia in AIDS-free, HIV-infected IVDUs, mainly due to *S. pneumoniae* and *H. influenzae*. A similar trend was observed by us in the seropositive IVDU cohort followed-up at the Milan University's Clinic of Infectious Diseases (Galli M, et al., *unpublished data*). In Milan, the lower mortality due to this cause may

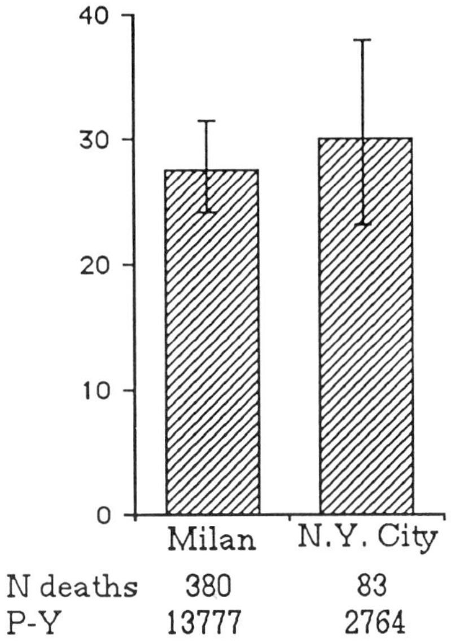

FIG. 3. Mortality (per 1,000 person-years) among intravenous drug users in Milan and New York City, 1984–1991.

be due in part to the different method of ascertaining the cause of death. In our study, investigation was not restricted to the examination of death certificates, and, moreover, a large number of the enrolled subjects were actively followed at the participating centers. It is probable that this greater availability of clinical data allowed us to make a diagnosis of AIDS in patients who would otherwise have been classified as deceased from pneumonia or sepsis. This methodological difference could also explain the higher percentage of deaths attributed to pneumonia in Rome than in our study. Furthermore, the different health-care systems in the US and Italy may also contribute towards the different patterns of mortality; health care in Italy is cost-free and easily accessible to drug users, while the US system does not encourage interaction between IVDUs and health services to the same extent.

The reasons for the large and increasing number of deaths due to overdose, and the different trend in comparison with New York City, may be highly complex. Firstly, the IVDUs studied in the US have a higher mean age than that of our cohort. The average age at enrollment (1969 to 1972) of the IVDUs studied by Joe and Simpson (14) was 24.9 years, the same as that recorded by us for subjects enrolled between 1980 and 1988. As of January 1984, the median age of the population studied by Selwyn et al. (9) was 32 years, the central three-fourths of the subjects being between 30 and 45. In our population, the median age at enrollment was 23.9 years, and 75% of the subjects were under 29. The mean age at death in Los Angeles reported by

Klatt et al. (13) was 39 years, about 10 years older than that recorded for our cohort. The differences in the age of our population may explain the differences in mortality for some causes, such as AIDS-unrelated tumors, which accounted for only 1.5% of deaths in our cohort, but for 6.6% in the autoptic case file of Klatt et al. Furthermore, overdose may be more frequent in a younger IVDU population, not only as a consequence of the higher risk behavior associated with younger age, but also (and mainly) as a consequence of the selection over time of survivors at a lower risk of dying from overdose. In many respects, our cohort is more similar to the populations described in the US during the 1970s and the early 1980s, which had a similar mean age at enrollment (14).

The mortality rate from overdose observed in our cohort closely reflects that observed in Milan (28), which ranged from 0.47 per 100,000 in 1978 to 4.6 in 1987, increasing to 8.1 in 1988 and 9.6 in 1989. These rates are higher than those observed in various US cities between the late 1960s and the early 1980s (16-19,29,30) and more recently in Denmark (where the rates range from 0.3 to 1.4 per 100,000; 31), but they resemble the rates observed in San Francisco between 1971 and 1975 (a mortality from acute narcotism of 6.2 per 100,000 white males and 11.3 per 100,000 black males; 32) and those recorded in the District of Columbia between April, 1979, and December, 1982 (which reached 17.4 per 100,000; 33). Furthermore, the deaths for acute narcotism reported by the Italian Ministry of Internal Affairs for 1989 (965 cases) allow us to calculate a rate of about 1.7 per 100,000 in Italy as a whole (lower than in Milan and in agreement with the higher mortality rate from overdose observed in our cohort than in Rome; 10).

In the province of Milan, 184 deaths for acute narcotism were reported among IVDUs in 1989, 25 involving subjects enrolled in our cohort (13.6%). Given that, during the same period, the number of active drug users in the province was estimated as being about 15,000 to 20,000, the mortality for overdose can be estimated as between 10.9 and 12.3%. In our cohort, the mortality rate for overdose was 12.2 per 1,000 p-y in 1989, a mortality which seems to be similar or only slightly higher than that in the general population of active IVDUs in the district of Milan.

The current explanations for the increase in the number of deaths by acute narcotism in Italy are mainly two. The first is the increased availability of street heroin, indirectly demonstrated by the increase in the amount of heroin seized and the number of police operations (data from the Ministry of Internal Affairs). The second is an increase in the number of IVDUs, although this cannot explain the increase in mortality due to overdose in our cohort (enrollment was stopped in 1988). A further possible explanation may derive from a changed attitude regarding methadone maintenance programs. As a consequence of a change in the therapeutic orientation of working staff, the proportion of subjects on methadone maintenance decreased from 94% in 1984 to 16% in 1989. During 1990, methadone was administered to 38% of the drug users attending the public centers in Italy (21% in the north, 71% in the center, 49% in the south, and 73% in Sicily and Sardinia; data from Ministry of Internal Affairs). During 1988, 30% of the centers in Lombardy did not administer any methadone at all, while the average proportion of treated patients in the other centers was 6% (range 1% to 68%). Furthermore, the mean administered dose during 1989 was generally low, with a median starting dose of 20 mg/die (34). In our cohort, the increase in the death rate from overdose is inversely correlated to the percentage of subjects under methadone treatment. Restrictions in the use of substitutive treatments may have played a role in causing the increase in the number of cases of overdose outside the cohort also, particularly in Northern Italy; in a recent study, we demonstrated the higher risk for death from overdose in IVDUs never treated with methadone (35).

Our data suggest that interventions aimed at modifying the behavioral habits of IVDUs are urgently needed. These interventions must not merely be limited to measures against the spread of HIV-1 infection, since the large excess of deaths among IVDUs can be attributed to causes unrelated to AIDS.

ACKNOWLEDGMENTS

This research was in part supported by grants 42051/89, 520503/90, and 6205007/91 from the Italian Ministry of Health—ISS (Progetto AIDS), and a grant from the Assessorato alla Sanità of the Lombardy Regional Government.

The authors thank Dr. Don C. Des Jarlais for having shared his data on mortality among intravenous drug users in New York City.

Members of COMCAT (Coorte Mortalità Centri Assistenza Tossicodipendenti): Maurizio Amendola, M.D., Mauro Carito, M.D., Danilo Ciaci, M.D., Gabriele Codini, M.D., Francesco Confalonieri, M.D., Susanna Conti, M.S., Mario Corbellino, M.D., Livia Corsi, Virgilio Cruccu, M.D., Isabella Currado, Ph.D., Gino Farchi, M.S., Simonetta Fracchia, M.D., Cristina Gervasoni, M.D., Gianfranca Lovicu, Franco Marozzi, M.D., Alfredo Nicolosi, M.D., Ph.D., Anna Lisa Ridolfo, M.D., Agostino Riva, M.D., Stefano Rusconi, M.D., Alberto Saracco, M.D., Antonio Villa, M.D., Luisa Zampini, M.D., and Mauro Moroni, M.D.

REFERENCES

1. Louria DB, Hensle T, Rose J. The major medical complication of heroin addiction. *Ann Intern Med* 1967;67:1–22.
2. White AG. Medical disorders in drug addicts: 200 consecutive admissions. *JAMA* 1973;223:1469–1471.

3. Mosley JW. The epidemiology of viral hepatitis: an overview. *Am J Med Sci* 1975; 270:253–270.
4. Cherubin CE. The medical sequelae of narcotic addiction. *Ann Intern Med* 1967;67:23–33.
5. Helpern M, Rho YM. Deaths from narcotism in New York City. *J Med* 1966;66:2391–2408.
6. Cherubin C, McCusker J, Baden M, Kavaler F, Amsel Z. The epidemiology of death in narcotic addicts. *Am J Epidemiol* 1972;96:11–22.
7. Musto FD, Ramos MR. Notes on American medical history: a follow-up study of the New Haven morphine maintenance clinic of 1920. *N Engl J Med* 1981;304:1071–1077.
8. Stoneburner RL, Des Jarlais DC, Benezra D, et al. A larger spectrum of severe HIV-1 related disease in intravenous drug users in New York City. *Science* 1988;242:916–919.
9. Selwyn PA, Hartel D, Wasserman W, Drucker E. Impact of the AIDS epidemic on morbidity and mortality among intravenous drug users in New York City methadone maintenance program. *Am J Public Health* 1989;79:1358–1362.
10. Perucci CA, Davoli M, Rapiti E, Abeni DD, Forastiere F. Mortality of intravenous drug users in Rome: a cohort study. *Am J Public Health* 1991;81:1307–1309.
11. Rothman KJ. *Modern epidemiology*. Boston: Little, Brown & Co; 1986.
12. Mientjes GH, van Ameyden EJ, van den Hoek AJAR, Coutinho RA. Increased morbidity without rise in non-AIDS mortality among HIV-1 infected intravenous drug users in Amsterdam. *AIDS* 1992;6:207–212.
13. Klatt EC, Mills NZ, Noguchi TT. Causes of death in hospitalized intravenous drug abusers. *J Forensic Sci* 1990;35:1143–1148.
14. Joe GW, Simpson DD. Mortality rates among opioid addicts in a longitudinal study. *Am J Public Health* 1987;77:347–348.
15. Zimney EL, Luke JL. Narcotic-related deaths in the District of Columbia, 1971–1979. *J Forensic Sci* 1981;26:462–469.
16. Alexander M. Surveillance of heroin-related deaths in Atlanta, 1971 to 1973. *JAMA* 1974;229:677–678.
17. Wetli C, Davis JH, Blackbourne BD. Narcotic addiction in Dade Country, Florida: an analysis of 100 consecutive autopsies. *Arch Pathol Lab Med* 1972;93:330–343.
18. Desmond DP, Maddux J, Trevino T. Street heroin patency and deaths from overdose in San Antonio. *Am J Drug Alcohol Abuse* 1978;5:39–49.
19. Garriot JC, Di Maio VJ, Petty CS. Death by prisoning: a ten-year survey of Dallas County. *J Forensic Sci* 1982;27:868.
20. Ghodse AH, Sheehan M, Stevens B, Taylor C, Edwards G. Mortality among drug users in Greater London. *BMJ* 1979;2:1742–1744.
21. Ingold FR. Study of deaths related to drug abuse in France and Europe. *Bull Narc* 1986;38:81–89.
22. Lazzarin A, Galli M, Geroldi D, et al. Epidemic of LAV/HTLV-III infection in drug addicts in Milan: serological survey and clinical follow-up. *Infection* 1985;13:216–218.
23. Lazzarin A, Crocchiolo P, Galli M, et al. Milan as possible starting point of LAV/HTLV-III epidemic among Italian drug addicts. *Boll Ist Sieroter Mil* 1987;53:9–13.
24. Galli M, Lazzarin A, Saracco A, et al. Clinical and immunological aspects of HIV infection in drug addicts. *Clin Immunol Immunopathol* 1989;50:s166–s176.
25. Istituto Superiore di Sanità—Centro Operativo AIDS. Aggiornamento dei casi di AIDS conclamato notificati in Italia al 30 settembre 1992. *Notiziario Ist. Sup. Sanità* 1992;5(12):S1–S8.
26. Centers for Disease Control. Increase in pneumonia mortality among young adults and the HIV epidemic, New York City, United States. *MMWR* 1988;37:593–596.
27. Selwyn PA, Feingold AR, Hartel D, et al. Increased risk of bacterial pneumonia in HIV-infected intravenous drug users without AIDS. *AIDS* 1988;2:267–272.
28. Caligara M, Gigli F, Lodi F, Marozzi E, Marozzi F, Zoja R. Mortalità da droga in Milano nel decennio 1978–1987. Nota I: Dati demoscopici. *Riv It Med Leg* 1990;12:141–161.
29. Caplan YH, Ottinger W, Park J, Smith T. Drug and chemical related deaths: incidence in the State of Maryland 1975–80. *J Forensic Sci* 1985;30:1012.
30. Froede SH, Byer JM, Froede AM, Jones AM, Henry T. An analysis of toxic deaths 1982–85, Pima County Arizona. *J Forensic Sci* 1987;32:1676.

31. Steentotf A, Worm K, Christensen H. Morphine concentration in autopsy material from fatal cases after intake of morphine and/or heroin. *J Forensic Sci Soc* 1988;28:87.
32. Hine CH, Wright JA, Allison DJ, Stephens BG, Pasi A. Analysis of fatalities from acute narcotism in a major urban area. *J Forensic Sci* 1982;27:372–384.
33. Ruttenber AJ, Luke JL. Heroin-related deaths: new epidemiologic insights. *Science* 1984;226:14–20.
34. Mainini F, Bertolini G, Grilli R, Liberati A. Il metadone nei servizi per le tossicodipendenze della regione Lombardia. *Practitioner* (Italian Ed) 1991;152:15–21.
35. Galli M, Musicco M, Zampini L, et al. Influence of long term therapeutic programs for opiate addicts and methadone treatment upon mortality and spreads of HIV-1 in intravenous drug users (IVDUs). In: Rossi GB, et al., eds. *Proceedings of the VII International Conference on AIDS, Florence,* 1991. Abstract WC 3351;II:383.

DISCUSSION

Dr. Halloran: You said there was no statistically significant difference between seropositives and the people of undetermined status. . . .

Dr. Galli: The mortality is only different for AIDS and infectious disease. By the way, the group of undetermined status is likely to include a number of infected individuals.

Dr. Rezza: In a similar study in Rome, we found a significant excess of mortality for overdose in seropositive over seronegative users. Of course, this may be just a case of differences in sample size, the power of the study, or different conditions (in Rome, we have a lower prevalence of HIV infection, and maybe the incidence of AIDS and AIDS mortality is different from that of Milan). But I would like to ask a question about the possible effect of methadone treatment. Are your findings in any way similar to those of the Amsterdam study? As I understand it, you didn't find any association between the duration of methadone treatment and HIV infection, but did you adjust your data for the duration of drug use?

Dr. Galli: That is something that we are developing now, and I think it may be a good way of establishing the function of methadone correctly. But the dosage of methadone, particularly in Milan, was very low in the majority of cases, and a lot of subjects continued intravenous drug use during methadone treatment (at least in some centers). Another problem is that the spread of the virus was more extensive and occurred 1 or 2 years earlier in Milan than in other parts of Italy. It's probable that methadone protection was greater in relation to overdose and acute narcotism because it decreased the number of injections and therefore the number of risk opportunities, but it wasn't sufficient to solve the problem.

Of course, newly enrolled subjects represent a completely different problem, and methadone remains a major tool, but, in the past, the Italian way of giving methadone wasn't sufficient.

Dr. Vall: Why was it that most of the people recruited in the study were from 1980 to 1985?

Dr. Galli: Because the centers were particularly active during this period; subsequently, their activities declined with the decline in methadone administration. At the same time, recruitment in these four centers also declined because other centers were opened.

Dr. Nicolosi: The way you classified the subjects according to HIV serology (seropositive versus undetermined) is a conservative way to estimate the excess of AIDS deaths. There are, obviously, a number of seropositive people among your subjects of undetermined serological status. If the distinction were clear, the excess of AIDS deaths would result [in] higher [mortality rates for AIDS]. Do you have any hypotheses as to what this misclassification implies for comparisons of other causes of death?

Dr. Galli: We can estimate that at least 20% to 30% of the undetermined cases were seropositive. We are trying to solve the problem of misclassification by using a smaller group of subjects whose serological status at enrollment we are absolutely sure about. It seems that the preliminary data are substantially similar, but we have to complete the analysis. We are using the same cohort that we used to give the data on methadone, and on overdose linked to the use of methadone.

Dr. Vlahov: Do you have any prospectively collected, pre-death information on the individuals in the group you are following?

Dr. Galli: Not for all of the cohort. But for a subgroup, we do have a good deal of prospectively collected data concerning behavior.

Dr. Vlahov: Sometimes, psychological measurements are made when people go into treatment; I was wondering whether you have any information about depression, anxiety, and so on, for the people in this cohort?

Dr. Galli: In general, yes, but the design of the study didn't include these items.

Dr. Susser: Are you suggesting a direct link between the withdrawal of methadone treatment and this phenomenal increase in the number of deaths from overdose? Or do you have any indirect hypotheses?

Dr. Galli: I don't think there is any link between AIDS and methadone. AIDS mortality is the result of the HIV epidemic present among intravenous drug users at the end of the 1970s, which became significant in Milan in the early 1980s. The increase in AIDS mortality is to be expected.

The problem of overdose is different, and we have no official explanation for the phenomenon in Milan, or anywhere else in Italy. Here, we have a problem of denominators (because we are not sure about the real number of drug users in Italy), but one possible explanation is the decrease in the use of methadone in some major cities. It is not so probable that it can be attributed to the drug (which in our case is almost always straight heroin because injecting cocaine is not frequent in Italy). We have no precise elements for thinking that the drug itself may be more toxic for certain individuals, but this is the only hypothesis we can make.

HIV Epidemiology: Models and Methods, edited by Alfredo Nicolosi. Raven Press, Ltd., New York © 1994.

5

Reliability and Validity in Cross-National Research on AIDS Risk Behavior Among Injecting Drug Users

*Don C. Des Jarlais, †Samuel R. Friedman, †Jo L. Sotheran, †John Wenston, ‡Manuel Carballo, §Kachit Choopanya, §Suphak Vanichseni

**Beth Israel Medical Center, New York, New York, 10003; †National Development and Research Institutes, Inc. (formerly Narcotic and Drug Research, Inc.), New York, New York, 10013; ‡Program on Substance Abuse, World Health Organization, Geneva, Switzerland; §Health Department, Bangkok Metropolitan Administration (BMA), Bangkok, Thailand*

The injection of illicit drugs has been reported from over 80 different countries, and HIV infection has been reported among injecting drug users (IDUs) in over 50 countries (1). Historically, different cultures have adopted widely varying patterns of use of psychoactive drugs (2). One might therefore expect that there would also be great variation in the social characteristics and behavior of injecting drug users in different societies. The rapid diffusion of injecting drug use into many different societies over the last 20 years, however, suggests that there may also be important cross-cultural similarities in the behavior of IDUs. The rapid spread of HIV among IDUs in some of these countries makes determination of cross-national similarities and differences in the behavior of injecting drug users a matter of immense and immediate practical importance. Sufficient prior knowledge of the similarities and differences would provide a basis for more rational design of AIDS prevention programs, without having to go through a trial-and-error learning process for each separate site.

Determining cross-cultural similarities and differences in the social characteristics of injecting drug users would be most efficiently done through multi-site comparative studies using the same methodology. Reliability and validity issues are always a major concern in the study of an illicit behavior, such as nonmedical injecting of psychoactive drugs, and are of even greater concern for a multi-site, cross-national study. Research techniques and strategies that are likely to produce highly reliable and valid results in one cul-

TABLE 1. *Participating sites and principal investigators*

City	Country	Principal investigator
Athens	Greece	M. Malliori
Berlin	Germany	W. Heckmann
Bangkok	Thailand	K. Choopanya
Glasgow	United Kingdom	D. Goldberg
London	United Kingdom	G. Stimson
Madrid	Spain	M. Zunzunegui
Naples	Italy	S. Salmaso
New York	USA	D. Des Jarlais
Rio de Janiero	Brazil	E. Lima
Rome	Italy	G. Rezza
Santos	Brazil	F. Mesquita
Sydney	Australia	A. Wodak

tural setting may be totally inappropriate in other cultural settings. This paper will address some of the cross-cultural reliability and validity issues in the multi-site study of HIV and drug injecting that was initiated by the World Health Organization (WHO). The paper will not attempt to address all relevant reliability and validity issues, but will focus on the validity of subject responses to critical questions for AIDS prevention.

Table 1 lists the different sites currently participating in the study and the principal investigator for each site. While many of the sites are from Western Europe, these sites nonetheless encompass substantial differences in terms of economic development, economic class structures, religion, prevalence of injecting drug use, provision of treatment for drug dependence, drug most frequently injected, and prevalence of AIDS among injecting drug users. These differences, then, should permit a good test of cross-cultural validity questions.

STUDY METHODS

To be eligible for the study, all subjects had to have injected illicit drugs within the 2-month period prior to data collection. In each site, potential subjects were recruited from two different sources: drug-abuse treatment programs and a nontreatment site. The types of treatment programs varied from detoxification to residential to outpatient drug-free to methadone maintenance programs. Recruiting subjects for the nontreatment sample included use of the following: (a) an established research storefront in a drug-user neighborhood; (b) roving teams of outreach workers; and (c) "snowball" sampling (including the payment of active drug users to recruit new subjects). In addition, in one city (Bangkok), it was necessary to recruit subjects who were newly entering the treatment system.

The study was explained to the potential subject, informed consent was obtained, a standard questionnaire (translated into the local language) was administered by a trained interviewer, HIV pre-test counseling was administered, and a blood or saliva sample was obtained for HIV testing. In some cities, it was also necessary to refer subjects to a separate location because HIV testing could not be performed in the field setting.

The study was reviewed by a research ethics committee in each of the separate sites.

RESULTS

Table 2 shows the ranges for selected demographics, drug histories, and AIDS risk behaviors among subjects from the different sites participating in the study. The relatively narrow ranges for these important variables suggest substantial validity in the subjects' responses at the group level. The similarity must be due either to similar valid answers or to similar cross-cultural factors that would produce uniform distortion in the responses. It is inter-

TABLE 2. *Ranges for selected demographic, drug history, and AIDS risk behaviors among IDUs participating in the WHO multi-site study*

	Lowest	Highest
Gender (% male)	<60 (Berlin)	95 (Bangkok)
Age at first injection	17.5 (Glasgow)	21.7 (Bangkok)
Freq. of injection[a]		
reporting "daily"	19.1 (Rio)	88.5 (Rome)
reporting "weekly"	9.2 (Rome)	43.1 (Rio)
reporting "monthly"	2.3 (Rome)	37.7 (Rio)
Freq. of sharing injection equipment in last 6 months		
reporting "daily"	1 (Naples)	18 (Santos)
reporting "weekly"	1 (Naples)	12 (Bangkok)
reporting "monthly"	11 (Rome)	36.6 (Sydney)
reporting "never"	46 (Santos)	81 (Naples)
Freq. of condom use with primary partners in last 6 months		
reporting "always/mostly"	11 (3 sites)	31 (Rome)
reporting "half the time"	1 (Rio)	6 (2 sites)
reporting "occasionally"	4 (Santos)	17 (Bangkok)
reporting "never"	50 (Rome)	77 (Rio)
Freq. of condom use with casual partners in last 6 months		
reporting "always/mostly"	13 (Rio)	49 (New York)
reporting "half the time"	2 (Athens)	12 (London)
reporting "occasionally"	6 (Athens)	26 (Santos)
reporting "never"	31 (New York)	73 (Rio)
Sharing outside of study area in last 2 years		
reporting "yes"	6 (Naples)	50 (Santos)
reporting "no"	50 (Santos)	93.6 (Naples)

From Carballo (6).
[a]Frequency, expressed as percent, of site's most frequently injected drug.

esting to note that the question with the greatest variation, i.e., gender, is also the question with the highest face validity.

The questions reflected in Table 2, however, are relatively straightforward items. They involve reporting on facts that are relatively clear (e.g., gender) or behaviors that are relatively easy to remember and to report.

More difficult validity problems are likely to arise when the behaviors addressed by the question involve reflection, judgments, and attributions about behavior rather than simple reporting of behavior. These more complicated questions are likely to be susceptible to memory lapses and social desirability effects.

The goal of almost all AIDS prevention programs for injecting drug users is to influence and enable IDUs to change their behavior in order to reduce their chances of becoming infected with HIV and to reduce their chances of transmitting HIV to others if they have already been infected. Injecting drug users are educated, peer influenced, fear aroused, and often even provided with the means to reduce their AIDS risk behaviors. Almost all of the models upon which these programs have been based, from common sense to the health belief model to the theory of reasoned action to self-organizing, presume that injecting drug users can comprehend what constitutes the various AIDS risk behaviors and are capable of sufficient self-monitoring to know when they have changed those behaviors.

Despite the importance of AIDS-related behavior change among injecting drug users, and the implicit assumption on the part of most AIDS prevention programs that IDUs are capable of recognizing changes in their own behavior, relatively few studies, whether single- or multiple-site studies, have simply asked subjects, "Have you changed your behavior because of AIDS?" There are multiple threats to the reliability and the validity of such a question:

1. The responses may be highly subject to social desirability effects, because subjects would already know that researchers, public-health officials, and many drug-injecting peers strongly support behavior change and risk reduction.
2. The question does not suggest any specific type of behavior to be changed, and different subjects may apply it to numerous different behaviors, which may differ substantially in their relative efficiency of transmitting HIV.
3. Attribution of the cause of a behavior change to concern about AIDS may vary across subjects. Responses to attribution questions are particularly subject to variations in the specific wording of a question.
4. Coding answers to such an open-format question introduces another source of potential unreliability.
5. Many persons may have changed their behavior for a certain period of time in response to concerns about AIDS but then reverted back to pre-

AIDS behavior patterns. This reversion to previous behavior itself may have ranged from episodic lapses to a full relapse.

Despite all of these concerns, this question was utilized in the WHO standard questionnaire. A follow-up question of "How?" was asked of subjects who reported that they had changed their behavior. A rather long (two-and-one-half page) coding system was used to classify different responses. An additional follow-up question was used to probe the extent to which each of the mentioned behavior changes was maintained (coded into categories of completely, partially, or very little). In the remainder of this paper, we will examine the evidence for the validity of the answers to this question among injecting drug users in Bangkok, Thailand and New York City, USA, the two cities where extensive analyses of the responses have already been conducted.

BIOLOGICAL CRITERION VALIDATION

Strong correlations with biological measures often serve as a standard for validation of self-reported data in epidemiology. If the responses to a question are strongly associated with biological measures in theoretically predicted directions, then one presumes that the questions are reliably and validly elucidating some characteristic or behavior that is also reflected in the biological measures. (This presumes, of course, that the respondents did not have knowledge of the biological data prior to answering the relevant questions.) This biological validation can occur either at an individual level, where the individual's responses to particular questions are associated with a biological measure for the individual, or at a group level, where the responses of the group as a whole are associated with biological measures for the group as a whole.

In both Bangkok and New York, there is group-level validation for the responses to the "Have you changed your behavior since you heard about AIDS?" question. By 1985 in New York and by 1989 in Bangkok, a majority of injecting drug users were responding affirmatively to this question, reporting that they had changed their behavior. Indeed, HIV seroprevalence among injecting drug users is now known to have stabilized in the two cities at about those times. HIV seroprevalence stabilized at approximately 50% among IDUs in New York and approximately 40% among IDUs in Bangkok (3).

Behavior change in response to AIDS is, of course, only one possible factor in the stabilization of HIV seroprevalence among IDUs which occurred in the two cities at about those times. Saturation of very high-risk subgroups of IDUs in the two cities is another potential contributor to the stabilization. Nevertheless, the relationship between large-scale, self-reported behavior change and stabilization of HIV seroprevalence is an example of where the validity of the behavior change might have easily been disproved but was not.[1]

Individual-level biological validation (i.e., lack of disproof) was established regarding the behavior-change question in a study of HIV seroconversion among injecting drug users in Bangkok (4). As part of the 1989 data collection, subjects were asked if they had been tested for HIV previously, and, if yes, what the results were of the previous test. One hundred seventy-three of the subjects in Bangkok responded that they had previously tested negative. Seventeen of these were HIV positive as of the 1989 data collections; records of HIV testing in the Bangkok Metropolitan Administration were checked and a previous HIV-negative test was located for all 17 of these subjects.[2] They were thus considered to be true seroconverters and, in a case-control design, were compared with the other 156 subjects who reported a previous negative test and who were still HIV negative as of 1989.

Standard bivariate analyses followed by a multiple logistic regression analysis with backwards elimination were used to identify risk factors for remaining HIV seronegative (failing to seroconvert) among IDUs in Bangkok. The multiple logistic analysis showed two factors associated with failing to seroconvert: having a regular sexual partner and having responded "stopped sharing" in response to the question, "Have you changed your behavior in order to reduce the chance of developing AIDS?"

To our knowledge, this is the first instance where self-reported behavior change in response to concern about AIDS was significantly associated, on an individual level, with not seroconverting. It is important to note here that the period of seroconversion covered by this particular study—starting in 1987, when HIV-antibody testing began on a large scale among IDUs in Bangkok, up through 1989, the time of data collection—was a period during which both large numbers of HIV seroconversions and large-scale behavior change were occurring. This simultaneous occurrence of both large-scale seroconversions and large-scale behavior change would, of course, increase the statistical power for observing a relationship between the two variables.

---

[1]In brief, it is worth noting here Popper's philosophical argument that a scientific hypothesis can never be proved empirically, but only survive instances where it might have been disproved empirically. This argument may be particularly important for reliability and validity issues in cross-cultural studies, as the opportunities for disproving the reliability and validity of instruments may be very frequent in such research and may require careful analysis as to the underlying hypotheses about the reliability and validity of a particular instrument in a particular setting. Any generalized hypothesis, such as, "this instrument will be reliable and valid in these settings," may overlook important details as to which specific characteristics of the instrument are supposed to be valid or reliable, or both, in regard to each specific characteristic of the different settings.

[2]Because it was not possible to check on HIV-test records for subjects in New York, we did not conduct a parallel study for IDUs in New York.

CONSTRUCT VALIDATION

While biological criterion validation provides an important verification for cross-national studies of AIDS risk behavior among injecting drug users, studies that demonstrate construct validation are at least as important for designing effective prevention programs. Prevention programming needs to have sound, long-term conceptual bases rather than being limited to haphazard, eclectic empiricism.

However, construct validation (i.e., showing that a particular instrument produces responses that are associated in predicted ways within a conceptual framework) may be even more difficult to demonstrate than biological criterion validation for cross-cultural studies of AIDS risk behavior among injecting drug users. It is relatively easy to identify biological criteria, such as HIV serostatus, for criterion validation studies. Identifying what might be appropriate theories for construct validation studies is considerably more difficult. Theories of AIDS prevention among injecting drug users are still in a relatively early stage of development, and it is quite difficult to state which potential theories are relevant, which are irrelevant, and how the relevant theories should be integrated.

As part of the analyses of self-reported AIDS behavior change and risk reduction among IDUs in New York and Bangkok, we identified determinants of any self-reported, AIDS-related behavior change. These analyses were conducted on data collected in 1989 in Bangkok, at a time when 92% of the IDUs reported that they had changed their behavior because of AIDS, and on data collected from 1990 to 91 in New York City, at a time when 80% of the IDUs reported that they had changed their behavior because of AIDS. Bivariate analyses followed by multiple logistic regression analyses were used to identify possible determinants from among 40 demographic, drug-history, and behavioral variables. Table 3 presents the results from the final multiple logistic regression analyses for each city. Three factors were associated with self-reported behavior change in both cities: (a) talking with drug-using friends about AIDS; (b) having been tested previously for HIV; and (c) knowing that one can be infected with HIV/AIDS while still looking

TABLE 3. *Determinants of AIDS risk reduction among injecting drug users in Bangkok and New York City*

	Bangkok	New York
Talking with peers	×	×
HIV testing	×	×
Know HIV+ can look healthy	×	×
Education		×
Recruitment site		×

healthy. These results indicate that, in both cities, AIDS risk reduction is a social process that is further facilitated by HIV testing and a sophisticated understanding of the relationship between HIV exposure and developing disease (5).

The congruence of these findings across the two cities is impressive, particularly since the outcomes of multiple logistic regression can be highly sensitive to very small variations in the strength of the associations between the predictor and outcome variables. In assessing this congruence, it is important to note that both Bangkok and New York were in relatively similar stages of an HIV epidemic at the time of the respective studies. Both cities had previously undergone periods of very rapid transmission of HIV among IDUs and had entered periods of stable HIV seroprevalence by the time that the data were collected. In both cities, the great majority of IDUs reported that they had changed their behavior because of AIDS, and the regression analyses primarily enable us to identify the characteristics and behaviors of the small percentage of IDUs who had not changed their behavior despite the epidemics of HIV that had occurred among drug injectors in both cities.

CONCLUSION

There is considerable evidence for reliability and validity in the responses of IDUs in the WHO's multi-site study. Basic consistencies in responses across the 13 different sites suggest both reliability and validity for many of the questions. The additional analyses of data on self-reported behavior change among injecting drug users in Bangkok and in New York provide evidence for biological criterion and construct validity. Finding evidence for the biological criterion and construct validity in these two cities was facilitated by particular circumstances. In the Bangkok serconversion study, the data covered a period of high rates of both seroconversion and behavior change. The observed similarities in the determinants of risk reduction in the two cities occurred during similar stages of the HIV epidemic among IDUs in the cities. Knowing when the circumstances are favorable or unfavorable for observing criterion or construct validity may be a critical aspect of addressing validity concerns with respect to cross-national research on AIDS among injecting drug users.

The common stereotype of illicit drug users holds that they are so drugged out that they cannot accurately remember their behavior and so dishonest that they would not accurately report it, even if they could remember it. It is important to remember that, despite occasional periods of cognitive impairment due to acute drug effects or drug withdrawal, injecting drug users are sentient and competent human beings. Indeed, functioning within a drug-use subculture often requires a considerable degree of street smarts. Injecting drug users are clearly capable of monitoring their own behavior, including changes in behavior due to major concerns such as AIDS. Obtaining valid information from injecting drug users, therefore, may be mainly a question of developing a basis of trust between the researcher and the competent respondent.

ACKNOWLEDGMENTS

The authors would like to thank Thomas Ward for editorial assistance and expertise during the preparation of this manuscript. This research was supported by grant DA03574 from the National Institute on Drug Abuse, and by the World Health Organization's Multi-Site Study of Drug Injecting and the Risk of HIV Infection. The views expressed in this paper do not necessarily reflect the positions of the granting agencies or of the institutions by which the authors are employed.

REFERENCES

1. Stimson GV. Epidemiology of injecting drug use. Presented at the VIII International Conference on AIDS, Amsterdam, The Netherlands, 1992.
2. DuToit BM, ed. *Drugs, rituals and altered states of consciousness*. Rotterdam, The Netherlands: AA Balkema; 1977.
3. Des Jarlais DC, Choopanya K, Wenston J, et al. Risk reduction and stabilization of seroprevalence among drug injectors in New York City and Bangkok, Thailand. In: Rossi GB, et al., eds. *Science challenging AIDS: proceedings of the VII International Conference on AIDS, Florence*. Basel, Switzerland: Karger; 1992:207–213.
4. Choopanya K, Des Jarlais DC, Vanichseni S, et al. AIDS risk reduction and HIV seroconversion among drug injectors in Bangkok. Presented at the VIII International Conference on AIDS, Amsterdam, The Netherlands; 1992.
5. Des Jarlais DC, Choopanya K, Friedmann P, et al. Determinants of AIDS risk reduction among injecting drug users in New York City, USA and Bangkok, Thailand. Presented at the VIII International Conference on AIDS, Amsterdam, The Netherlands; 1992; (abstract #PoD 5490).
6. Carballo M. Prevention for injecting drug users. Presented at the VIII International Conference on AIDS, Amsterdam, The Netherlands; 1992.

DISCUSSION

Dr. Vermund: Can you comment on the recruitment-site difference in New York?

Dr. Des Jarlais: The people recruited coming into treatment on either the methadone or the detoxification program were more likely to report that they had changed their behavior than the people in the street-recruited sample. We don't exactly understand the significance of this, but, for example, there are data from Montreal showing higher seroconversion rates among street-recruited people than among treatment-recruited people, and there are some possible parallels there. But, if we want to do good prevention and good epidemiology, it certainly argues for the need to go out and do work in the streets and not just rely on the people coming into treatment programs.

Dr. Susser: Is it possible that there is a handle if we take the balance between the population recruited in treatment, the population on the streets, and the population recruited and not recruited across cities? I see you have a lot of similarities as far as these key issues are concerned.

Dr. Des Jarlais: We are trying to work on this question of who else is out there other than the people coming into treatment, the people entering jail, and the people you can easily recruit from street research settings. It looks like we're now moving towards two ways of identifying these very hard-to-reach populations. One possibility is when they develop AIDS and go into the hospital. There you can ask them whether they have ever been in treatment or ever been in jail and about the places where they bought drugs (whether they just bought and left immediately, whether they stayed and used the shooting galleries, whether they hung out in the neighborhood, and so on); although, of course, it's too late for prevention.

The other way in which progress is being made is through syringe exchange work, where you can briefly talk to a lot of hidden drug users who would not normally be recruited either in the treatment setting or by people hanging out in drug-user neighborhoods. In the US, these people are often white and employed in working class occupations. They come into a neighborhood, buy their drugs, go to a syringe exchange, and then leave. They don't hang out in that neighborhood, because they don't want to be known as drug users. But they will go to a syringe exchange, particularly to the group in Tacoma, where they have a mobile syringe exchange that accepts telephone orders and actually delivers the syringes. This is allowing us to get in touch with a lot of people who would otherwise be totally unknown to the system.

Dr. van den Hoek: Is there any difference in seroprevalence and injecting behavior between subjects in treatment and subjects recruited in the street?

Dr. Des Jarlais: That varies from city to city. In New York, the treatment samples had higher seroprevalence; in Bangkok, the in-treatment sample had higher prevalence than the group which was new to treatment. When there is a difference, it tends to be higher in the in-treatment groups, but in some cities there was no difference. So that seems to be an area where much more research is needed.

Dr. Nicolosi: In Italy, Stefania Salmaso at the National Institutes of Health did a study using saliva tests in street drug users, and the prevalence was lower in out-of-treatment people.

You mentioned the increasing number of deaths from overdose in Milan, and hypothesized that this might be due to the reduction in methadone treatment. You also said that there was a difference between New York and Milan as far as overdose deaths were concerned. Can you tell us about methadone treatment in New York; has its use been increasing?

Dr. Des Jarlais: It's been basically constant. Many people say that the use of methadone should be expanded in New York, but this has not been the case. It has remained at about 35,000 methadone treatment slots over the last 15 to 20 years. Most of these involve high-dose methadone, with average daily doses of between 50 and 60 mg. So it's not only a case of more methadone but also a very different type of methadone treatment. It's classic, high-dose, indefinite maintenance, as opposed to the Italian low-dose, extended detoxification treatment. Nevertheless, comparison would certainly support the interpretation that the availability of high-dose methadone treatment tends to reduce overdose deaths.

Dr. Moss: In San Francisco, we were able to compare our treatment study with John Watter's street study, and the rate of new infection in the street study was the same as the new infection rate in the people we picked up in 21-day short-term detoxification programs, about three-and-a-half percent per year. This is considerably higher than when methadone maintenance is used. We need to remember that treatment isn't just one thing, it's a spectrum of things; and this also means that you can get the same rates as in out-of-treatment situations.

Dr. Des Jarlais: Many people feel that methadone-assisted detoxification (whether it's 7, 21, or 180-day) is not drug-abuse treatment; it's perhaps more an entry into treatment or a needed immediate medical service.

Dr. Moss: What I'm saying is that this is a way of picking up a population which isn't really a treatment population.

Dr. Vlahov: The validity of self-reports has been questioned in several earlier sessions. Here we see the question, "Have you changed your behavior in response to the AIDS epidemic?" and the degree to which people will admit that they haven't. This leads to the problem of getting at recent past data both cross-sectionally and prospectively (when you're providing counseling to individuals who come back later). Would you like to make any comments about this?

Dr. Des Jarlais: I can give you some more specific information about the Bangkok study. That study included the question, "Have you changed your behavior? If so, how? And have you maintained the change?" More than 90% of the people said that they had changed their behavior; 60+% said they had simply stopped sharing injection equipment, which was by far the dominant response, and so we classified that as a variable.

We also had the question, "Have you been previously tested for HIV? If so, what were the results?" One hundred and seventy-three people said that they had previously been tested HIV negative. Out of those, 17 were HIV positive at the time of the interview. As we went back and found the previous HIV-negative test results for these 17 subjects, we knew they were accurately reporting a previous HIV-negative test result, and that they had actually seroconverted since that time. We then did a standard risk factor analysis comparing those 17 with the 159 who had reported a previous negative test and were still HIV negative. The two factors which emerged were whether or not they had a regular sexual partner and whether or not they said that they had stopped sharing injection equipment. We took that as validating, because the seroconverters didn't know their HIV status at the time they answered the question, and so it wasn't a matter of social desirability or anything like that.

HIV Epidemiology: Models and Methods, edited by Alfredo Nicolosi. Raven Press, Ltd., New York © 1994.

6

Differences Between African and Western Patterns of Heterosexual Transmission

Peter Piot

WHO Collaborating Centre on AIDS, Institute of Tropical Medicine, 2000 Antwerp, Belgium; currently at the Global Programme on AIDS, World Health Organization, Geneva, Switzerland

Though the AIDS epidemic was originally perceived as a problem largely confined to homosexual men and injecting drug users, it has now become clear that, on a global scale, HIV is mainly spread by heterosexual intercourse. However, the relative contribution of heterosexual contact to the spread of HIV infection varies greatly among continents and populations. Thus, whereas in Europe in 1992, 11.4% of all reported cases of AIDS were thought to be acquired heterosexually, this was the case for approximately 90% of patients with AIDS in sub-Saharan Africa (1,2). On the other hand, even within Europe there are large variations in the importance of heterosexual spread of HIV, with as few as 5% of AIDS cases in Germany being heterosexually acquired, as compared to well over 20% of cases in Belgium, Greece, and Portugal (1).

In the United States, the percentage of AIDS cases attributed to heterosexual contact has increased steadily from 0.9% to 4% in 1989 (3). However, as in Europe, there are major geographic differences in HIV epidemiologic patterns, with inner city minority populations, and even poor rural communities, at highest risk for heterosexual spread of HIV (3–5).

THE SIZE OF THE AIDS EPIDEMIC IN AFRICA

As of July 1, 1992, over 152,000 cases of AIDS had been reported from Africa, but the World Health Organization estimates that by 1992 approximately 1 million adults had developed AIDS (6). It is thought that over 6 million people in Africa are now infected with HIV.

The epidemic is still expanding and has clearly not reached an equilibrium point as yet, although there is some evidence from Zaire of a relatively stable HIV seroprevalence at 3% to 6%, implying that the incidence does not exceed the loss of deaths of HIV infected people (7,8). The highest HIV infection rates are found in East and Central Africa, and in Ivory Coast, with urban populations usually more affected than rural ones. In cities such as Kampala, Kigali, and Lusaka, one-fifth to one-fourth of adults in the general population are now infected. Among high-risk populations, such as female prostitutes, as many as 90% may be infected with HIV-1. There is a marked heterogeneity in the spread of HIV, with as many epidemiologic differences within Africa as between Africa and Europe. Thus several countries, particularly in their rural areas, have still very low HIV prevalence rates, with less than 1% of the adult population infected (e.g., Madagascar, and several West African countries).

The sex ratio is usually around one to one, though women make up the majority of cases in countries such as Ghana, Uganda, and Zaire, and male cases predominate in the Ivory Coast.

Mother-to-child transmission is the second most common route of transmission of HIV-1 in Africa, with transmission rates as high as 30% to 40%. This has resulted in hundreds of thousands of children with HIV infection and AIDS. In addition, most children born to HIV-positive mothers and who escaped HIV infection will become orphans.

DETERMINANTS OF HETEROSEXUAL TRANSMISSION IN AFRICA

Table 1 lists various variables which influence the sexual transmission of HIV-1 in Africa (9). These include biological, behavioral, and societal factors, none of which is unique to Africa.

In general, the spread (or reproductive rate, Ro) of a sexually transmitted disease, such as HIV infection, is determined by the equation, $Ro = \beta c D$, where β is the average probability that infection is transmitted from an infected person to a suspectible individual, c is the average rate at which new sexual partners are acquired, and D the average duration of infection (2,10). It is the (often subtle) mix and interaction of risk determinants influencing directly (i.e., biological or behavioral variables) or indirectly (i.e., demographic and social parameters) these three factors that define how and where HIV-1 infection spreads in population. Similarly, interventions affecting any of these factors will decrease the reproductive rate.

Virologic Parameters

African isolates of HIV-1 exhibit an unusually high degree of genetic variability (11). Its epidemiologic significance, if any, is unclear, but may result from strain differences in infectivity and virulence and their capacity to reach higher viremic levels. In addition, the efficiency of sexual transmission at the population level probably increases over time after the introduction of the virus. This should result in higher average viremic levels, which in turn

TABLE 1. *Variables influencing the spread of HIV-1 infection in Africa*[a]

Virological parameters
Infectivity and virulence of HIV-1 strains
Level of viremia (and immunodeficiency)
Local genital factors
Presence of other sexually transmitted diseases
Lack of male circumcision
Use of certain vaginal products
Sexual behavior
Rate of partner change
Sexual mixing patterns
Type of sexual intercourse (e.g., receptive anal intercourse, sex during menses)
Size of and rate of contact with core groups
Level of condom use
Demographic variables
Proportion of sexually active age groups to other age groups
Male-to-female ratio in the population
Proportion of urban population to rural population
Migration patterns
Economic and political factors
Poverty
War and social conflicts
Status of roads and mobility of population
Performance of the health-care system
Response to the epidemic

[a]Adapted from Piot et al., ref. 9.

are associated with a higher rate of transmission of HIV-1 (12). This phenomenon may explain why, in general, higher HIV-1 infection rates are found in partners of HIV-1 positive persons in Africa than in Europe (13,14).

Local Genital Factors

There is good, though not conclusive, evidence that other sexually transmitted diseases (STDs) enhance the risk of sexual transmission of HIV-1 by increasing both the infectiousness of an HIV-1–infected individual and the susceptibility of a noninfected sex partner to HIV-1 (15,16). This is best documented for genital ulcers, which are mainly caused by chancroid in Africa, but increasingly also for nonulcerative STDs, such as gonorrhea, chlamydial infection, and trichomoniasis. The complex interrelationship between STDs and HIV infection is reviewed elsewhere in this volume. As STD prevalence and incidence are generally high in sub-Saharan Africa, particularly in urban populations, this may significantly contribute to a more intensive heterosexual spread of HIV-1 than in Europe.

Lack of circumcision in men was independently associated with an increased prevalence and incidence of HIV-1 in several, but not all, studies in Africa (15,17–19). This association seems biologically plausible and may operate through an increased risk for genital ulcer disease, particularly chancroid, as well. However, its contribution to the spread of HIV-1 in Africa is unclear. In any case, lack of male circumcision has not resulted in an accelerated spread of HIV-1 in Europe (where the overwhelming majority of men are uncircumcised), nor has the generalized practice of circumcision in men prevented the rapid spread of HIV-1 in populations such as that in Burkina Faso.

In women, vaginal abrasions or trauma, desiccating vaginal products, and a vaginal sponge containing nonoxynol-9 have been associated with an increased risk of HIV-1 infection (20). This possibility is not well explored and offers opportunities for prevention, at least in some countries.

Sexual Behavior

HIV infection is, in the first place, a sexually transmitted disease, and sexual behavior is without doubt the most important determinant for its spread. The heterogeneity of sexual behavior among and within populations can be enormous and probably plays an important role in the heterogeneity of the AIDS epidemic in Africa, as well as in Europe (21).

High rates of partner change increase the risk of HIV-1 infection, and rapid spread of HIV-1 has been documented in female prostitutes, clients of prostitutes, and long distance truck drivers in Africa, just as in homosexual men in some major cities in North America and Western Europe (16,22,23). In addition, the sexual mixing patterns largely define how rapidly HIV-1 spreads in a population, particularly in the early stages of the epidemic (22,24). Thus, in cities with a high male-to-female ratio, such as Harare or Nairobi, the rate of casual and commercial sex is increased, resulting in high HIV-1 prevalence rates in prostitutes and their clients and in fairly rapid spread in the general population. In contrast, sexual patterns involving roughly equal numbers of men and women may imply a slower spread of HIV. However, as the prevalence of infection increases in the general population, an increasing number of people, particularly women, become infected without practicing high-risk sexual behavior themselves. This is illustrated by data from Kenya, Rwanda, and Zaire, showing that an increasing proportion of women with HIV-1 infection have a regular partner or husband as their only sexual contact (25–27).

In contrast to the West, in several African countries women have higher HIV-1 infection rates than men (28). It is not clear whether this is due to a more efficient transmission from men to women, earlier onset of sexual activity in women, a higher degree of exposure of women to infected men, or a longer survival among infected women.

Condoms are becoming increasingly popular in Africa, mainly as a result of social marketing programs (29). The reduction in HIV-1 incidence following condom use has been well documented in prostitutes in Zaire and Kenya

(30,31), and in discordant couples in Kinshasa. It is probable that massive condom use will further slow down the spread of HIV. Unfortunately, governments of several countries are still not supportive of an aggressive promotion of condom use.

Demographic Variables

A major difference between Europe and Africa is the proportion of the most sexually active age group, which is much higher in sub-Saharan Africa. This by itself implies higher incidence rates of STDs. As a result of continuing high birth rates, this population of young adults will become even larger in the near future.

As mentioned earlier, a distorted male-to-female ratio in the population may lead to an increased frequency of casual and commercial sexual encounters and is associated with high levels of HIV spread. Similarly, large urban concentrations and migratory populations have been linked historically with above average rates of sexually transmitted diseases. In 1965, only 16% of Africans lived in large cities, as compared to 25% in 1983 (32). Whereas significant rural to urban migration is occurring all over Africa, some regions also experience extensive transnational migration, such as to the Ivory Coast from its neighboring countries. It is unclear if and how the recent migration waves to Eastern Europe have any impact on the spread of HIV.

Economic and Political Factors

Poverty is one of the most powerful drives of epidemics, not just a consequence, and is the most difficult factor to change. It engenders prostitution, homeless adults and street children, poorly educated citizens, migration and separated families, all fertile ground for the spread of HIV.

War in Uganda has probably greatly contributed to this country's AIDS epidemic. In Kinshasa, most preventive efforts, such as social marketing of condoms and interventions among prostitutes and their clients, were interrupted in September, 1991, following major political unrest.

As a result of poor management, low political priority to health and social services (as compared with military expenditure), and structural readjustment plans, in many African countries the health-care system has severely deteriorated. This has been accompanied by declining access to health services and control of sexually transmitted diseases, as well as less opportunities for preventative activites.

Last, but not least, society's response to the epidemic will ultimately determine the extent of HIV spread. Clearly there are success stories of HIV prevention, both in Africa and Europe, but it is uncertain whether they can be extended to larger populations.

CONCLUSIONS

In general, similar risk factors for heterosexual transmission have been identified in Africa and Europe, and under comparable conditions the risk of heterosexual transmission is of the same order of magnitude. However, most determinants of heterosexual HIV transmission are much more frequent in many parts of Africa, which could explain the different epidemiologic patterns between the two continents.

To continue purely descriptive studies on risk factors of heterosexual transmission is hard to justify today in Africa. It is time to focus our efforts on the development and evaluation of interventions to prevent the further spread of HIV.

REFERENCES

1. European Centre for the Epidemiological Monitoring of AIDS. *AIDS Surveillance in Europe*. Paris: 1992; Quarterly Report no 35.
2. Anderson RM, May RM. Transmission dynamics of HIV infection. *Nature* 1987;26:137–142.
3. Holmes KK, Karon JM, Kreiss J. The increasing frequency of heterosexually acquired AIDS in the United States, 1983–88. *Am J Public Health* 1990;80:858–862.
4. Ellerbrock TV, Lieb S, Harrington PE, et al. Heterosexually transmitted HIV infection among pregnant women in a rural Florida community. *N Engl J Med* 1992;327:1704–1709.
5. Rosenberg PS, Levy ME, Brundage J, et al. Population-based monitoring of an urban HIV/AIDS epidemic: magnitude and trends in the District of Columbia. *JAMA* 1992; 268:495–503.
6. World Health Organization. AIDS-data as of 1 July 1992. *Wkly Epidemiol Rec* 1992; 67:201–203.
7. Magazani K, Laleman G, Perriëns JH, et al. Low and stable HIV seroprevalence in pregnant women in Shaba province, Zaire. *J AIDS [in press]*.
8. Ryder RW, Ndilu M, Hassig SE, et al. Heterosexual transmission of HIV-1 among employees and their spouses at two large businesses in Zaire. *AIDS* 1990;4:725–732.
9. Piot P, Laga M, Ryder R, et al. The global epidemiology of HIV infection: continuity, heterogeneity and change. *J AIDS* 1990;3:403–415.
10. Yorke JA, Heathcote HW, Nold. Dynamics and control of the transmission of gonorrhea. *Sex Transm Dis* 1978;5:51–57.
11. Peeters M, Piot P, van der Groen G. Variability among HIV and SIV strains of African origin. *AIDS* 1991;6[Suppl 1]:S29–S36.
12. Laga M, Taelman H, Van der Stuyft P, et al. Advanced immunodeficiency as a risk factor for heterosexual transmission of HIV. *AIDS* 1989;3:361–369.
13. European Study Group. Comparison of female to male and male to female transmission of HIV in 563 stable couples. *BMJ* 1992;304:809–813.
14. Johnson AM, Laga M. Heterosexual transmission of HIV. *AIDS* 1988;2[Suppl 1]:S49–S56.
15. Cameron DW, Simonsen JN, D'Costa LJ, et al. Female-to-male transmission of HIV-1: risk factors for seroconversion in men. *Lancet* 1989;ii:403–407.
16. Laga M, Manoka A, Kivuvu M, et al. Non-ulcerative sexually transmitted diseases as risk factors for HIV-1 transmission in women: results from a cohort study. *AIDS* 1993;7:95–102.
17. Borgdorff MW, Barongo LR, Mosha FF, et al. HIV infection in Mwanza region, Tanzania: prevalence and risk factors. Presented at the VI International Conference on AIDS in Africa, Dakar, 1991; (Abstract 265).

18. Caraël M, Van de Perre P, Lepage P, et al. HIV transmission among heterosexual couples in Central Africa. *AIDS* 1988;2:201–205.
19. Moses S, Bradley JE, Nagelkerke NJD, et al. Geographic patterns of male circumcision practices in Africa: association with HIV seroprevalence. *Int J Epidemiol* 1990;19:693–697.
20. Dellabeta G, Miotti P, Chiphangwi J, et al. Vaginal agents as a risk factor for acquisition of HIV-1. Presented at the V International Conference on AIDS in Africa, Kinshasa, 1990; (Abstract FOA2).
21. Caraël M, Cleland J, Andeokun L. Overview and selected findings of sexual behavior surveys. *AIDS* 1991;5[Suppl 1]:S65–S74.
22. Anderson RM, May RM, Bioly MC, et al. The spread of HIV-1 in Africa: sexual contact patterns and the predicted demographic impact of AIDS. *Nature* 1991;352:581–589.
23. Plummer FA, Nagelkerke NJD, Moses S, et al. The importance of core groups in the epidemiology and control of HIV-1 infection. *AIDS* 1991;5[Suppl 1]:S169–S176.
24. Larson A. Social context of HIV transmission in Africa: historical and cultural bases of East and Central African sexual relations. *J Rev Infect Dis* 1989;11:71–73.
25. Allen S, Lindan C, Serufilira A, et al. HIV infection in urban Rwanda. *JAMA* 1991;266:1657–1663.
26. Kamenga M, Ryder RW, Jingu M, et al. Evidence of marked sexual behavior change associated with low HIV-1 seroconversion in 149 married couples with discordant HIV-1 status: experiences at an HIV counseling center in Zaire. *AIDS* 1991;5:61–67.
27. Temmerman M, Mohamed Ali F, Ndinya-Achola J, et al. Rapid spread of both HIV-1 infection and syphilis among pregnant women in Nairobi, Kenya. *AIDS* 1992;6:1181–1185.
28. Berkley S, Namaara W, Okware S, et al. AIDS and HIV infection in Uganda: are women more infected than men? *AIDS* 1990;4:1237–1242.
29. Lamptey P, Goodridge GAW. Condom issues in AIDS prevention in Africa. *AIDS* 1991;5[Suppl 1]:S183–S191.
30. Laga M, Alary M, Nzila N, et al. Condom promotion and STD treatment leading to a declining incidence in a cohort of high risk women. [submitted for publication].
31. Moses S, Plummer FA, Ngugi E, et al. Controlling HIV in Africa: effectiveness and cost of an intervention in a high-frequency STD transmitter core group. *AIDS* 1991;5:407–411.
32. The World Bank. *Sub-African Africa: from crisis to substainable growth.* Washington, DC: The World Bank; 1989.

DISCUSSION

Dr. Padian: First a comment: although a strong effect of the lack of male circumcision was found in a study involving UCSF, among others, there was also an interaction with age. The kinds of associations found when considering men circumcised later were not the same as those found in people circumcised at birth. That's something to think about.

But I'd like to know what's going on in Western Africa. I was wondering if you attributed the lower rates there to the more recent introduction of the virus, the lower rates of other STDs, or something else. How commonly are prostitutes used there? Is there perhaps a lack of a core group?

Dr. Piot: If you take Abidjan, there are about 70% more men than women; that's where there is a really explosive epidemic and a pattern which is more similar to that of Eastern Africa.

I think all three of your suggestions may be involved. Sexual behavior patterns are different in West and East Africa. The status of women is very different; a lot of businesses are completely controlled by women, and not just on behalf of men, but because it's their own money. I think that this is also reflected in personal relationships and so on. The only good survey which has been done on STDs was done in Dakar, and it showed a very low prevalence of STDs, which was also the case in Kinshasa. And there's also the later introduction.

Dr. Susser: Cameroon looked a bit out of line, with a high rate of STDs.

Dr. Piot: I'm not sure how representative the Cameroon sample was. But, in any case, there's something interesting when you see review papers on STDs in Africa: The authors tend not to cite studies where the rate of presence of STDs is low. There's an incredible bias; they want to make a point, and so they always take the high prevalence rates.

Dr. Vlahov: Two quick points. In your last slide about the risk factors for heterosexual transmission, you didn't mention the number of different sex partners. Is there some reason why this is not a risk factor in Africa?

Dr. Piot: Yes and no. It obviously relates to an increase in exposure risk, but, as the prevalence of infection in the population increases, you don't need to have a high number of sex partners to become infected; the difference in risk is no longer measurable.

There are also several studies showing that, in East Africa (but not West Africa), most of the women with HIV infection had no obvious risk in terms of their own sexual behavior; their risk is really determined by the risk behavior of their male partner, which is incredibly difficult to put into studies.

Dr. Vlahov: In one of your early slides, you made an urban versus rural comparison. What I noted was the typical bimodal distribution in the urban part; but in the rural part, the slide showed 0% in those under the age of 6, and then there was a change in the curve in the range 6 to 15. Can you comment on that?

Dr. Piot: It probably has something to do with the fact that only 3% to 4% of the women of child bearing age in rural Rwanda are HIV-positive, which means that you would expect 1% to 2% of infected children under the age of five. It may be a sample problem, or something.

Dr. Nicolosi: At the beginning of your talk, you showed a slide comparing the characteristics of HIV prevalence in different parts of the world. The sex ratio of cases in Africa was 1:1. Why do you think it is different in the Western world?

Dr. Piot: First of all, it needs to be said that the sex ratio is not the same throughout Africa. In countries like Uganda and Zaire, there are more women with AIDS or HIV infection than men, and women are infected at an earlier age. In the Ivory Coast in Western Africa, there are about 30% more men than women. We don't know why this is. It may be a reflection of the initial phase of the epidemic, and the fact that a lot of men have been traveling around; and you can't exclude the prevalence of homosexual contacts in this initial small group. If the efficiency of transmission at a population level were much higher from men to women than from women to men, we would see many more women than men with HIV infection. But the problem is that many different factors need to be put into the model (exposure, networks, mixing, and so on). And in any case, I'm not so convinced that man-to-woman transmission is necessarily that much more efficient.

The major difference between Africa and Europe is not the risk markers or determinants themselves, but their prevalence. We should pay more attention to trying to estimate what's attributable to what, because that is obviously more important from a public health point of view.

Dr. Musicco: I believe that the efficiency of man-woman transmission is greater than that from woman to man, but if you are right in your hypothesis that the dynamics of transmission is from a core group mainly represented by prostitutes to the rest of the population, you can have a different level of efficiency in terms of transmission and the same rate of infection. One woman can infect a larger number of men, while the sexual partners of infected men are always in the same group. That may be an explanation.

Dr. Piot: That is only true if the core group only consists of women, which is not the case.

Dr. Musicco: You have also hypothesized that some viral strains may be more sexually infective in Africa, and that the rate of transmission among steady couples is as low as in developed countries. Is this supported by data, or is it just a feeling?

Dr. Piot: I have no data about viral strains, but, as far as couples are concerned, I think it depends on how they are recruited. If, as in most studies, you recruit people from clinics or people who are ill, you find much higher transmission rates. But several hundred discordant couples were recruited in a study done in various businesses in Kinshasa (including a bank and a textile factory), which gave a cross-sectional picture of the situation, and there were as many couples with only the man infected as there were couples with only the woman infected. Concordant couples made up only a small minority. The rate of seroconversion in the discordant couples was extremely low, less than one new infection per 100 couple-years, although, of course, the study also included a prevention program. In Nairobi, they recruited couples including one partner with an STD, and they found a tremendous transmission rate among the couples.

It is also important that comparisons are made between comparable groups. In many couples, there is a complete absence of risk determinants. This has been a problem in several intervention studies where they found that the sample size was just too small.

Dr. Rezza: One of the issues about Western Africa is the question of international travel, migration, and tourism. In Senegal, for example, there is a very low prevalence of HIV infection in Dakar, but the rates are relatively high in the rural tourist areas in the south. We did a study in Guinea and found that almost all of the AIDS cases involved subjects who had traveled to Abidjan. Do you think that any intervention strategy is applicable without limiting international travel?

Dr. Piot: Well, I don't think that limiting international travel would be desirable.

HIV Epidemiology: Models and Methods,
edited by Alfredo Nicolosi. Raven Press, Ltd.,
New York © 1994.

7

Partner Studies in the Heterosexual Transmission of HIV

Nancy S. Padian and Stephen C. Shiboski

Department of Epidemiology and Biostatistics, University of California, San Francisco, California 94110

The likelihood of sexual tranmission of human immunodeficiency virus (HIV) depends first on the likelihood of exposure or choosing HIV-infected partners and then on the likelihood of transmission given exposure. The likelihood of exposure is driven by the probability that a random partner is infected (and infectious) and depends on the rate of new partner acquisition and the risk group of the partners (1). The more partners a susceptible person has, the more likely it is that one partner is infected. Conversely, the more partners an infected person has, the more likely it is that transmission will occur with at least one partner. However, the significance of number of partners depends on the prevalence of infection within a community. For example, in the U.S. homosexual community of San Francisco, California, where the infection rate may be as high as 50% (2), it might require fewer partners to select an infected partner than in communities characterized by lower infection rates. In addition, number of partners is also mediated by the risk group of the partner. Large numbers of low-risk partners are less significant than a few high-risk partners. For example, selecting partners who are intravenous drug users or prostitutes obviously increases the risk that the partner is infected. Thus, how partners are selected (mixing between high-risk and low-risk groups) moderates the direct effect of rate of new partner acquisition.

Variables that measure the likelihood of selecting an infected partner, such as numbers of partners, knowledge of partner's risk history, and information about how and where partners meet (surrogate measures of mixing), are probably best assessed in surveys of sexual behavior in various samples within the population. However, variables that measure risk of transmission subsequent to exposure are best assessed in partner studies that enroll an infected individual and his or her sexual partners. Partner studies are tools that can be used to study transmission probabilities by examining the efficiency of transmission and concomitant risk factors.

The general protocol for heterosexual partner studies is to enroll individuals known to have acquired immunodeficiency syndrome (AIDS) or to be infected with HIV and their opposite-sex partner(s). Couples in whom transmission has occurred are then compared with couples in whom transmission has not occurred to ascertain risk factors that either may be protective or may increase the likelihood of transmission. Extraneous sources of exposure (other than sexual transmission from the identified index case) are ruled out through risk histories and a variety of laboratory tests (e.g., toxicity tests that may reveal recent drug use, or tests for other sexually transmitted diseases that may provide evidence of other high-risk partners).

Of course, a more rigorous type of partner study would be a prospective design where couples who are discordant for HIV are enrolled and where transmission events can then be observed during the course of the study. This design enhances the ability to rule out other sources of exposure and eliminates problems associated with uncertainty regarding the direction of transmission (i.e., determining who was infected first in couples concordant for HIV).

In this chapter, we will present results from our own partner study and review results from other studies. We will also discuss methodological strengths and weaknesses of partner studies. Finally, we will examine outstanding questions about the heterosexual transmission of HIV that can best be answered through a partner study design.

STUDY METHODS AND RESULTS

Since 1985, we have been conducting a study of the heterosexual transmission of HIV in which we enroll the opposite-sex partner of individuals with AIDS or HIV. Although discordant couples are enrolled in a prospective phase of the study, to date, we have observed high rates of behavior change over time and no seroconversions. Thus, we have only been able to examine transmission rates and risk factors from the cross-sectional component of the study. Here, we report on baseline results for participants recruited through December 1991.

Couples were recruited without regard to the sex of the index case, and over 75% of the sexual partners did not know their serostatus at entry into the study. More than 70% of the recruited couples were monogamous since 1978, and more than 90% of participants reported only 1 partner in the 6 months prior to enrollment (3). The direction of transmission in concordantly infected couples was determined through risk histories; in all couples, the infected index case had a well-established source of risk. If the source of infection, and hence the direction of transmission, could not be established with certainty, couples consisting of two infected partners were eliminated from the study. Eighteen such couples were recruited but eliminated from analysis. All but one of these couples were eliminated because the putative susceptible partner reported recent intravenous drug use.

Infected individuals were passively recruited from a variety of sources throughout California (e.g., confidential test sites, local departments of public health, physicians, and research studies). They were counseled to refer their heterosexual partners for HIV testing and counseling and were informed about the study. At the time of recruitment, the serostatus of the presumed originally uninfected partners was ascertained together with a retrospective risk history of sexual pratices for both partners, as well as other behavioral, medical, and demographic factors for each partner in the couple. After the risk assessment, couples received extensive counseling and education about HIV risk reduction. Participants were interviewed in their homes or in local clinics. Study protocol and data collection methods have been previously described (4,5).

Four hundred four couples were recruited through December 1991. Of these, 328 couples consisted of female partners of HIV-infected men and 76 consisted of male partners of HIV-infected women. Forty percent of the male index cases were bisexual men, and the most common risk group of the female index cases was that they (44%) were the heterosexual partner of an HIV-infected man in the study. These women had acquired new male partners subsequent to their HIV infection. Over 70% of the couples were white and in their 30s and 96% of the couples were concordant for race.

Sixty-four or 19.5% of the female partners were infected (95% confidence limit, 15–24%), compared to 1% or 1.3% of the male partners (95% confidence limit, 0.3–7%). There were no differences in transmission rates stratified by gender according to risk group of the index case.

Table 1 presents results from a logistic regression analysis examining risk factors for male-to-female transmission. All of the factors in the model, with the exception of log number of contacts, were significant in a univariate analysis. Although not significant, we added this latter factor in the multivariate model for two reasons. First, it makes biological sense to assume that repeated exposure increases the chance of transmission. Second, its presence modifies the effect of other risk factors that were in the model (6). Anal intercourse was defined as ever practicing this behavior during the relationship, no condoms was defined as no use prior to entry into the study,

TABLE 1. *Logistic regression (male-to-female transmission) (n = 328)*

Factor	Odds ratio	P value	95% confidence interval
Anal intercourse	2.27	0.01	1.2–4.1
No condoms	2.63	0.005	1.3–5.2
Bleeding	2.07	0.05	1.0–4.2
Log number of contacts	1.10	0.27	0.9–1.4

and bleeding was defined as noticeable bleeding from trauma immediately following intercourse. These risk factors have remained the only variables independently associated with transmission since the inception of the study.

Because there was only one instance of female-to-male transmission, we could not examine risk factors for this direction of transmission. Thus, although there were several salient characteristics of the couple in whom female-to-male transmission occurred, the following brief description of their risk history (a more detailed report has been previously described [5]) must be viewed as a case history, and not something that can be generalized to others.

The female index case became infected through heterosexual contact. She knew of at least three previous partners from identified risk groups. She had had 2000 contacts with a bisexual man, an unidentified number of contacts with an intravenous drug user, and over 1000 contacts with a man she knew to be HIV positive. The couples reported an average of 15 sexual contacts a month for the last 7 years. Almost all of these contacts consisted of unprotected penile–vaginal intercourse. They practiced anal intercourse twice, and never used condoms for any sexual activity.

Both partners reported vaginal or penile bleeding after intercourse. Among all couples, observed bleeding during sex was usually of either vaginal or rectal origin. However, there were six other couples with a female index case who reported penile bleeding, and the average number of times this was observed was 4 with a range of 1 to 20 times. In contrast, both partners in this couple reported over 100 episodes of both vaginal and penile bleeding. The cause of this bleeding could not be established. Medical data were available only by history. Over the last 5 years, the women reported four cases of vaginal yeast infections, both reported one case of trichomoniasis, and the man reported one case of urethral gonorrhea. In addition, the woman reported a history of endometriosis and had a hysterectomy during the year prior to entry into the study. The bleeding was not associated with menses as both partners reported vaginal–penile intercourse only rarely when the woman was menstruating.

RESULTS FROM OTHER STUDIES

Table 2 presents results from a sample of similar partner studies that have examined both directions of transmission. Not all such studies are included. For example, several studies have observed no female-to-male transmission (19,20). These are results from studies with fundamentally similar designs. Still, transmission rates differ across studies and some attempt must be made to reconcile differences.

The first most obvious difference can be attributed to a different distribution of risk factors in the study samples. A reasonable prevalence level of any factor is required in order to detect an effect. In addition, the varied prevalence and distribution of identified risk factors in different study sam-

TABLE 2. *Number possible/total (%)*

Index risk group	Female-to-male	Male-to-female	Place	Reference
Mixed	19/159 (12)	82/404 (20)	Europe	7
	5/15 (33)	36/58 (62)	Belgium	8
	10/64 (16)	30/135 (22)	Italy	9
	8/90 (9)	99/368 (27)	Italy	10
	12/17 (71)	14/28 (50)	U.S.	11
	3/33 (9)	12/41 (23)	Martinique	12
Transfusion-associated	2/25 (8)	10/55 (18)	U.S.	13
IDU[a]	1/19 (5)	3/54 (16)	Edinburgh	14
	7/14 (50)	51/114 (45)	U.S.	15
	2/12 (16)	29/61 (48)	Italy	16
Haiti	23/38 (61)	73/136 (54)	Haiti	17
Central Africa	55/78 (73)	92/150 (61)	Zambia	18

[a]IDU, intravenous drug user.

ples will also result in different transmission rates. Although in our study we have only identified three independent risk factors for male-to-female transmission, a variety of other factors have been revealed in other studies. Table 3 represents a summary of these risk factors. Obviously, the prevalence of such risk factors drives transmission rates. For example, in our study, the prevalence of other sexually transmitted diseases (STD) in both the men and

TABLE 3. *Factors associated with heterosexual transmission of HIV[a]*

	Transmission	
Factor	Male-to-female	Female-to-male
Sexual practices		
Anal intercourse	Yes	No
Sex during menses	No	Yes
Number of sexual contacts	Yes	Yes
Biological factors		
Lack of male circumcision	Possibly	Yes
Advanced disease state (as measured by CD4, p24 antigen, or AIDS[b] diagnosis)	Yes	Yes
Variations in viral strains	Possibly	Possibly
Host immunological profile	Possibly	Unknown
Genital sores, infections, or inflammations	Yes	Yes
Cervical ectopy	Yes	Unknown
Contraceptive practices		
Lack of condoms	Yes	Yes
Oral contraceptives[c]	Yes	Unknown
IUD[d] use	Possibly	Unknown
Spermicides[c]	Possibly	Possibly
Zidovudine (AZT)	Yes	Unknown

[a]HIV, human immunodeficiency virus.
[b]AIDS, acquired immunodeficiency syndrome.
[c]Whether oral contraceptives and spermicide use are protective or increase the likelihood of transmission is controversial.
[d]IUD, intrauterine devices.

the women is approximately 3%. If STD in either the infected or susceptible partner increase the likelihood of female-to-male transmission, then the low prevalence of this risk factor could contribute to our observed low rates of female-to-male transmission. Similarly, in several studies, transmission probabilities increase with progression to disease and individuals who are sicker, as measured by low CD4 counts, presence of p24 antigen, or AIDS diagnoses, are more likely to transmit than individuals who are asymptomatic. Significantly more female index cases in our study were asymptomatic than male index cases. Perhaps this also contributed to low rates of female-to-male transmission in our study.

Transmission probabilities are heterogeneous, with some individuals becoming infected after only a few contacts while others remain uninfected in spite of thousands of unprotected contacts (6). Thus, there are variations in both infectiousness and susceptibility that cannot be entirely explained by the presence of identified risk factors; these variations could also contribute to varied transmission rates. For example, differences in the prevalence of high efficiency transmitters in different samples would affect results.

PROBLEMS INHERENT IN PARTNER STUDY DESIGNS

In addition to the differences across studies discussed above, there are also problems inherent in the design of partner studies that also might contribute to observed variation in transmission rates across studies. No partner study has reported results from a random probability sample of HIV-infected individuals and their heterosexual partners; all partner studies are fundamentally volunteer samples. Thus, although such studies highlight the biological plausibility of particular risk factors and give indications as to transmission efficiencies, generalizing results from one study to other studies or populations is probably inappropriate. In addition, the extent to which other potential biases (discussed below) contribute to any one study may also effect the resulting observed transmission rate.

Problems common to both cross-sectional and prospective studies include the fact that in a partner study there are two sources of potential error for recall and response bias. Furthermore, couples do not necessarily agree on reports of joint practices. Although reliability studies between partners are one way to examine this phenomenon, unless there is close to perfect agreement, researchers may have to rely solely on the reports of one sex.

Another generic problem is selection bias: in a cross-sectional study, it may be easier to identify concordantly infected couples, thus inflating transmission rates. Recruiting couples with partners of unknown serostatus is one way to control for this bias. However, even in a prospective study, AIDS cases may be easier to recruit than asymptomatic cases, and if transmission probabilities increase with progression to disease, this may bias transmission rates upwards.

In both designs, there is also limited ability to control for other sources of exposure leading to possible misclassification. This is a more fundamental problem in cross-sectional studies where inability to control for extraneous sources of exposure (e.g., intravenous drug use or multiple sexual partners) may confound ascertainment of the true index case in concordantly infected couples. Obviously, couples without a clear index case, such as concordantly infected couples in whom both partners are intravenous drug users, should be eliminated. Nevertheless, this is still a problem in prospective designs where one must be certain that seroconversion can be traced back to the enrolled index case. For example, if transmission rates are higher among intravenous drug users and their partners in either design, one must at least consider the possibility that risk factors other than those associated with sexual transmission are present. The cleanest design for any partner study would restrict recruitment to monogamous couples consisting of one HIV-infected partner. However, such couples are not easy to identify and if recruitment were restricted in such a fashion, numbers would be small, thus decreasing the power to examine the effect of more than a few risk factors.

Finally, in both designs, unless the index case was infected by a contaminated blood transfusion, it is difficult to estimate the time of infection of the index case. This makes estimates of true exposures, as measured by behavior subsequent to infection of the index case, subject to substantial measurement error. Of course, this problem is further exacerbated in a cross-sectional design where time of infection of the partner of a concordant couple is also unknown.

There are also several problems unique to each design. In cross-sectional studies, as stated above, the fundamental challenge is to identify the true index case. In concordantly infected couples, investigators rely mainly on risk histories to ascertain the true index case and thus the direction of transmission. Sometimes this is obvious, as in the case of a monogamous female partner of bisexual men, but even this scenario must be derived retrospectively. Likewise, it is not always possible to link data collected from a retrospective risk history with the transmission event, thus limiting the ability to identify risk factors proximal to transmission.

The greatest problem in prospective studies is also their greatest source of success. All prospective studies include counseling aimed at risk reduction along with ascertainment of interval risk histories. Thus, seroconversion is limited by the effects of behavior modification. Although a partner study provides a natural cohort in which to observe behavioral change over time, power to detect effects of risk factors associated with observed seroincidence is severely limited. In addition, longitudinal studies are expensive and difficult to conduct. Issues associated with attrition and maintenance of the cohort are foremost in these designs to insure that loss to follow-up is not affected by risk status. Intensive follow-up of lost couples must be built into all prospective designs.

Biases such as those discussed above may affect transmission rates as well as estimates of risk factor effects. Although such biases are often inherent in partner study designs, there are ways to quantify their effects so that their influence on infectivity, transmission probabilities, and measures of association can be gauged. These methods are not the subject of this chapter, but are the goals of future methodologic studies. Meanwhile, investigators need to be aware of potential biases in their study and should consider them when interpreting and comparing study results.

CONCLUSIONS

These problems notwithstanding, partner studies have provided some of the most convincing data about risk factors associated with transmission, and they still remain the most powerful design to examine the efficiency of transmission and risks of transmission given exposure. For example, although transmission rates may differ depending on the study, the fact that male-to-female transmission is more efficient than female-to-male transmission is an almost universal finding, even though the magnitude of this asymmetry may not be certain.

Now that a variety of risk factors associated with transmission have been identified, partner studies could switch their focus from couples in whom transmission has occurred to couples in whom, in spite of well-defined exposure, transmission has not occurred. The study of seronegative partners with long-term exposure might reveal data about variations in viral strain or host immunological profiles that could explain heterogeneous transmission rates or that might provide data relevant for vaccine development. Partner studies also provide the best source of information about the mechanism of transmission, including the importance of cell-free virus and target cells for HIV, that would also be relevant for treatment or prophylaxis.

In epidemiology, disease does not occur randomly, but varies according to person, place, and time. Our charge then is not to make results come out identically in each study, but rather to understand why results may vary. Perhaps through comparisons across studies, additional risk factors or the significance of known risk factors will be elucidated.

REFERENCES

1. Padian N. Heterosexual transmission: infectivity and risks. In: Alexander N, Gabelnick H, Spieler J, eds. *Heterosexual transmission of AIDS*. New York: Wiley-Liss; 1990.
2. Winkelstein W, Lyman D, Padian N, et al. Sexual practices and risk of HIV infection by the human immunodeficiency virus: The San Francisco Men's Health Study. *JAMA* 1987;257:321–325.
3. Padian N. Sexual histories of heterosexual couples with one HIV-infected partner. *Am J Public Health* 1990;80:990–991.
4. Padian N, Marquis L, Francis D, et al. Male-to-female transmission of human immunodeficiency virus. *JAMA* 1987;258:788–790.

5. Padian N, Shiboski S, Jewell N. Female-to-male transmission of human immunodeficiency virus. *JAMA* 1991;266:1664–1668.
6. Padian N, Shiboski S, Jewell N. The effect of number of exposures on the risk of heterosexual HIV transmission. *J Infect Dis* 1990;161:883–887.
7. European Study Group on Heterosexual Transmission of HIV. Comparison of female to male and male to female transmission of HIV in 563 stable couples. *Br Med J* [*Clin Res*] 1992;304:809–813.
8. Laga M, Taelman H, Bonneux L, et al. Risk factors for HIV infection in heterosexual partners of HIV-infected Africans and Europeans. Fourth International Conference on AIDS, June 13, 1988, Stockholm, Sweden.
9. Costigiola P, Ricchi E, Marinacci G, et al. Risk factors in heterosexual transmission of HIV. Fifth International Conference on AIDS, June 6, 1989, Montreal, Canada.
10. Nicolosi A, and Italian Partners' Study. Different susceptibility of women and men to heterosexual transmission of HIV. Sixth International Conference on AIDS, June 21, 1990, San Francisco, California.
11. Fischl M, Dickinson G, Scott G, et al. Evaluation of heterosexual partners, children, and household contacts of adults with AIDS. *JAMA* 1987;257:640–644.
12. Neisson-Vernant C, Quist D, Delaunay C. Seroconversion in heterosexual partner of HIV infected patients in Martinique. Eighth International Conference on AIDS, July 1992, Amsterdam, The Netherlands.
13. Peterman T, Stoneburner R, Allen J, et al. Risk of human immunodeficiency virus transmission for heterosexual adults with transfusion-associated infections. *JAMA* 1988; 259:55–58.
14. Davidson S, Robertson J, Brettle R. Transmission of HIV in Edinburgh amongst heterosexual injection drug users (IDU). Fifth International Conference on AIDS, June 6, 1989, Montreal, Canada.
15. Steigbigel N, Maude D, Feiner C, et al. Heterosexual transmission of infection and disease by the human immunodeficiency virus (HIV). Fourth International Conference on AIDS, June 13, 1988, Stockholm, Sweden.
16. Castelli F, Casari S, Donisi, et al. Risk factors for heterosexual transmission. Eighth International Conference on AIDS, July 1992, Amsterdam, The Netherlands.
17. Pape J, Stanback M, Pamphile M, et al. Seroepidemiology of HIV in Haiti. *Clin Res* 1987;35:486 (abst).
18. Hira S, Wadhawan D, Nikkowane B. Heterosexual transmission of HIV in Zambia. Fourth International Conference on AIDS, June 13, 1988, Stockholm, Sweden.
19. Stewart G, Typer J, Cunningham A, et al. Transmission of human T-cell lymphotropic virus type III (HTLV-III) by artificial insemination by donor. *Lancet* 1985;2:581–584.
20. Sion F, Signodini D, Santos E. Absence of female-to-male transmission of HIV in stable couples in Rio De Janeiro, Brazil. Eighth International Conference on AIDS, July 1992, Amsterdam, The Netherlands.

DISCUSSION

Dr. Piot: The results of these kinds of studies are probably heavily influenced by the mix of determinants, and the problem is that you end up with cells containing only four or five couples. What I found interesting about the European collaborative studies on transmission was that the effect of the sex of the index case disappeared only when the case was symptomatic. This suggests to me that one risk may be so great that it overwhelms the others, which might explain some of the disparities among different studies.

Dr. Padian: The distribution of risk factors is, of course, very important. Although the rates of transmission from intravenous drug users were not higher when you looked at the number of intravenous drug users in the denominator, 65% to 75% of partners of intravenous drug users seroconverted.

We are beginning a U.S. collaborative study precisely in order to fill out the cells a little more.

Dr. Johnson: I wonder whether partner studies are the best way to look at the biology of transmission, unless you can use a case control design to compare seroconverters with nonconverters on a national basis. But, if the European study is right in relation to woman-to-man transmission, it does seem that infectivity may be extremely important in these partnerships: that could be sufficient to explain the differences between your study and the European study.

We really need to involve biologists now that the methods exist for measuring variability and viral load, but, so far, they've largely been used in drug trials rather than in epidemiological studies. Even large-scale cross-sectional studies of variability and viral load among asymptomatic subjects at a particular point in time, followed by follow-up studies of the same individuals to see how their viral load varies, may make a very important contribution to our understanding of why we see these enormous differences in transmission probabilities among individual couples.

In terms of the probability of female-to-male transmission, I think it is important to explain the differences between your study and the European study, if only for public health reasons. If you study female-to-male transmission in drug-using couples, there is a tendency to be so surprised at finding a positive male that you grill him until he owns up to something, and then you assume that that is how he became infected. But unless you treat all of the negative people in the same way, you are introducing a bias that throws up the positives, and, although somebody has very clear transmission exposure to an HIV-positive person as a result of unprotected sex, the cause is often attributed to the fact that they shot up once in 1982. We need to think of statistical methods that overcome this problem.

Dr. Padian: I agree that we need to understand exactly what the differences are, but I still think that partner studies are stronger than surveys over time, although I agree that we need to involve biologists in order to compare viral load in cases where transmission did or did not occur.

I don't want to go into the results of particular studies because I don't think that there is any one right answer. We need to consider the factors underlying these differences.

Dr. Detels: I wonder whether the fact that you found only one female-to-male transmission is a result of recruitment bias. In the U.S., we have very little evidence of heterosexual transmission and, if the man and the woman are in exactly the same disease stage, the man is much more likely to be tested before the woman. This means that he is often considered the index case simply because you have documentation of his seroconversion, and it's only as his disease advances that we look at the status of the woman.

Dr. Padian: I agree. But to put it in a slightly different way, the pool of infected women is smaller, and this means that you have less opportunity to study it, let alone recruit it. Even if the odds are lower, as the number of infected women increases we will be able to see more.

Dr. Detels: I think that you are seeing no seroconversions because you are selecting against seroconversion. I believe that the amount of virus entering through sexual intercouse is relatively small in comparison with that deriving from transfusion. When you take a couple in which the index case has a long-standing infection and the "susceptible" partner has been repeatedly exposed and resisted, you have obviously selected by resistance. I suggest that these resistant people make up a very interesting group, because I'd like to know what this resistance is. We are doing some studies in the MACS to identify the characteristics of resistance, and I believe that at least part of it is host-related. It also seems to me that you could stratify your couples. If I were you, I would vigorously recruit couples in whom the index case has been recently infected because this would mean that you are not selecting for resistance. In this way, you could compare long-standing, uninfected or "resistant" partners with seroconverters and recently infected partners.

Dr. Padian: I agree with you. Although we see behavioral change, there is a feeling that we've exhausted the group of susceptibles. It's a wonderful idea to recruit these people, but it's very hard to recruit them into this study. We take everybody who meets the criteria, and we don't always know when the index case seroconverted. But certainly, I would prefer to have someone who has not developed AIDS.

Dr. Nicolosi: In our cross-sectional study of female-to-male sexual transmission among stable couples, we found that 19 of 201 (9.5%) men, who presented no other risk factors than sexual exposure to the HIV-infected female partner, were HIV positive. At logistic regression, the highest risks of transmission were for men practicing peno–anal intercourse (the odds ratio was almost 8) and for men whose partner had AIDS or detectable p24 antigen (the odds ratio was higher than 6). But, when we study male-to-female transmission in comparison with female-to-male transmission, there is also the problem of bias in measuring exposure. For example, the duration of intercourse is a potentially very important variable. Since HIV is carried in cervicovaginal secretions (free or within HIV-infected cells), the exposure of the man is greater the longer the duration of sexual intercourse and the greater the quantity of the woman's vaginal and cervical secretions and the number of HIV-infected cells. In man-to-woman transmission, HIV-carrying semen remains in the woman's genital apparatus after ejaculation until it is fully absorbed, regardless of the duration of intercourse. The duration of intercourse is a variable that has never been measured, but that I think is crucial.

Dr. Musicco: In the cross-sectional phase of our study, we found that the prevalence of HIV-infected males is three times greater than that of females in stable couples. In the longitudinal phase, during which we followed about 100 men exposed to infected women, we observed no seroconversion, while there was a 4% annual rate of seroconversion in woman.

Another thing we need to think about is our assumption that each sexual intercourse carries the same risk, regardless of the duration of the relationship. In your study, you have demonstrated that the relationship between the risk of infection and the number of episodes of sexual intercourse is not simply linear but log-linear. I believe this means that the risk of transmission involved in the first intercourse with an infected person is higher than that in subsequent episodes. Consequently, in our longitudinal study, we are considering a selected group of couples who escaped infection during their first intercourse, which is perhaps not very representative of what happens in terms of sexual transmission.

Dr. Padian: You can find as many studies showing no female-to-male transmission as those showing equal rates of transmission. The problem is to understand the reasons for these differences.

Dr. Biggar: Nobody has raised the issue of the possible virus that is more likely to be spread heterosexually than, for example, in drug use. This was suggested in a

CDC [Centers for Disease Control] study from Thailand. I don't know if we will find a biological basis for this in the future, but it will be interesting to see whether some viruses are more suited to heterosexual transmission. The example that Dr. Piot gave yesterday of the man who infected 11 of his 19 partners indicates that there is something happening in the disseminator of the virus, not just in the receiving host. I can't believe that all 11 of those 19 people were of the same background. There is certainly something connected with the man himself and/or the virus he has.

HIV Epidemiology: Models and Methods,
edited by Alfredo Nicolosi. Raven Press, Ltd.,
New York © 1994.

8

Epidemiological Methods to Investigate the Role of Sexually Transmitted Diseases as Risk Factors in HIV Transmission

Marie Laga

Department of Infection and Immunity, Institute of Tropical Medicine, Nationalestraat 155, 2000 Antwerp, Belgium

Human immunodeficiency virus (HIV) infection has been spreading through sexual contact at strikingly different rates in different parts of the world and within continents. Factors that influence the speed of this spread are on one hand the susceptibility of the host to the virus, the infectiousness of the infected individuals, and maybe the virulence of the HIV strain, and on the other hand HIV prevalence in the community, the sexual behavior of the individuals, and the mixing patterns of subgroups in the populations. Host susceptibility and infectiousness could both be influenced by biological risk factors such as sexually transmitted diseases (STD).

Since the beginning of the acquired immunodeficiency syndrome (AIDS) epidemic, researchers from different geographic areas have been struck by the high rates of current STD or a history of STD among HIV-positive individuals compared to HIV-negative controls, as well as high prevalences of HIV infection among people attending STD clinics.

In search for an explanation for these observations and for the rampant HIV epidemic among heterosexuals in Africa and recently in Asia, it was hypothesized that STD were facilitating the sexual transmission of HIV (1).

Since then, it has become clear that the relationship between HIV and STD is much more complex, and several types of interactions have been postulated:

(a) The presence of STD enhances the transmission of HIV.
(b) HIV infection and consequent immunodeficiency alter the natural history, diagnosis, and response to treatment of other STD.
(c) STD may influence the natural history of HIV infections.

This chapter will examine the available data on the first hypothesis, with special emphasis on the epidemiologic methods used.

THE IMPACT OF STD ON HIV TRANSMISSION: EPIDEMIOLOGIC EVIDENCE

When analyzing the relationship between STD and HIV, several methodologic problems must be considered. First, such studies are complicated by the fact that HIV infection is itself an STD. STD and HIV are transmitted in the same way and share the same behavioral risk factors (e.g., number of partners, type of sexual contact, prostitute contact, use of barrier methods, and being single and/or young). Not only the risk behavior of the infected person but also that of his or her partners are important confounders in this relationship. Controlling for these confounders is therefore essential in establishing whether STD are independent risk factors for HIV transmission, instead of just markers for high risk behavior. However, obtaining accurate and reliable information on sexual behavior around the presumed time of seroconversion from both the index patient and the partner is complex and often not possible at all.

A second problem arises from the potential impact of HIV infection and related immunodeficiency on other STD, such as increased frequency of genital herpes lesions in HIV-infected people. Without prospective studies documenting the temporal sequence, it is impossible to determine whether a higher rate of STD among HIV-infected individuals indicates that STD facilitate HIV transmission or whether STD are simply markers for HIV-related immunosuppression.

As discussed by Cameron and Padian (2) even prospective studies may not establish a temporal sequence of events with certainty because of the varying delay between HIV infection and development of antibodies.

Cross-sectional Studies

Numerous epidemiologic studies have been addressing the issue of STD as cofactors in HIV transmission, and many have attempted to control for confounders.

Over 50 cross-sectional studies have been published, showing an association between past or present STD and HIV infection. Although the strength of association is high in some of these studies, their interpretation is sometimes difficult. It is impossible to determine the temporal sequence of events in such a design and the information about sexual behavior may be inaccurate because the time of acquisition of the virus is unknown. Some of these studies have, however, contributed to the recognition and understanding of other interactions between STD and HIV, such as increased susceptibility for genital herpes or genital warts in HIV-infected persons.

Longitudinal Studies

Several carefully conducted longitudinal studies have shown an increased risk of seroconversion when STD are present, both in men and women (Table 1).

This design is much more powerful and convincing because the temporal sequence of events is clear, and the sexual behavior information relates to the time of seroconversion. However, accurate controlling for all possible confounders remains a challenge.

The majority of these studies have focused on the role of genital ulcer disease. The most convincing evidence that genital ulcer disease facilitates the transmission of HIV comes from a cohort study of male clients of prostitutes in Nairobi reported by Cameron et al. (3). They showed that men who acquired an ulcer from a group of female prostitutes with a very high HIV infection rate had a fivefold increased risk for subsequent HIV seroconversion than those men who did not acquire an ulcer. This illustrated that genital ulcer disease in women increased infectiousness of HIV to the male partner.

Cohort studies among homosexual men in the U.S. also documented a strong association between herpes simplex virus seroconversion and syphilis (the two main causes of genital ulcer in the industrialized world) and HIV seroconversion (4,5).

Data on nonulcerative STD and HIV are far more limited than those on genital ulcers, but evidence that these syndromes also facilitate HIV transmission is accumulating. In a cohort of gay men in Vancouver, gonorrhea and syphilis were reported more frequently among seroconverters than among men who remained negative after controlling for unprotected sexual

TABLE 1. *Selected prospective studies documenting STD[a] as risk factors for HIV[b] transmission*

Study population [ref.]	STD studied	Relative risk[c]
Heterosexual men, Kenya [3]	Genital ulcer[d] (clinical diagnosis)	4.7
Homosexual men, U.S. [4]	Syphilis (serology self-reported)	1.5–2.2
Homosexual men, U.S. [5]	Herpes (serology)	4.4
Heterosexual women, Kenya [6]	Genital ulcer[c] (clinical diagnosis)	3.3
	Chlamydial infection (culture)	2.7
Heterosexual women, Zaire [7]	Gonorrhea (culture)	4.8
	Chlamydial infection (chlamydiazyme)	3.6
	Trichomoniasis (direct examination)	1.9

[a]STD, sexually transmitted disease.
[b]HIV, human immunodeficiency virus.
[c]Relative risk adjusted after multivariate analysis.
[d]The majority of genital ulcer disease in Kenya and Zaire was chancroid, confirmed by culture for *Haemophilus ducreyi*.

exposure. As part of Project SIDA in Kinshasa, 430 HIV-negative female prostitutes were followed monthly for STD diagnosis and treatment and HIV testing was performed every 3 months. To identify potential risk factors occurring around the time of acquisition of HIV, a nested case-control study within the cohort was performed. Cases were women who seroconverted and controls were those remaining HIV negative (7).

A window period of 2 to 5 months prior to the first HIV-positive test was defined. The incidence of STD, sexual exposure, and other potential risk factors occurring during this window period in the cases were compared to a concurrent period in the controls. During the presumed period of acquisition of HIV, seroconverters had a much higher incidence of gonorrhea, chlamydial infection, and trichomoniasis than controls.

After controlling for sexual exposure, the adjusted odds ratios were 4.8, 3.6, and 1.9 for gonorrhea, chlamydial infection, and trichomonas, respectively. Genital ulcers were also more frequent in seroconverters, but their overall incidence was very low.

Discordant Couple Studies

Comparison of HIV seroconversion rates in stable discordant couples (one partner HIV negative) with and without STD offers several methodologic advantages because of the certainty of 100% exposure of the partner to HIV and the exclusion of other potential confounders. However, the incidence of STD among stable couples is generally low, and the low HIV seroconversion rates among the partners require a large sample size. This approach therefore has not been very useful in establishing whether STD facilitate the transmission of HIV.

Intervention Trials

Descriptive epidemiologic studies only cannot prove causality beyond any doubt, especially for a relationship as complex as that of STD and HIV. If community-based intervention trials (considered by some as the ultimate proof of the enhancing effect of STD and HIV transmission) could demonstrate the reversible effect of STD on HIV incidence, this would be a strong and convincing argument. The design would randomize communities to STD intervention and monitor HIV incidence in those with and without intervention (8,9). These studies are not only enormous undertakings (in terms of time and money), but also are extremely complex in terms of (a) identifying representative study populations with high enough STD and HIV incidence; (b) avoiding contamination of the control group; and (c) monitoring the impact of STD interventions on STD levels and HIV incidence. There are also several ethical considerations.

These intervention trials therefore may only be completed in several years and may not yield definitive conclusions, as has been the case with other large intervention trials in the area of cardiovascular disease.

THE IMPACT OF STD ON HIV TRANSMISSION: BIOLOGICAL PLAUSIBILITY

The body of biological evidence supporting the enhancing effect of STD on HIV transmission is also growing (10). It has been shown that the pool of T-lymphocytes and macrophages is increased considerably in the male and female genital tracts when STD are present. These cells are either target cells for HIV in an uninfected person, or HIV-infected cells in an HIV-positive person.

STD lesions can be associated both macroscopically and histopathologically with a disruption of the normal epithelial barrier of the genital mucosa in the form of overt ulcerations, microulceration, cervical erosion, or cervical friability.

Several new quantitative measures of infectious virus levels in blood, semen, or vaginal secretions, such as quantitative culture and PCR, have now become available. Although standardization of the techniques is still a problem, they have added to the biological evidence of STD as risk factors for HIV. Not only has the virus been isolated directly from the ulcer base in men and women, but viral shedding in vaginal and urethral discharge is also increased in cases of female cervicitis or male urethritis.

CONCLUSION

Although the perfect epidemiologic study has not yet been performed and may never be performed, several prospective studies that controlled for behavioral risk factors now strongly support the hypothesis that both ulcerative and nonulcerative STD facilitate transmission of HIV and its biological plausibility is accumulating.

Meanwhile, HIV is spreading rapidly in several parts of the world and the need to intervene on modifiable risk factors for sexual transmission of HIV is urgent.

The decision to implement STD control as part of HIV control activity should not await additional research. The question is no longer whether STD control should be done, but rather how it should be done. Also, which STD interventions can be most effectively implemented and where? Due to their much higher prevalence and incidence, nonulcerative STD may have a higher impact worldwide on the transmission of HIV than genital ulcers. STD interventions should therefore focus on all locally prevalent STD and not only on genital ulcers.

REFERENCES

1. Laga M, Nzila N, Goeman J. The interrelationship of sexually transmitted diseases and HIV infection: implications for the control of both epidemics in Africa. *AIDS* 1991; 5[Suppl 1]:S55–S63.
2. Cameron DW, Padian NS. Sexual transmission of HIV and the epidemiology of other sexually transmitted diseases. *AIDS* 1990;4[Suppl 1]:S99–S103.
3. Cameron DW, Lourdes JD, Gregory MM, et al. Female to male transmission of human immunodeficiency virus type 1: risk factors for seroconversion in men. *Lancet* 1989; ii:403–407.
4. Darrow WW, Echenberg DF, Jaffe HW, et al. Risk factors for human immunodeficiency virus (HIV) infection in homosexual men. *Am J Public Health* 1987;77:479–483.
5. Holmberg SD, Stewart JA, Gerber AR, et al. Prior herpes simplex virus type 2 infection as a risk factor for HIV infection. *JAMA* 1988;259:1048–1050.
6. Plummer FA, Simonsen JN, Cameron DW, et al. Co-factors in female-to-male sexual transmission of HIV. *J Infect Dis* 1991;163:233–239.
7. Laga M, Manoka A, Kivuvu M, et al. Non-ulcerative sexually transmitted diseases as risk factors for HIV-1 transmission in women: results from a cohort study. *AIDS* 1993;7:95–102.
8. Nkowane BM, Lwanga SK. HIV and design of intervention studies for control of sexually transmitted disease. *AIDS* 1990;4[Suppl 1]:S123–S126.
9. Mertens TE, Hayes RJ, Smith PG. Epidemiologic methods to study the interaction between HIV infection and other sexually transmitted diseases. *AIDS* 1990;4:57–65.
10. Wasserheit J. Epidemiological synergy: interrelationships between human immunodeficiency virus infection and other sexually transmitted diseases. *Sex Transm Dis* 1992;19:61–77.

DISCUSSION

Dr. Susser: I assume that the attributable risk estimates you have given are not adjusted.

Dr. Laga: You are right, they are not adjusted, but I used them to indicate the role of the relative risk of STD (which are very strongly associated, but also rare in some communities).

Dr. Biggar: You spoke about the incidence of various venereal diseases in these prostitutes, but earlier you said how effective condom use was. I was struck by this disparity. Am I correct in assuming that this was a prospective study and that, despite the fact that they were supposedly using condoms, the women were getting venereal disease at such a tremendous rate?

Dr. Laga: These were rates in seroconverted women. I have to say that when we started the study in 1988, less than 5% of women had ever used a condom in their lives and most of them didn't even know what a condom was. So, there was quite an intensive intervention with a lot of educational sessions and the distribution of free condoms. In this way, we raised the use of condoms until, at every visit, about 50% of the women claimed that they had always used a condom. But, of course, the other 50% were still exposed to STD.

Dr. Padian: I would like to know whether you also tried to get the men clients to use condoms.

Second, considering the biological plausibility of STD increasing the likelihood of HIV transmission, I wonder what is the level of STD infection due to the pH of the vagina? That is an issue that has come up when looking at contraceptives.

Dr. Laga: Yes, we did try to do something with the men. Most of the women in

Kinshasa have what they call occasional clients and what they call regular clients. We started the project with their so-called stable clients, and we reached about 200 of them with a condom intervention program. But, it is very hard to make women use condoms with their so-called stable partners because they perceive them as more personal, more or less like a husband for at least 2 or 3 months. Even after two and a half years, only 15% to 20% of the women said that their partners agreed to use condoms with them. It's very difficult because many of these men are also at high risk. We did a prevalence study and 15% of them were HIV positive, which is more than double the prevalence in the general population of Kinshasa. Some of the women were certainly infected by these men; in fact, some of the women who seroconverted declared that their only sexual relationships at the time were with these partners.

STD do influence pH. Candidiasis is probably the only one that decreases the level of pH; most of the others increase the pH of the vagina.

Dr. Susser: With the intervention on STD by means of treatment and condoms, you decided you could not segregate those factors in your cohort study, and, from everything you have just said, it is clear that they are deeply confounded. But, didn't you have a reasonable distribution of STD-treated women who didn't use condoms versus STD-treated women who did? Were they not segregated out, or is it that these histories of regular partners with whom they don't use any protection would simply wreck the analysis?

Dr. Laga: The big problem with these kinds of studies is that condom use is not a constant risk or protective factor over time. In other words, women will say that they have been regular condom users for 3 months and then that they have not. It's true that you can give a final score to every woman after two and a half years (a good condom user, so-so, etc.), but it's very difficult to find a difference between them because the women who have had a lot of STD control are normally the better condom users. They're more motivated to come to the clinic and so they receive more condoms and educational messages. It's virtually impossible to separate these things out.

Dr. Des Jarlais: Nancy Padian was talking about the need to study monogamous couples in order to look at the efficiency of HIV transmission, and you pointed out that there are few or no STD in such couples. Perhaps we need to develop further the idea of a methodological trade-off in our studies; by which I mean trying to move towards a methodology that allows us to answer one question (such as the efficiency of heterosexual transmission in monogamous couples) even though it may mean a dramatic decrease in our ability to study other issues, such as STD.

I'd also like to comment on the idea of STD control. You mention clinical services and the screening of high-risk populations, but, if you look at the developed world over the last 8 years or so, the places where we've seen increases or decreases in STD were not related to clinical services or screening. They were community organizations built around AIDS as an issue and in which there was a dramatic reduction in STD, or they involved crack use in the inner cities of the U.S. where we saw a dramatic increase in STD. Perhaps we need to broaden our idea as to what constitutes STD control by looking at communities as a whole and what is happening inside them and should move away from the traditional idea of providing medical services to individuals.

Dr. Laga: I couldn't agree more.

HIV Epidemiology: Models and Methods,
edited by Alfredo Nicolosi. Raven Press, Ltd.,
New York © 1994.

9

Oral Contraceptives and the Risk of HIV

Studies Among Heterosexual Women in Nairobi

*Pierre J. Plourde and †Francis A. Plummer

**Departments of Internal Medicine and Medical Microbiology, University of Manitoba, Winnipeg, Manitoba, Canada R3EOW3; and †WHO Centre for Research and Training on Sexually Transmitted Diseases, Department of Medical Microbiology, University of Nairobi, Kenya*

The majority of new infections of human immunodeficiency virus type 1 (HIV-1) worldwide are acquired by heterosexual intercourse. Transmission of HIV-1 to female sex partners of infected men in North America continues to increase. It is likely that more women than men are infected with HIV-1 in developing countries and that these women are seropositive for HIV-1 at a younger age than men (1). Several behavioral and exogenous risk factors have been linked to the increased risk of HIV-1 infection in women. Behavioral factors include receptive anal intercourse (2), multiple sexual partners (3), and the sale of sex (3). Several exogenous factors, including genital ulcer disease (4) and chlamydial cervicitis (4), enhance a woman's susceptibility to HIV-1. Oral contraceptive use has also emerged as a potential risk factor in studies from Nairobi and Rwanda. We have hypothesized that cervical ectopy, induced by oral contraceptives, may render women more susceptible to HIV-1 infection through the more friable cervical columnar epithelium. However, the true relationship between cervical ectopy and HIV-1 susceptibility is likely very complex.

The initial studies from Nairobi of Simonsen et al. (5) and Plummer et al. (4) were conducted entirely with women who sell sex. Since then, studies by Plourde et al. (6,7) and Pattullo et al. (8) have duplicated the initial findings in women who are not prostitutes. This chapter summarizes the studies from Nairobi, which have examined the interaction of various cofactors in the male-to-female sexual transmission of HIV-1 and discusses them in the context of other studies on the relationship between oral contraceptive use and HIV-1 (9,10).

METHODS

Study Population

Cross-sectional studies were the first of two study designs used in Nairobi to examine factors associated with male-to-female transmission of HIV-1. In this particular design, seropositive women and otherwise comparable seronegative women presenting to sexually transmitted diseases (STD) clinics were compared with respect to several variables chosen prior to study enrollment. Seropositive women enrolled in this fashion therefore represent prevalent cases. The major drawback with this design is that it is virtually impossible to determine the time of HIV-1 seroconversion. Therefore, determining exposure status to any particular variable at the time of HIV-1 infection is equally difficult. For example, use of oral contraception is often intermittent and historical recollection of oral contraceptive use is probably inaccurate. Hence, in a cross-sectional study, it is impossible to definitely establish whether or not oral contraceptives were used at the time of HIV-1 infection. This type of misclassification will decrease the ability of the study to demonstrate a significant association between a particular variable and HIV-1 infection.

To overcome this problem, prospective studies were performed by obtaining initial exposure data in HIV-1 seronegative women who were then followed to seroconversion. Due to the high efficiency of male-to-female transmission of HIV-1 in Nairobi, initial cohorts of 100 to 200 women have been sufficiently large to obtain adequate numbers of seroconverting women in a relatively short time span of 6 to 12 months. However, the major obstacle in these studies has been achieving high follow-up rates. Thus far, the prospective studies (4,6,8) have managed to achieve follow-up rates of 60% to 65%. Although this rate of follow-up is remarkable in a STD clinic setting, significant bias can occur if women lost to follow-up are more or less likely to seroconvert to HIV-1.

The Nairobi male-to-female HIV-1 transmission studies have been performed in two very different populations of women. The first group of women was largely Tanzanian immigrants enrolled from January 1985 to August 1985 and subsequently followed to June 1987. They were enrolled at a research clinic established within a lower socioeconomic residential section of Nairobi at a Nairobi City Commission facility. This residential section, known as Pumwani, houses a population of approximately 10,000 and occupies an area of less than 1 km^2. It is widely known for its association with prostitution. The second group of women were recruited from among those attending the Nairobi City Comission Special Treatment Clinic (STC) between February 1988 and September 1989. In the prospective arm of this study, a cohort of women were followed until February 1990. The STC is located in the central core area of Nairobi, approxiately 2.5 km from Pumwani. This STD clinic is not usually frequented by women who practice prostitution.

The study designs were similar for both groups of women, including the use of comparable standard questionnaires and the performance of identical physical examinations and laboratory procedures. In the prospective studies, women were followed at monthly intervals and complete re-evaluations were performed at each visit. Since all interview and physical examination data were collected prior to seroconversion, observers were blinded to the eventual HIV-1 serostatus at the time of data collection.

Analysis of Data

The analysis of the relationship between several different variables, including use of oral contraceptives and HIV transmission, is highly susceptible to confounding. Univariate analyses were initially performed on selected variables to determine which factors to include in multivariate analyses. Chi-square tests were performed for categorical variables and Student's t tests were performed for continuous variables. Stratified data were analyzed with Mantel–Haenszel chi-square testing. Multivariate analyses used logistic regression for cross-sectional study data and Cox proportional hazards modelling for prospective data. Variables that continued to show statistical significance after multivariate analysis in the prospective studies were also subject to survival analysis using Kaplan–Meier survival curves and log rank testing to determine statistical significance. All reported tests of significance were two-tailed.

RESULTS

The initial studies enrolled a cohort of 595 prostitutes. One hundred ninety-six (33%) were HIV-1 seronegative and were enrolled in the 12-month follow-up study. Seroconversion occurred in 83 of the 124 (67%) women who returned for follow-up. The cross-sectional study performed at the STC enrolled 600 women. One hundred thirty-four women with genital ulcers who were HIV-1 seronegative were entered into the 6-month follow-up study. Seroconversion occurred in 10 of 81 (12%) women. The HIV-1 seroconversion rate in both prospective studies was 4.0 per 100 woman-months of follow-up (95% confidence interval [CI], 1.9–7.3). More recent data from STC document 13 seroconversions in 113 (12%) women followed for a mean of 3.3 months, with a seroconversion rate of 3.4 per 100 woman-months of follow-up (8).

The study by Simonsen et al. (5) found that age ($P < 0.001$), duration of prostitution ($P < 0.001$), and the presence of genital ulcers (odds ratio [OR], 3.3; 95% CI, 1.9–5.4; $P < 0.001$) were strongly associated with HIV-1 seropositivity. A weaker association was found between current use of oral contraception and HIV-1 seropositivity (OR, 1.8; 95% CI, 1.1–2.9; $P < 0.05$). No significant demographic or sexual behavior differences were found between oral contraceptive users and nonusers. Further analysis of the relationship between oral contraceptive use and HIV-1 seropositivity revealed a moderate duration-response relationship with a frequency of HIV-1 infection increasing from 58% in those not using oral contraceptives to 76% in those reporting more than 1 year of use. Current oral contraceptive use remained associated with HIV-1 infection after stepwise logistic regression analysis (OR, 2.02; 95% CI, 1.22–3.35; $P = 0.006$).

The prospective study by Plummer et al. (4) found oral contraceptive use prior to seroconversion and the presence of genital ulcer disease to be the strongest cofactors associated with HIV-1 seroconversion. Thirty-nine percent of seroconverting women had used oral contraceptives before seroconversion compared to 17% of women who remained seronegative (risk ratio [RR], 3.1; 95% CI, 1.4–6.7; $P = 0.005$). Comparison of women using and not using oral contraceptives revealed minor differences. Women using oral contraceptives reported a slightly higher number of daily sex partners compared to nonusers (4.46 ± 2.73 versus 3.63 ± 1.97; $P = 0.06$). Once again, a duration-response relationship of the risk of HIV-1 seroconversion with consistency of oral contraceptive use was demonstrated. Sixty percent of women who never used oral contraceptives seroconverted compared with 76% of women who used oral contraceptives intermittently during the study period and 89% of women who used oral contraceptives continually throughout the study period ($P < 0.05$; chi-square test for trend). Oral contraceptive use remained associated with an increased risk of HIV-1 seroconversion when controlling for condom use, genital ulcers, and chlamydial cervicitis in stratified analysis. A survivorship analysis also showed that women who were using oral contraceptives during the study period seroconverted to HIV-1 at a higher rate ($P < 0.05$; log rank test). Finally, multivariate analysis found oral contraceptive use and genital ulcer disease to be the only variables that remained associated with HIV-1 seroconversion.

The cross-sectional study by Plourde et al. (7) of women from STC determined that being unmarried (OR, 3.2; 95% CI, 1.9–5.4; $P < 0.001$), early age at first sexual intercourse ($P = 0.01$), number of lifetime sexual partners ($P < 0.001$), current prostitution (OR, 9.5; 95% CI, 4.8–18.8; $P < 0.001$), history of genital ulcers (OR, 2.3; 95% CI, 1.3–4.1; $P = 0.003$), and current genital ulcers (OR, 5.5; 95% CI, 3.2–9.4; $P < 0.001$) were most strongly associated with HIV-1 seroprevalence. In this study, contraceptive use was analyzed in greater detail. Interestingly, ever use of oral contraception was not associated with HIV-1 seroprevalence ($P = 0.34$). This is likely related to the fact that of women reporting any use of oral contraception, 15% reported only 1 to 2 months of use and 30% reported less than 6 months of use. If duration of oral contraceptive use is significantly associated with risk of HIV-1 infection, then oral contraceptive data that are presented as ever/never use may not always reveal an association with HIV-1 seroprevalence. A duration-response relationship between oral contraceptive use and HIV-1 seropositivity was found in this study, with the greatest effect being observed in women with genital ulcers. In these women, HIV-1 seroprevalence increased from 27% in those who used oral contraceptives for less than 12 months, to 50% in those who reported 12 to 24 months of use, to greater than 95% for those taking oral contraceptives more than 24 months ($P < 0.001$; chi-square test for trend). This association with genital ulcers was unexpected. A comparison of women currently using oral contraceptives with nonusers in this study revealed some differences. Oral contraceptive users were more likely to be practicing prostitution (OR, 2.98; 95% CI, 1.5–5.9; $P = 0.001$) and to have genital ulcers (OR, 2.0; 95% CI, 1.1–3.6; $P = 0.017$). However, these women were also more likely to be using condoms (OR, 2.9; 95% CI, 1.4–5.9; $P = 0.002$). Cervical ectopy was more commonly seen in women using oral contraceptives (OR, 2.6; 95% CI, 1.4–4.8; $P = 0.002$). Due to the complex interactions between contraceptive use, sexual behaviors, and STD, the data were further analyzed using stratified and multivariate analyses. In stratified analysis, oral contraceptive use remained associated with an increased risk of HIV-1 infection when controlling for lifetime sex partners and condom use. However, a strong relationship was demonstrated once again between oral contraceptive use and genital ulcers. Therefore, in multivariate analysis, a combined oral contraceptive use and current genital ulcer variable was included. This analysis found that lifetime number of sex partners ($P < 0.001$) and current genital ulcers (OR, 3.8; 95% CI, 2.9–5.1; $P < 0.001$) remained associated with HIV-1 infection. The strongest association, however, was found in women with genital ulcers who had used oral contraceptives for 12 months or longer (OR, 25.7; 95% CI, 7.3–90.2; $P < 0.001$). Since a strong association was noted between prostitution and use of oral contraceptives, multivariate analysis was repeated for the 404 nonprostitutes presenting to STC with STD. This analysis revealed that lifetime number of sex partners was no longer associated with HIV-1 infection ($P = 0.46$) and that current genital ulcers remained associated (OR, 4.0; 95% CI, 2.8–5.7; $P < 0.001$). As in the previous analysis, a very strong association remained between HIV-1 infection and a combination of genital ulcers with 12 months or longer of oral contraceptive use (OR, 22.4; 95% CI, 5.5–90.7; $P < 0.001$). Use of oral contraception alone was no longer associated with HIV-1 infection in both multivariate analyses. The inclusion of cervical ectopy had no effect on these results.

The study by Plourde et al. (6) followed 81 women with genital ulcers who were HIV-1 seronegative at enrollment for a duration of 1 to 6 months. Since women with genital ulcers were enrolled, the effect of this factor on HIV-1 seroconversion could not be analyzed. The reason for this inclusion criteria was an assumption that a higher seroconversion rate in women with genital ulcers would require a smaller study population to show a significant association between other cofactors and HIV-1 seroincidence. Univariate analysis found a history of prostitution at enrollment (RR, 3.9; 95% CI, 1.2–12.2; P = 0.05), the presence of cervical ectopy at enrollment (RR, 4.9; 95% CI, 1.5–15.6; P = 0.001), and cervicitis (RR, 4.5; 95% CI, 1.5–13.7; P = 0.001) or pelvic inflammatory disease (RR, 6.5; 95% CI, 2.4–17.8; P = 0.001) at enrollment to be signficantly associated with HIV-1 seroconversion during the follow-up period. Forty percent of seroconverting women had used oral contraceptives prior to seroconversion versus 25% of women who remained seronegative (RR, 2.1; 95% CI, 0.7–6.0; P = 0.18). During follow-up, seroconverting women were more likely to be practicing prostitution (RR, 9.3; 95% CI, 1.9–46.4; P = 0.006) and had higher rates of recurrent genital ulcers (RR, 3.5; 95% CI, 1.01–12.1; P = 0.05) and gonococcal cervicitis (RR, 5.3; 95% CI, 1.8–15.9; P = 0.003). The prevalence of cervical ectopy differed only at enrollment between the two groups of women and was not significantly different during the follow-up period (P = 0.10). The only difference detected between women with cervical ectopy and those without was current use of oral contraceptives. Women with cervical ectopy were more likely to be oral contraceptive users (OR, 4.6; 95% CI, 1.2–18.5; P = 0.03). A survivorship analysis of the incidence of HIV-1 seroconversion in women with and without cervical ectopy demonstrated a probability of seroconversion at 20 weeks of approximately 0.5 among women with cervical ectopy at the time of enrollment (P = 0.05, log rank statistic). Age at first sexual intercourse, number of years in Nairobi, prostitution, condom use, duration of oral contraceptive use, cervical ectopy, and pelvic inflammatory disease were entered as variables into a Cox proportional hazards model. The only two variables that remained significantly associated with HIV-1 seroconversion were cervical ectopy (RR, 2.8; 95% CI, 1.3–6.0; P = 0.05) and pelvic inflammatory disease (RR, 6.5; 95% CI, 2.9–14.6; P = 0.02).

Thirty-two more women were enrolled in this study and follow-up has detected three more seroconversions (8). The association of oral contraceptive use prior to enrollment with HIV-1 seroconversion has now attained statistical significance (RR, 3.8; 95% CI, 1.1–13.4). Cox proportional hazards analysis once again demonstrates an association between HIV-1 seroconversion and cervical ectopy (RR, 3.2; 95% CI, 1.03–9.7) as well as gonococcal cervicitis (RR, 8.9; 95% CI, 2.1–37.8), rather than pelvic inflammatory disease.

CONCLUSION

Since 1985, all of the studies from Nairobi examining male-to-female transmission of HIV-1 have raised the possibility that use of oral contraceptives may facilitate HIV-1 transmission. Approximately 20% to 25% of the women enrolled in these studies have reported use of oral contraceptives at any time in their lives. Calculated attributable risks of contraceptive use in the Nairobi studies, as it relates to risk of HIV-1 infection in exposed women, have been between 0.13 and 0.22. Since oral contraceptives form the backbone of most family planning programs in Africa, it is vital to know whether or not oral contraceptives can be a cofactor for HIV-1 transmission. This potential association stresses the importance of including barrier contraceptive promotion in family planning programs as well as in programs dedicated to the control of STD. It follows that an important priority should be the integration of STD control programs with family planning services (9).

Several potential biological mechanisms may explain the interaction between oral contraceptives and HIV-1 infection. Oral contraceptives may increase the susceptibility of the female genital tract to HIV-1 through an estrogenic effect on the genital mucosa, increasing the area of cervical ectopy and exposing the cervix to a greater likelihood of mucosal disruption during sexual intercourse. Cervical ectopy is a physiologic condition defined as an extension of the endocervical columnar epithelium beyond the external os onto the vaginal surface of the cervix. It is known to be more frequent in younger women, present in a large percentage of adolescent women at the onset of menarche and gradually declining through young adulthood. It is also more commonly seen in pregnant women. Oral contraceptives may also act through an indirect effect by increasing the risk of *Chlamydia trachomatis* cervicitis or possibly genital ulcers as suggested in the study by Plourde et al. (7). *Chlamydia trachomatis* cervicitis is known to produce an intense mononuclear cell infiltration of the cervix that could potentially lead to the presence of activated HIV-1 susceptible immunocompetent cells in the genital tract. Finally, oral contraceptives may mediate steroid-like immunologic changes that render women more susceptible to HIV-1 infection.

The mechanisms of altered susceptibility to HIV-1 with cervical ectopy are unknown. However, several possibilities have been postulated. Recent data (10a,11) suggest that the Langerhans cell (dendritic cell) may be the initial target cell infected in the female genital mucosa. These cells are present in the submucosa of both columnar and squamous cervical epithelium. The columnar epithelium, characteristic of cervical ectopy, may be more susceptible to trauma during sexual intercourse, leading to mucosal breaks that could facilitate viral penetration to these potential HIV-1 target cells. Another possibility is that the columnar epithelium itself could be susceptible to HIV-1 infection.

Data demonstrating the association of oral contraceptives with cervical ectopy are somewhat limited. The data have usually been provided by cross-sectional studies performed at STD clinics. No prospective study has been able to clearly establish an association between oral contraceptive use and cervical ectopy. There also exists a difficulty in standardizing the classification of cervical ectopy. Several studies record the presence or absence of cervical ectopy, whereas others use a percentage term to grade the degree of ectopy. There is also a problem of misclassification bias when the presence of cervical ectopy is determined using visual inspection of the cervix instead of colposcopy. The direction of such bias would be to misclassify small degrees of ectopy as negative. This bias would likely be towards the null hypothesis as the effect of ectopy on susceptibility is most plausibly related to the size of the area of ectopy.

The association of HIV-1 transmission with cervical ectopy implies that the cervix may be the primary portal of entry for HIV-1 in the female genital tract. Since the prevalence of ectopy is greater in younger women, enhanced susceptibility of such could explain the observed higher prevalences of HIV-1 in younger African women (1). The postulated effect of oral contraceptives and chlamydial cervicitis on the induction of ectopy could help to explain the observed association that has been noted between these factors and HIV-1 infection. The association of pregnancy with ectopy also suggests that pregnancy may be an HIV-1 hypersusceptible state. However, pregnancy has not been found to be associated with HIV-1 seroconversion to date. The reason for the association between oral contraceptive use and genital ulcer disease as they relate to HIV-1 susceptibility is not fully understood. It is evident from these and other studies that genital ulcers have a very profound effect on male-to-female transmission of HIV-1. It is plausible that genital ulcers may be a marker of increased exposure to HIV-1. Women with genital ulcers in Nairobi may have sex partners at increased risk of HIV-1 infection since 25% to 30% of men who present to STC with chancroid are HIV-1 positive. Therefore, women who are exposed to an HIV-1–positive man with a genital ulcer and who have cervical ectopy at the time of this exposure may be highly susceptible to HIV-1 infection.

Of all other studies that have examined male-to-female transmission of HIV, those performed in Rwanda (12,13) are the only ones demonstrating an association of oral contraceptives with HIV-1 infection. Several other studies have failed to confirm this association, reporting OR ranging from 0.4 to 1.4 (14–21). All of these studies have been either cross-sectional or case-control in design and all have compared ever or current oral contraceptive use versus never or noncurrent use (Table 1). Duration of oral contraceptive use has not been analyzed in any of these studies. Further HIV-1 transmission studies will need to give more attention to the duration of oral contraceptive use and to the association of oral contraception with other HIV-1 transmission cofactors. Recent data from Brazil suggest that oral contraceptives may strongly interact with STD, facilitating male-to-female HIV-1 transmission (19). Markers of sexual behaviors that may be associated with oral contraception will also need to be taken into consideration.

The current evidence for an increased HIV-1 transmission risk associated with oral contraceptive use is confusing. Oral contraceptives by themselves probably play a minor role in increasing women's susceptibility to HIV-1 as is suggested by attributable risks of less than 0.20 in exposed women. However, the interaction of different HIV-1 transmission cofactors in concert may be additive or even multiplicative. Therefore, although oral contracep-

TABLE 1. *Oral contraceptive use and HIV[a] status*

Country/year	Study population	Comparison	Measure of effect
Cohort studies			
Kenya, 1992 (8)	STD[b] clinic	Ever/never	3.8 (1.1–13.4)
Kenya, 1991 (4)	Commercial sex workers	Ever/never	4.5 (1.4–13.8)
Case-control studies			
Rwanda, 1991 (13)	Antenatal clinic	Ever/never	5.0 (2.1–11.3)
Rwanda, 1988 (12)	Discordant couples	Past 2 yrs	4.3 (1.4–15.4)
Thailand, 1991 (14)	Commercial sex workers	Use/nonuse	0.7 (0.3–1.6)
Kenya, 1991 (15)	Family planning clinic	Use/nonuse	1.0 (0.7–1.3)
U.S., 1988 (16)	Commercial sex workers	Past 5 yrs	1.0 (0.4–2.2)
Zimbabwe, 1989 (17)	Discordant couples	Current/nonuse	1.1 (0.4–3.3)
Cross-sectional studies			
Kenya, 1992 (17)	STD clinic	≥12/<12 mos	1.1 (0.7–1.7)
Kenya, 1990 (15)	Commercial sex workers	Current/nonuse	2.0 (1.2–3.4)
Zambia, 1990 (18)	AIDS[c] clinic	Current/nonuse	1.1 (0.9–1.3)
Discordant couples studies			
Brazil, 1992 (19)	Couples	≥12/<12 months	2.4 (1.1–5.3)
Italy, 1990 (20)	Couples	Current/nonuse	0.4 (0.3–1.8)
Europe, 1989 (21)	Couples	Use/nonuse	1.4 (0.4–5.9)

Revised and updated from Hunter (10) and Cates (9).
[a]HIV, human immunodeficiency virus.
[b]STD, sexually transmitted disease.
[c]AIDS, acquired immunodeficiency syndrome.

tives alone may minimally increase a woman's susceptibility to HIV-1 infection, a combination of this cofactor with others such as genital ulcer disease may greatly facilitate male-to-female HIV-1 transmission.

Clearly, more data are needed to further substantiate this association between oral contraceptives and HIV-1 infection. Ideally, this association should be investigated in well-designed prospective studies. Until more data are available, any potential cofactor that can cause cervical ectopy should be considered as possibly enhancing women's susceptibility to HIV-1. The need to promote barrier contraceptives such as male or female condoms in STD control and family planning counselling programs cannot be overemphasized. A closer merger between health care workers interested in reproductive health from both a STD and a contraceptive point of view will be paramount to the successful control of heterosexual HIV-1 transmission (9).

REFERENCES

1. Berkley S, Naamara W, Okware S, et al. AIDS and HIV infection in Uganda: are more women infected than men? *AIDS* 1990;4(12):1237–1242.

2. Padian N, Marquis L, Francis DP, et al. Male-to-female transmission of human immunodeficiency virus. *JAMA* 1987;258:788–790.
3. Guinan ME, Hardy A. Epidemiology of AIDS in women in the United States. *JAMA* 1987;257:2039–2042.
4. Plummer FA, Simonsen JN, Cameron DW, et al. Co-factors in male-female sexual transmission of HIV-1. *J Infect Dis* 1991;163:233–239.
5. Simonsen JN, Plummer FA, Ngugi EN, et al. HIV infection among lower socioeconomic strata prostitutes in Nairobi. *AIDS* 1990;4:139–144.
6. Plourde PJ, Plummer FA, Pepin J, et al. Incidence of HIV-1 seroconversion in women with genital ulcers. In: *Program and abstracts of the sixth International Conference on AIDS*. San Francisco: University of California; 1990.
7. Plourde PJ, Plummer FA, Pepin J, et al. Human immunodeficiency virus type 1 infection in women attending a sexually transmitted diseases clinic in Kenya. *J Infect Dis* 1992;166:86–92.
8. Pattullo ALS, Plourde P, Ndinya-Achola JO, et al. Prospective study of HIV-1 seroconversion in women with genital ulcers attending an African STD clinic. In: *Program and abstracts of the eighth International Conference on AIDS/Third STD World Congress*. Amsterdam: Harvard University/Dutch Foundation; 1992.
9. Cates W, Stone KM. Family planning: the responsibility to prevent both pregnancy and reproductive tract infections. In: Germain A, Holmes KK, Piot P, Wasserheit JN, eds. *Reproductive tract infections global impact and priorities for women's reproductive health*. New York: Plenum Press; 1992:93–129.
10. Hunter DJ, Mati JK. Contraception, family planning, and HIV. In: Chen LC, Amor JS, Segal SJ, eds. *AIDS and women's reproductive health*. New York: Plenum Press; 1991:93–107.
10a. Langhoff E, Terwilliger EF, Poznansky MC, et al. Prolific HIV-1 growth in human dendritic cells. In: *Program and abstracts of the seventh International Conference on AIDS*. Florence, Italy: Istituto Superiore di Sanità; 1991.
11. Zambruno G, Mori L, Marconi A, et al. HIV-1 proviral DNA is present in epidermal Langerhans cells of HIV-infected patients: detection using the polymerase chain reaction. In: *Program and abstracts of the seventh International Conference on AIDS*. Florence, Italy: Istituto Superiore di Sanità; 1991.
12. Carael M, Van de Perre PH, Lepage PH, et al. Human immunodeficiency virus transmission among heterosexual couples in Central Africa. *AIDS* 1988;2:201–205.
13. Bulterys M, Saah A, Chao A, et al. Is oral contraception use associated with prevalent HIV infection in Rwandan women? In: Program and Abstracts of the Fifth Congress on AIDS and Associated Cancers in Africa, Kinshasa, Zaire, 1991.
14. Siraprasiri T, Thanprasertsuk S, Rodklay A, et al. Risk factors for HIV among prostitutes in Chiangmai, Thailand. *AIDS* 1991;5:579–582.
15. Mati J, Maggwa N, Hunter D, et al. Reproductive events, contraceptive use, and HIV infection among women users of family planning in Nairobi, Kenya. In: *Program and abstracts of the seventh International Conference on AIDS*. Florence, Italy: Istituto Superiore di Sanità; 1991.
16. Darrow WW, Bigler W, Deppe D, et al. HIV antibody in 640 U.S. prostitutes with no evidence of intravenous-drug abuse. In: *Program and Abstracts of the Fourth International Conference on AIDS*, Stockholm, Sweden, 1988.
17. Latif AS, Katzenstein DA, Bassett MT, et al. Genital ulcers and transmission of HIV among couples in Zimbabwe. *AIDS* 1989;3:519–523.
18. Hira SK, Kamanga J, Macuacua R, et al. Oral contraceptive use and HIV infection. *Int J Sex Transm Dis AIDS* 1990;1:447–448.
19. Guimaraes M, Castilho E, Sereno A, et al. Heterosexual transmission of HIV-1: a multicenter study in Rio de Janeiro, Brazil. In: *Program and abstracts of the eighth International Conference on AIDS/Third STD World Congress*. Amsterdam: Harvard University/Dutch Foundation; 1992.
20. Musicco M, The Italian Partners' Study. Oral contraception, IUD, condom use and man to woman sexual transmission of HIV infection. In: *Program and abstracts of the sixth International Conference on AIDS*. San Francisco, University of California; 1990.
21. European Study Group. Risk factors for male to female transmission of HIV. *Br Med J* [*Clin Res*] 1989;298:411–415.

DISCUSSION

Dr. Biggar: Who uses oral contraceptives in the population of Kenya? I can make the hypothesis that these are people who have better socioeconomic status, education, etc., and that the population of men to whom these woman are exposed are also of higher class and therefore have a higher risk of HIV infection. These women may be exposed to a group of men who are simply more infectious.

Dr. Plourde: It's certainly very possible. In the follow-up study where we looked at women with genital ulcers, we knew that they were exposed to men who were more likely to be infectious. But, at least in Kenya, family planning clinics distribute oral contraceptives free of charge, so the economic factor should not figure so much. I don't know whether David Hunter and his colleagues have looked at socioeconomic status in their family planning clinic data, but women do have access to these clinics without having to pay for their oral contraception; so, women of lower socioeconomic status would also have access.

But, you may be right that women are more likely to know about oral contraceptives simply by virtue of the fact that they are more educated.

Dr. Biggar: And the population to which they are exposed would be men of a similar, higher educational background.

Dr. Plourde: Yes, we heard about men with higher education and their risk for HIV from Dr. Piot yesterday.

Dr. Biggar: So this needs to be looked at as a confounding factor?

Dr. Plourde: Yes, I agree.

Dr. Muñoz: You indicate that you have a very interesting group of 133 women who had no history of STD, and 4 of them were HIV positive.

Dr. Plourde: Well, some of them had STD in the past.

Dr. Muñoz: But, even granted that it's a very small number, do you know about their oral contraceptive use?

Dr. Plourde: It was the same in all of the women across the board: roughly 20% to 25% of them (whether prostitutes or pregnant women) were either using oral contraceptives or had done so in the past.

Dr. Stein: Did you establish the relationship of oral contraceptive use and duration of oral contraceptive use with cervical ectopy? Is this a well-known association? And, what about its relationship with STD in other studies?

Dr. Plourde: There are several studies (although most of them are not prospective) that suggest an association between oral contraceptive use and cervical ectopy, but I don't know of any studies that look at the duration of oral contraceptive use and cervical ectopy (when cervical ectopy comes in, how long it lasts during and after, whether it's intermittent during a cycle, and so on).

Dr. Stein: What do we know about cervical ectopy in relation to other STD?

Dr. Plourde: We know that it is associated with chlamydial cervicitis, which we think may explain some of the data showing an association between chlamydial cervicitis and HIV incidence in follow-up studies. But, we don't see such a close association with gonococcus cervicitis. Oral contraceptive use has been associated with gonococcal cervicitis in some studies, while others have found no association. Except for the example I found in my study, I know of no association between oral contraceptive use and genital ulcer disease; so, I don't know how to explain that.

Dr. Cameron: I don't think that anybody would argue that oral contraceptive use is not an epidemiological marker or an ecological risk factor for exposure to STD and HIV, particularly in unmarried women of any class. My question is about the nature of oral contraceptive pills in the biology of cervical ectopy. We believe that cervical ectopy is an estrogen-mediated effect that is increased in high-estrogen physiological states; some oral contraceptive pills have a predominance of estrogen, some a predominance of progesterone (which I think has an opposite effect on the presence of cervical ectopy). Is there any information about the selection of estrogen- or progesterone-based oral contraceptive agents in any of these studies that might be amenable to meta analysis, or any validation of the idea that we have about cervical ectopy and estrogen- or progesterone-based oral contraceptives?

Dr. Plourde: Very little, unfortunately. This was not initially designed into my study either because we didn't expect that there would be an association. It was something we looked at after the fact, and so not much data were collected. Where it was collected, the large majority of women using oral contraceptives were using the estrogen predominant preparations, which are the ones mainly distributed in family planning clinics in Kenya. However, there were some intriguing data showing an association between HIV seroprevalence and deproprovera, a progestational agent. Depro use was very uncommon (only about 5% of women were given it), but I don't know how to explain the association because it's strictly a progestational agent.

Dr. Cameron: The ecological risk (oral or injectional contraceptives, or anything else) is a marker for sexual activity and biases towards exposure. We're never going to escape that fact.

Dr. Plourde: I agree. It's what makes the data that much more confusing.

Dr. Piot: I'd like to return to the Chairman's comment because there are some data on that from the Kenya multistudy. Pierre mentioned that it's a cross-sectional study, but, in the meantime, they have followed up a cohort and they didn't find any association between HIV infection and the use or non-use, or the duration of use of deproprovera. The most interesting finding was that this was a population of women recruited in family planning clinics, and they had a 4% HIV incidence rate over 1 year, which I think is enormous. They found that women who opted for oral contraception in the family planning setting were very different from women who chose other contraceptive methods, such as intrauterine contraceptive devices, deproprovera, or barrier contraception, the choice mainly depending on the social status of the women. But, when they controlled for that, nothing came out in terms of oral contraception as a risk factor. Once again, I think it really shows that the way study populations are recruited may extensively determine the findings.

One final comment, in the cohort study of female prostitutes in Kinshasa, there was no association between HIV seroconversion and oral contraception.

Dr. Biggar: Before you leave the microphone, can you explain two things? Where was the study? And, when you say that nothing came out, do you mean to say that there was no association or that it didn't remove the association?

Dr. Piot: This was the study in a Nairobi family planning clinic done by Mattie and Hunter from Harvard. The relative risk was basically 1. It had no effect in terms of seroconversion.

Dr. Plourde: Just in answer to your comment, I followed Mattie and Hunter's data with great interest. If you followed the presentation of the data from one AIDS international conference to the next, you saw that one time they showed an association, the next time they didn't. I think we're starting to learn something about this phenomenon where the data at one point in time, or from one study, show an association and then they don't. It may be because the risk is lower; the OR may only be somewhere between 1.5 and 2. It may not necessarily be that different study designs or different types of analysis are playing a role, but rather that the attributable risk relating to that particular factor is low and, depending on the study population and the prevalence of that factor in the population, you may get measures of the effect that bounce back and forth between the renewed unity. It's something that the math modellers in our unit are trying to look at in a little more detail.

Dr. Padian: I'm curious about the independence of the effect of PID from cervicitis. Although you had PID in the slide, you lumped them together in your discussion. What is the independent association, and what's the biological mechanism that you postulate?

Dr. Plourde: Perhaps I gave the wrong impression. They are not independent; the two are strongly associated and often go together. What we did was a random multivariable analysis including PID and excluding cervicitis, and vice versa, and we found that the two remained associated. But, when we put them both together, they cancelled each other out, probably because they are so strongly associated with one another. I only showed one because, whichever one you show, you get the same effect. I'm not sure why that is. We suspect that women who come to the clinic with PID or cervicitis may be much more exposed to the risk of HIV, but we don't have any data on that.

HIV Epidemiology: Models and Methods,
edited by Alfredo Nicolosi. Raven Press, Ltd.,
New York © 1994.

10

The Role of Contraceptive Practices in HIV Sexual Transmission from Man to Woman

*Massimo Musicco, *†Alfredo Nicolosi, ‡Alberto Saracco, and ‡Adriano Lazzarin for the Italian Study Group on HIV Heterosexual Transmission

**Department of Epidemiology and Medical Informatics, Institute of Advanced Biomedical Technologies, National Research Council, 20131 Milan, Italy; †Gertrude H. Sergievsky Center, School of Public Health, Columbia University, New York, New York 10032; and ‡Institute of Infectious Diseases, University of Milan, Scientific Institute "Ospedale S. Raffaele," 20157 Milan, Italy*

In the era of acquired immunodeficiency syndrome (AIDS), contraception strategies are important in both developed and developing countries. If some contraceptive practices interact with mechanisms of human immunodeficiency virus (HIV) sexual transmission and increase the risk of infection, family planning campaigns in developing countries (where the prevalence of HIV infection is high and HIV is primarily transmitted through heterosexual contacts) can potentially contribute to the spread of the epidemic. In developed countries, HIV infection is now spreading from the high-risk groups to the non-intravenous drug user (IVDU) heterosexual population (1). In Italy, where the prevalence of seropositivity is high among IVDU, stable couples consisting of a non-IVDU seronegative woman and an HIV-infected current or former IVDU are not uncommon (2,3). These couples often request contraception, either spontaneously or after counseling about the risks of HIV transmission to the woman and child. In this situation, it is important to offer an effective contraceptive that does not increase the risk of infection for the woman.

Condom use can reduce the sexual transmission of HIV (4–9), but condoms are less than optimal as a contraceptive (10). Intrauterine devices (IUD) have been reported to increase the risk of pelvic inflammatory diseases, genital infections, and sexually transmitted diseases (11–15). Since IUD induce inflammatory modification of the uterine mucosa, thus increasing the number of lymphocytes and macrophages (the target cells of HIV) on the genital mucosa, they might also increase the risk of HIV sexual transmission from man to woman (16). Oral contraceptives were found to be associated with an increased risk of male-to-female transmission in two studies carried out in Nairobi among prostitutes (17) and clients of a sexually transmitted diseases clinic (18), while others did not find any association (19–22).

In a previous study on the risk factors for HIV sexual transmission from man to woman among 368 stable couples, among other findings we observed that the woman's susceptibility to HIV was influenced by the use of contraceptives, taking risk factors into account. The study of monogamous, stable couples offers an opportunity to control for confounding factors. The sexual behavior of two stable partners can be assessed over time and its influence on the risk of HIV transmission more easily investigated than in people with multiple partners. There is the methodological advantage that each sexual contact potentially exposes the uninfected partner to the virus. The infected partner can be clinically examined and his or her infectiousness graded in terms of CD4+ cell number or clinical stage.

In this presentation, we describe the results of an analysis of the risk for HIV infection associated with contraceptive practices from the above mentioned study with an increased population of 524 couples.

SUBJECTS AND METHODS

Couples were recruited from 1988 through 1989 in 19 participating centers: 11 hospital departments of infectious diseases, 5 drug dependence treatment services, and 3 HIV surveillance centers (23). The HIV-infected men attending the centers were asked about their heterosexual partners. Each female partner not already known to be HIV infected was invited for an interview and screening tests. We excluded women with infections that were already recognized in order to minimize both recall bias and the confounding of risk factors and disease correlates. Women reporting intravenous drug use, sexual intercourse with other subjects, blood transfusion, blood derivate therapies, or prostitution, as well as women reporting a relationship lasting less than 6 months, were also excluded.

Serum antibodies against HIV were assessed by immunoenzymatic methods using commercially available kits from Abbott Laboratories, North Chicago, Illinois, and Organon Teknika, Holland. Positive samples were repeat-tested and confirmed by Western blot techniques. The HIV-infected man was considered to have been infectous since his first potential exposure to the virus (first intravenous drug use, first homosexual contact, first blood transfusion, or blood derivate therapy), although in no case before 1979, when HIV was first detected in Italy (24). The first sexual contact with the infectious man or the last seronegative test of the woman was considered the starting point of the risk of seroconversion of the woman.

A structured interview was conducted by the treating physician who was blind to the subject's HIV antibody status. The number and type of different contraceptive practices adopted by the woman during the period at risk were investigated. Women were considered condom users when they used this device during 50% or more of sexual intercourse with the infected man; the couple were considered to be practicing "coitus interruptus" when this was used in all sexual intercourse. The use of condoms, oral contraceptives, and IUD was defined as "always" when the woman reported having used one or the other of them for the entire duration of the period at risk of seroconversion, "not always" when use covered only part of the risk period, and "never." We also investigated the use of spermicides and vaginal mechanical barriers, but, because of their very rare use, no analysis was made of the data.

All of the interviewees were asked to report the date when they learned about the HIV positivity of their partner. Information was obtained regarding the frequency and nature of sexual intercourse with the infected partner. In the case of women unaware of their partner's seropositivity, and for women who had been aware since the beginning of their relationship with the infected partner, the information collected related to the preceding year. For the others, it related to the year preceding the moment when the woman learned of the woman's HIV seropositivity. Every woman was asked to describe her weekly frequency of sexual intercourse (≤ 2 or >2) and to report whether she had practiced anal sex and whether she had had any sexually transmitted diseases or genital infections at any time during the relationship. Information on the clinical stage of the infected man (the presence of AIDS at last visit) was collected from standard medical records used by all centers.

Crude odds ratios (OR) and the confidence intervals (CI) for each factor were calculated in order to estimate the risk for HIV infection of the exposed women (25). Interaction terms were built in order to test the presence of interaction between different contraceptive practices, but they were excluded (26). Logistic regression analysis was used to estimate the unconfounded association of each variable with the risk of infection (27). In the univariate analysis, confidence intervals were calculated by the log method; in the logistic model, they were based on the standard error of the regression coefficient (28,29). Data analysis was performed using the statistical software SPSSPC+ and Epilog.

RESULTS

Of the 690 women eligible for the study, 166 were excluded (28 had used intravenous drugs, 6 had had previous transfusions, 51 reported only occasional sexual contact, and 81 had a relationship lasting less than 6 months). The general characteristics of the 524 women included, their male partners, and their sexual behavior are presented in Table 1. One hundred fifty six

TABLE 1. *Characteristics of the women and their male partners*

	Number	HIV[a]-positive women (%)
Total	524	156 (29.8)
Characteristics of the women		
Age 21–30 years	403	123 (30.5)
Risk duration > 1 year	269	104 (38.7)
History of sexually transmitted diseases or genital infections	115	53 (46.1)
Characteristics of the HIV-positive men		
Intravenous drug user	408	125 (30.6)
With AIDS[b]	48	22 (45.8)
Sexual behavior		
Anal sex	130	59 (45.4)
More than twice weekly intercourse	356	121 (34.0)

[a]HIV, human immunodeficiency virus.
[b]AIDS, acquired immunodeficiency syndrome.

women (29.8%) were seropositive. A higher frequency of sexual intercourse, longer duration of sexual exposure, and the practice of anal sex were more frequent among seropositive women. Seropositive women also more frequently had a history of sexually transmitted diseases or genital infections, and their partners more frequently had symptoms of AIDS.

One hundred seventy-seven women (33.8%) had never practiced contraception during their relationship with the infected man, and 280 (53.4%) had used only one contraceptive method (Table 2). The remaining women had used different contraceptive practices, either in temporal sequence or in association. Only eight women reported the use of vaginal spermicides with or without vaginal mechanical barrier.

TABLE 2. *Contraception patterns and proportion of HIV[a]-positive women*

Contraceptive	Number of women	Number HIV positive	Percent HIV positive
None	177	79	45%
OC[b]	114	25	22%
Condom	97	12	12%
Coitus interruptus	40	9	23%
IUD[c]	29	16	55%
Condom and OC	38	5	13%
Condom and IUD	4	1	25%
Coitus interruptus and OC	14	3	21%
Coitus interruptus and IUD	11	6	55%
Total	524	156	30%

[a]HIV, human immunodeficiency virus.
[b]OC, oral contraceptives.
[c]IUD, intrauterine device.

TABLE 3. *Relative risk estimates of male-to-female HIV[a] sexual transmission by contraceptive use in women using only one or no contraceptive during the period at risk of seroconversion (crude odds ratios)*

	HIV positive	HIV negative	OR[b]	95% CI[c]
No contraceptive	79	98	1	
Condom				
Not always	9	61	0.2	0.1–0.4
Always	3	24	0.2	0.1–0.5
OC[d]				
Not always	4	14	0.4	0.1–1.1
Always	21	75	0.3	0.2–0.6
IUD[e]				
Not always	3	1	3.7	0.4–35.6
Always	13	12	1.3	0.6–3.1
Coitus interruptus	9	31	0.4	0.2–0.8

[a]HIV, human immunodeficiency virus.
[b]OR, odds ratio.
[c]CI, confidence interval.
[d]OC, oral contraceptive.
[e]IUD, intrauterine device.

The large majority of the women (457, 87.2%) reported only one or no contraceptive practice during the period at risk of seroconversion (Table 3). In this group, taking as the referent category women never practicing contraception, the risk of infection for women was reduced 80% in couples who had used condoms during part of or the entire duration of the relationship. The risk reduction was 60% in women who had used oral contraceptives during part of the relationship and 70% in those who had used them during

TABLE 4. *Relative risk estimates of male-to-female HIV[a] sexual transmission by contraceptive use in women using one or more contraceptives during the period at risk of seroconversion (crude odds ratios)*

	HIV positive	HIV negative	OR[b]	95% CI[c]
No contraceptive	79	98	1	
Condom				
Not always	17	92	0.2	0.1–0.4
Always	3	37	0.1	0.0–0.3
OC[d]				
Not always	9	39	0.3	0.1–0.6
Always	27	126	0.3	0.2–0.4
IUD[e]				
Not always	8	7	1.4	0.5–4.1
Always	16	17	1.2	0.6–2.5
Coitus interruptus	14	45	0.4	0.2–0.8

[a]HIV, human immunodeficiency virus.
[b]OR, odds ratio.
[c]CI, confidence interval.
[d]OC, oral contraceptive.
[e]IUD, intrauterine device.

TABLE 5. *Relative risk estimates of male-to-female HIV[a] sexual transmission by contraceptive use (odds ratios adjusted by logistic regression)*

	HIV positive	HIV negative	OR[b] (95% CI[c])
Condom			
Never	136	239	1
Not always	17	92	0.3 (0.2–0.6)
Always	3	37	0.2 (0.1–0.5)
OC[d]			
Never	120	359	1
Not always	9	39	0.6 (0.3–1.4)
Always	27	126	0.4 (0.3–0.7)
IUD[e]			
Never	132	476	1
Not always	8	15	4.0 (1.3–12.6)
Always	16	33	1.7 (0.8–3.5)
Coitus interruptus			
Never/sometimes	142	323	1
Always	14	45	0.6 (0.3–1.1)

[a]HIV, human immunodeficiency virus.
[b]OR, odds ratio.
[c]CI, confidence interval.
[d]OC, oral contraceptive.
[e]IUD, intrauterine device.

the entire period. Of the 29 women who had used IUD as the unique contraceptive, 16 (55.4%) were seropositive. Of the 4 women who had used IUD during only part of the relationship, 3 were seropositive, yielding a relative risk estimate of 3.7 (95% CI, 0.4–36.5). In couples who had used only coitus interruptus as contraceptive practice, the risk reduction for women was 60%. Women who had used different contraceptive practices during the relationship essentially presented the same risk estimates, except for IUD use, and this risk was somewhat diluted (Table 4).

TABLE 6. *Relative risk estimates of male-to-female HIV[a] sexual transmission—analysis of contraceptive practices and of factors influencing the risk of HIV sexual transmission (odds ratios adjusted by logistic regression)*

	Odds ratio	95% CI[c]
Contraceptive[b]		
Condom	0.3	0.2–0.5
Oral contraceptive	0.4	0.3–0.7
Intrauterine device	2.2	1.1–4.3
Coitus interruptus	0.6	0.3–1.2
More than twice a week sexual intercourse	1.9	1.1–3.1
Risk duration longer than 1 year	2.1	1.4–3.3
History of sexually transmitted diseases or genital infections	3.0	1.8–4.8
Anal sex	1.9	1.2–3.1
Partner with AIDS[d]	2.1	1.1–4.2

[a]HIV, human immunodeficiency virus.
[b]Reference category is women never users.
[c]CI, confidence interval.
[d]AIDS, acquired immunodeficiency syndrome.

When we used multiple logistic regression analysis to reach a risk estimate for each contraceptive, adjusting for use of other contraceptives (Table 5), the adjusted relative risks were consistent with the crude analyses. The risk associated with IUD use during part of the relationship was more evident (OR=4.0; 95% CI, 1.3–12.6).

Finally, we performed a multiple logistic regression analysis of the risk associated with each contraceptive, controlling for other factors that influenced the risk of HIV sexual transmission: frequency of sexual intercourse, duration of the exposure period, history of sexually transmitted diseases or genital infections during the relationship, anal intercourse, and the partner's clinical stage (Table 6). This analysis confirmed the risk estimates reached by the previous analyses, showing that the risks and the preventive effects associated with contraceptive practices were independent of other factors.

CONCLUSION

In agreement with previous studies, our cross-sectional study of 524 women who were steady partners of HIV-infected men shows that the risk of seroconversion is reduced by the use of condoms. The practice of coitus interruptus was also associated with a reduction in the risk of transmission. These results suggest that the avoidance of contact between semen and the female genital mucosa reduces the risk of the sexual transmission of HIV.

In this study, IUD use seems to increase the risk of HIV transmission from man to woman, which is consistent with a European study that investigated the role of contraception in HIV heterosexual transmission (30). Our data showed that women who used IUD during the whole relationship with the infected partner had a small increase in risk of infection, whereas women who inserted or removed the device while exposed to the infected man had a fourfold, statistically significant, increased risk of acquiring HIV infection. Recent data from the World Health Organization's IUD clinical trial indicate an increased risk of pelvic inflammatory disease limited to the first 20 days after IUD insertion (31). This finding parallels the results of our study, which suggest that the introduction or removal of IUD causes cervical or uterine lesions that may facilitate the penetration of free virus and/or HIV-infected cells.

In this study, oral contraceptive use was associated with a 60% risk reduction. Although one of the proposed reasons for the apparent increase in risk of HIV infection observed among the women using oral contraceptives in the African studies was that oral contraceptives may impair the immune system, there is no firm biological evidence to prove it. On the contrary, a number of studies have shown that there is no difference between oral contraceptive users and non-users in terms of the percentage or absolute number of total T cells, helper cells, suppressor/cytotoxic cells, or natural killer cells (32), nor in terms of alterations of the humoral immunoregulation (33,34).

Our result, which needs further confirmation, has a possible biological explanation. The progestine component of oral contraceptives induces a thickening of the cervical mucus that may block the penetration of HIV infected cells into the uterus, and thus limit HIV exposure to the vaginal mucosa (35). The stratified, squamous epithelium of the vaginal mucosa is probably more resistant to HIV entry than the thin layer of the uterine mucosa, which is also highly vascularized and richer in HIV-target cells than the vagina. Also, mucus acts as a support medium for a variety of antimicrobial secretions and is a proper environment for phagocytic cells and cell-mediated immune actions (36).

The crude relationship between HIV sexual transmission and contraception may be confounded by extraneous factors (37). Women using contraceptives generally have a higher frequency of sexual intercourse and a greater likelihood of exposure to potentially infective sexual encounters. Women using IUD and oral contraceptives are not concerned about unwanted pregnancies and may therefore be less attentive in avoiding contact between semen and genital mucosa; furthermore, women using IUD and oral contraceptives do not use condoms for contraceptive purposes. Although both oral contraceptive and IUD use is expected to be more prevalent among women at higher risk of acquiring HIV infection through sexual transmission, the fact that we found the risk of HIV transmission to be increased in IUD users and decreased in oral contraceptive users strengthens the internal validity of the results.

In this study on stable, monogamous couples, we were able to control for both the use of different types of contraceptive and all other factors known to influence HIV sexual transmission. We could not control for possible confounding due to education or socioeconomic status. We cannot exclude that oral contraceptive users were the most educated women, thereby adopting safer sexual behavior. However, the most effective factor of safe sexual intercourse (i.e., condom use) was controlled for, thus leaving little room for additional confounding by socioeconomic status.

Our study underlines the importance of contraceptive practices in the transmission of HIV to sexually exposed women. Waiting for further research to confirm these findings, we conclude that the only contraceptive that prevents HIV transmission is the condom and that, if a stable couple desire more effective contraception, oral contraceptives are the preferred choice.

ACKNOWLEDGMENT

This research was supported by a grant from the Ministry of Health (Istituto Superiore di Sanità-Progetto AIDS).

Members of the Italian Study Group on HIV Heterosexual Transmission include: Gioacchino Angarano, M.D. (Bari), Claudio Arici, M.D. (Bergamo), Maria Léa Corrêa Leite, M.D. (Milan), Paolo Costigliola, M.D. (Bologna), Sergio Gafà, M.D. (Reggio Emilia), Maddalena Gasparini, M.D. (Milan), Giovanna Gavazzeni, M.D. (Bergamo), Cristina Gervasoni, M.D. (Milan), Adriano Lazzarin, M.D. (Milan), Roberto Luzzati, M.D. (Verona), Giacomo Magnani, M.D. (Parma), Mauro Moroni, M.D. (Milan), Massimo Musicco, M.D. (Milan), Alfredo Nicolosi, M.D., Ph.D. (Milan), Raffaele Pristerà, M.D. (Bolzano), Francesco Puppo, M.D. (Genova), Bernardino Salassa, M.D. (Turin), Alessandro Sinicco, M.D. (Turin), Roberto Stellini, M.D. (Brescia), Umberto Tirelli, M.D. (Aviano), Giuseppe Turbessi, M.D. (Rome), Gian Marco Vigevani, M.D. (Milan), Roberto Zerboni, M.D. (Milan).

REFERENCES

1. Johnson AM. Heterosexual transmission of human immunodeficiency virus. *Br Med J [Clin Res]* 1988;296:1017–1020.
2. Nicolosi A, Correa Leite ML, Musicco M, Molinari S, Saracco A, Lazzarin A. Prevalence and incidence trends of HIV infection in intravenous drug users attending treatment centers in Milan and Northern Italy, 1986–1990. *J AIDS* 1992;5:365–373.
3. Nicolosi A, Correa Leite ML, Musicco M, Molinari S, Lazzarin A. Parenteral and sexual transmission of human immunodeficiency virus in intravenous drug users: a study of seroconversion. *Am J Epidemiol* 1992;135:225–233.
4. Peterman TA, Stoneburner RL, Allen JR, Jaffe HW, Curran JW. Risk of human immunodeficiency virus transmission from heterosexual adults with transfusion associated infections. *JAMA* 1988;259:55–58.
5. European Study Group. Risk factors for male to female transmission of HIV *Br Med J [Clin Res]* 1989;298:411–415.
6. Roumeliotou A, Papautsakis G, Kallinikos G, Papaevangelou G. Effectiveness of condom use in preventing HIV infection in prostitutes. *Lancet* 1988;2:1249.
7. Mann J, Quinn TC, Piot P. Condom use and HIV infection among prostitutes in Zaire. *N Engl J Med* 1987;316:345.
8. Smith GL, Smith KF. Lack of HIV infection and condom use in licensed prostitutes. *Lancet* 1986;1:1392.
9. Perlman JA, Kelaghan JK, Wolf PH, at al. HIV risk difference between condom users and nonusers among US heterosexual women. *J AIDS* 1990;3:155–165.
10. Sherris JD, Lewison D, Fox G. Update on condoms: products, protection, promotion. Population Reports, Series H, Number 6. Baltimore: Johns Hopkins University, Population Information Program, 1982: p H-129.
11. Faulkner WL, Ory HW. Intrauterine devices and acute pelvic inflammatory disease. *JAMA* 1976;235:1851–1853.
12. Westrom L, Bengtsson LP, Mardh P. The risk of pelvic inflammatory disease in women using intrauterine contraceptive devices as compared to non users. *Lancet* 1976;2:221–224.
13. Buchan H, Villard-Mackintosh L, Vessey M, Yeates D, McPherson K. Epidemiology of pelvic inflammatory disease in parous women with special reference to intrauterine device use. *Br J Obstet Gynaecol* 1990;97:780–788.
14. Wright EA, Aisien AO. Pelvic inflammatory disease and the intrauterine contraceptive device. *Int J Gynaecol Obstet* 1989;28(2):133–136.
15. Avonts D, Sercu M, Heyerick P, Vandermeeren I, Meheus A, Piot P. Incidence of uncomplicated genital infections in women using oral contraception or an interuterine device: a prospective study. *Sex Transm Dis* 1990;17:23–29.
16. Fornari ML. Cellular changes in the glandular epithelium of patients using IUCD: a source of cytologic error. *Acta Cytol (Baltimore)* 1974;18:341–343.

17. Plummer FA, Simonsen JN, Cameron WD, et al. Cofactors in male-female transmission of human immunodeficiency virus type 1. IV. *J Infect Dis* 1991;163:233–239.
18. Plourde PJ, Plummer FA, Pepin J, et al. Human immunodeficiency virus type 1 infection in women attending a sexually transmitted diseases clinic in Kenya. *J Infect Dis* 1992;166:86–92.
19. Goedert JJ, Eyster ME, Ragni MV, Biggar RJ, Gail MH. Rate of heterosexual transmission and associated risk with HIV antigen. International Conference on AIDS, 1988.
20. Darrow WW, Bigler B, Deppe D, et al. HIV antibody in 640 US prostitutes with no evidence of intravenous drug abuse. International Conference on AIDS, 1988.
21. Mati J, Maggwa A, Chewe D, et al. Contraceptive use and HIV infection among women attending family planning clinics in Nairobi Kenia. International Conference on AIDS, 1990.
22. Meirik O, Farley TMM. Oral contraceptives and HIV transmission. In: Alexander NJ, Gabelnick HL, Jeffrey MS, eds. *Heterosexual transmission of AIDS*. New York: Alan R. Liss, Inc; 1990:247–254.
23. Lazzarin A, Saracco A, Musicco M, Nicolosi A. Man-to-woman sexual HIV transmission: risk factors related to sexual behavior, man's infectiousness and woman's susceptibility. *Arch Intern Med* 1991;151:2411–2416.
24. Lazzarin A, Crocchiolo P, Galli M, et al. Milan as possible starting point of LAV/HTLV-III epidemic among Italian drug addicts. *Boll Ist Sieroter Milan* 1987;66:9–13.
25. Mantel N, Haenszel W. Statistical aspects of the analysis of data from retrospective studies of disease. *J Natl Cancer Inst* 1959;22:71948.
26. Breslow NE, Day NE. Stastistical methods in cancer research. In: *The analysis of case-control studies*. Lyon: IARC Scientific Publications, 1980.
27. Schlesselman JJ. *Case-control studies: design, conduct, analysis*. New York: Oxford University Press, 1982:227–290.
28. Rothman KJ. *Modern epidemiology*. Boston: Little, Brown & Co.; 1986.
29. Hosmer DW, Lemeshow S. *Applied logistic regression analysis*. New York: J Wiley & Sons; 1989.
30. European Study Group. Risk factors for male to female transmission of HIV *Br Med J* [*Clin Res*] 1989;298:411–415.
31. Farley TM, Rosenberg MJ, Rowe PJ, Chen JH, Meirik O. Intrauterine devices and pelvic inflammatory disease: an international perspective. *Lancet* 1992;339:785–788.
32. Baker DA, Hameed C, Tejani N, et al. Lymphocyte subsets in women on low dose oral contraceptives. *Contraception* 1985;32:377–382.
33. Bisset LR, Griffin JFT. Humoral immunity in oral contraceptive users. I. Plasma immunoglobulin levels. *Contraception* 1988;38:567–572.
34. Bisset LR, Griffin JFT. Humoral immunity in oral contraceptive users. II. *In vitro* immunoglobulin production. *Contraception* 1988;38:573–578.
35. Moghissi KS, Syner FN, McBride L. Contraceptive mechanism of microdose norethindrone. *Obstet Gynecol* 1978;41:585–591.
36. Cohen MS. Vaginal mucosal defenses. In: Horowitz BJ, Mardh PE, eds. *Vaginitis and vaginosis*. New York: Wiley-Liss, 1991:33–37.
37. Meirik O, Farley TMM. Oral contraceptives and HIV transmission. In: Alexander NJ, Gabelnick HL, Jeffrey MS, eds. *Heterosexual transmission of AIDS*. New York: Alan R. Liss Inc; 1990:247–254.

DISCUSSION

Dr. Padian: Do you recommend that women have their IUD removed? You made a very good point that it could be the insertion or removal of an IUD that causes the risk. When you look at the PID studies, that seems to be the general consensus. It may therefore be better to leave it in, because otherwise you may be introducing virus or some kind of trauma. You seem to have reached that conclusion, but you still recommend they should be removed.

Dr. Musicco: At the centers participating in the study, we recommend removing IUD and then abstaining from sexual contact for at least 1 month.

Dr. Detels: I'm a little concerned about the strong dependence on p values. In the previous presentation, there was a slide looking at potential confounders in which confounders were rejected if they didn't reach a p value of 0.05. I think we need to be careful because, if all of the confounders are going in the same direction and none of them reaches 0.05, it may be a fallacy to reject all of them out of hand. In terms of this presentation, I was a little concerned because you showed risk ratios of around 3.5, which were not statistically significant, and I wonder whether that was caused by extreme variability in the data or if it was a problem of sample size. If it's a problem of sample size, we have to be very concerned about rejecting something because it doesn't reach statistical significance.

Dr. Musicco: I completely agree with you. For the sake of completeness, I also tried to present raw data contrasting the three contraceptive patterns. You will remember, I presented women using only one contraceptive against women using no contraceptive, women using condoms and another contraceptive against women using only condoms, and women using coitus interruptus and IUD against women using oral contraceptives and coitus interruptus. Now, for the oral contraceptives, IUD, and coitus interruptus, we have enough evidence from the first group of the supposed protective effect. Because it seems that few women use IUD, and about half of them use them in association with another contraceptive, I have presented the strata values. In none of the single strata was there any significant increase in the risk for IUD users, which only becomes apparent in the multivariable analysis.

The problem of sample size is enormous, because we are not planning a study here. We are simply dealing with the men and women attending various centers who agree to participate in the study. We have to take what arrives spontaneously.

Dr. Biggar: Although we obviously can't reject something just because it doesn't reach statistical significance, you also can't accept something just because it looks high. I would only go so far as to say that anything that looks high is interesting, but I won't believe it until it has been confirmed.

Dr. Nicolosi: I'm not a statistician, but p values have nothing to do with confounding. Confounding comes from the sampling frame, so you can't just simply adjust using p values. Furthermore, some funny things can happen with p values. For example, in Pierre Plourde's presentation, some slides showed a significant difference in age at first intercourse (16.1 years for seropositives and 16.9 years for seronegatives), but I don't think this is substantially significant.

I would also like to make a couple of points concerning the differences between the African and Italian studies presented today, because these have wide-ranging implications for health policies. First of all, the African studies are based on promiscuous women, while the Italian study only involves monogamous couples. In the African prospective study, there was an incidence that was exactly ten times higher than that of the Italian study. This means that so many risk components are working together that it is difficult to make any comparison, and perhaps that the two situations cannot be compared at all.

Bill Cameron said that the majority of oral contraceptives used in Africa were estrogen based. In Italy, the majority have become progesterone based. If it is so, this can make a difference in terms of production of mucus and cervical ectopy.

There is also the issue of internal validity. Like most epidemiologic studies on

HIV, the study that Massimo presented was an exploratory (the old "fishing expedition"), in both the good and the bad sense of the term. We found several risk factors, but the study was not explicitly designed to study the effects of oral contraceptives, and this is a limitation that, at this stage of HIV research, affects all other studies that raised the issue of HIV infection and oral contraceptives. However, some internal validity was offered in our study because there was control for other factors (particularly, control for other contraceptives and markers of the infectiousness of the partner), and we saw that their effects are consistent with the reports of other studies and that they are biologically plausible.

Unfortunately, this control was not attainable in Africa. Some of the findings of the African studies are also puzzling in terms of internal validity. One of Pierre Plourde's slides showed univariate analyses in which condom use had an odds ratio of more than 3, which makes me wonder whether there is some misclassification or something else going on. Further, it was not possible to control for the stage of the partner in the African studies because it was a multipartner setting.

I think that both studies should be considered as suggestive, giving a lead for further studies explicitly designed for oral contraceptives. Pierre was right when he said the African studies must not be viewed as providing definitive answers.

Dr. Plourde: I agree that the difference between 16.1 and 16.9 years doesn't appear to be clinically significant. But, if you take the age at which the subjects presented at the clinic and the age at which they reported starting sexual behavior, subtract the two, and then look at the duration of sexual activity in months, you find that HIV-positive women had been sexually active almost a year longer than HIV-negative women. It's true that 0.9 may not look like a lot, but 12 months of sexual activity is a significant amount of time.

As far as African women being more promiscuous is concerned, that was an argument that we accepted until I started seeing the same associations in nonprostitutes who, although they are still promiscuous (but this depends on your definition of promiscuous), had had about six lifetime partners and very few of them had had more than ten. By our standards, that may be a lot, but I don't know what parameter can be used to call it promiscuous behavior or not (it probably depends on the investigator's personal number of lifetime sexual partners).

The interesting finding about condom use was that it was so strongly associated with prostitution. If you look at our Nairobi studies, you see condom use being quite effective in preventing transmission over the short-term. But, if you follow prostitutes long enough, they eventually seroconvert whether or not they are using condoms. Of course, this may be related to a failure to use condoms 100% of the time and may mean that 95% use is just not good enough.

Dr. Muñoz: I would like to bring up the question of interaction. Plourde's data suggested a ridiculously high interaction between GUD and OC use. With no GUD, the odds ratio was 1.1 with respect to oral contraceptive use. In your analysis, even though you throw both the history of sexually transmitted diseases and oral contraceptive use into the logistic regression, a qualitative interaction may provide false peace of mind with respect to confounding because it may prevent you from seeing the change.

I say this not only from a methodological point of view, but also on the basis of the data that are beginning to emerge from Brazil. Brazil has an interesting convergence: there is anal sex, sexually transmitted diseases and oral contraceptive use.

The Rio de Janeiro data presented in Amsterdam indicate that, if you have no sexually transmitted diseases, oral contraceptives may be protective; but if you have sexually transmitted diseases, oral contraceptive use may be a risk factor.

Dr. Musicco: I think you are completely right. In reference to our results showing a protective effect of oral contraceptives, the problem is that the frequency of sexually transmitted diseases is very low in our population; we have only 15 women who report a history of syphilis or genital herpes, and 10 who report a history of papillomavirus infection. The others were women who reported vaginitis. When we tried to analyze the possible interaction, we had so few numbers that our analysis couldn't support any conclusion. But I think that your suggestion is also important because in women using oral contraceptives with a genital infection, the vaginal environment itself may be particularly favorable for transmission and, consequently, you don't see any protective effect. If the vaginal environment is normal and doesn't favor transmission, blocking the passage of infected cells into the uterus and the cervix may exert a protective effect.

Dr. Cameron: I think the major distinction between the two studies is the study population itself. The Nairobi study population could not be standardized in terms of the amount of sexual exposure, and therefore the use of oral contraceptives and genital ulcers are very strongly confounded by the risk of exposure to HIV. In the Italian study, the monogamous selection and 100% sexual exposure to HIV meant that it was possible to measure potential confounders such as condom use and enter them into the regression models. I would suggest that the Nairobi study contains a tremendous amount of confounding, and it is this that produces the multiplicative synergy of risk factors that doesn't come out in the other study.

Dr. Biggar: I'm very tempted to ask for a show of hands as to how many people believe that oral contraceptives are really associated with an increased risk of transmission.

Dr. Cameron: I'd put the question more precisely: "Do you believe that oral contraceptives represent a biological risk factor that increases the susceptibility of a woman to HIV, given HIV exposure?"

Dr. Biggar: Does anyone believe that oral contraception has been proved to be protective? . . . I see that basically we have a very noncommittal group here, so let's go onto the next question. Based on what you know, would you advise or not advise your patient population and/or wife, girlfriend, or whatever? What would you recommend to the population that you serve or yourself?

Dr. Detels: I think you have to say a patient. After all, you have to assume that your wife doesn't have any other risk exposures?

Dr. Plourde: If the woman wants to avoid sexually transmitted diseases and pregnancy, I would recommend barrier contraception in combination with oral contraception, at least until more data are available.

Dr. Stein: Everybody is talking about oral contraceptives, but deproprovera and injected hormonal substances represent what is really happening across the world, and we have nothing on them. We need much more study about ectopy and the GU before anybody can make any Delphic comments about their safety or nonsafety.

Dr. Johnson: My comment concerns public health policy. The real issue concerning the oral contraceptive message is that it's not just a question of HIV prevention, but of population—maternal mortality, population control, and women's health. Making a public health statement about contraceptive use on the basis of data that we are clearly all uncertain about (including the people who have presented it and who put it up for discussion) is really an issue that needs to be put into any equation about the effectiveness of changing public health policy on recommending oral contraception.

Dr. Vermund: I was going to make the same point Anne just made, so I'll just add a corollary. Although AIDS is taking over in some countries, there are still a lot of others in which maternal or childbirth-related mortality is the number one killer of women of child-bearing age. Any recommendations of this kind are made prematurely and, just as Anne said, could be counterproductive from the public health point of view. I remember reading a paper published in *Lancet* about 4 years ago by some former colleagues with a title that was something like, "Where is the M in MCH?," referring to maternal child health. I think that paper is worth rereading if we want to avoid sweeping statements about the inadvisability of oral contraceptive use.

Dr. Musicco: We have two problems: the first concerns developed and the other concerns developing countries. In developed countries, I think that there is no problem in making a contraceptive recommendation now in order to avoid occasional infection during occasional sexual intercourse. The usual recommendation to use condoms achieves both goals: it is a reasonable contraceptive and a good preventive practice for avoiding HIV infection. In developing countries, the problem is somewhat more worrying because it is probably impractical to think in terms of family planning being based only on oral contraceptives, and it is probably too expensive to promote the use of condoms. The third method, even though it cannot be considered the method of choice, is the use of IUD, which are highly suspected of increasing the risk of transmission. This is a true problem of health policy.

In other countries, the problem arises when a woman is exposed to the risk of HIV transmission (and we cannot assume now that every woman who has sexual intercourse is highly exposed). We have estimated the risk from a single sexual intercourse to be around 1 per 1,000 or 1 per 500. To make a specific recommendation for occasional intercourse based on the data for contraception seems to me to be nonsense. The problem is when you have a woman who says that she has a sexual partner who is HIV positive and that she doesn't want to become pregnant. There, you have to combine the two requests: not to increase the risk of transmission and not to have an unwanted pregnancy.

We advised using oral contraceptives, with condoms, instead of IUDs.

Dr. Plourde: I didn't mean to give the impression that I would scrap hormonal contraceptives in family planning programs, but I would like to use the data we have. We know that condoms are 60% to 70% effective. They're as good as some vaccines that we have for the prevention not only of HIV transmission, but also of any other sexually transmitted diseases. What I'm suggesting is that, in existing family planning programs, we should continue to use whatever methods are best for population control (which I agree is an urgent problem in the Southern world) and that barrier contraceptives should be promoted more vigorously. Furthermore, maybe more research needs to be done in terms of female conduct because if men are unable or unwilling to take the responsibility, it should be put into the hands of women.

Dr. Biggar: In closing, I don't have much to say except that this has been a session devoted to the biological factors influencing the risk of transmission within a setting of individuals. The thing that has been missing from this discussion is a sense of how widespread exposure-promoting behaviors are. I hope that we shall be able to investigate this with Anne Johnson's work this evening. It's not an unknown area, but I'd say that it is at least as important as the individual risk of transmission that we, as biologists, like to study. There are issues of sociology and sexology that are hard to get at and probably uncomfortable for some of us who are more used to the hard sciences.

HIV Epidemiology: Models and Methods, edited by Alfredo Nicolosi. Raven Press, Ltd., New York © 1994.

11

Seroprevalence, Seroconversion, and the History of the HIV Epidemic Among Drug Injectors

Samuel R. Friedman, *Don C. Des Jarlais, Benny Jose, Alan Neaigus, and Marjorie Goldstein

*National Development and Research Institutes, Inc., New York, New York 10013; *Beth Israel Medical Center, New York, New York*

In previous papers, we have discussed the histories of the human immunodeficiency virus (HIV) epidemic in different cities as indicated by serial cross-sectional studies among drug injectors (1,2). We and others have studied the risk factors for seropositivity in cross-sectional studies (3–22). We and others have also examined the risk factors for seroconversion in cohort studies (23–34).

In this paper, we consider some issues in the interpretation of cross-sectional seroprevalence risk factor studies in light of (a) the fact that, in many cities, the HIV epidemic among drug injectors is now a decade or more old (2); and (b) the findings of our studies of seroconversion in a 14-city data set from the U.S.

MODEL

To begin with, it will be helpful to present a model of the relationship of seroprevalence to seroconversion. Equation 1 is definitional:

$$\text{Seroprevalence} = \frac{\text{Number of seropositives}}{\text{Number of seropositives} + \text{Number of seronegatives}} \qquad [1]$$

Equation 2 presents a "naive" equation for seroprevalence as a function of seroconversions from the start of an epidemic:

$$\text{Seroprevalence} = \frac{\int \text{seroconversions}}{\text{Number of drug injectors}} \qquad [2]$$

In reality, however, drug injectors enter and depart from the scene for a host of reasons, which are presented in Table 1. Thus, it is necessary to adjust the equations to take account of arrivals and departures. Equation 3 presents formulas for changes in the numbers of seropositives and seronegatives over time:

$$\begin{aligned}\Delta\text{Seropositives} &= \text{arriving seropositives} + \text{seroconversions}\\ &\quad - \text{departing seropositives}\\ \Delta\text{Seronegatives} &= \text{arriving seronegatives} - \text{seroconversions}\\ &\quad - \text{departing seronegatives}\end{aligned} \qquad [3]$$

Thus, if we assume that time 0 is the time at which HIV arrives among drug injectors in a given locality, we arrive at equation 4, which relates seroprevalence to seroconversion and to arrivals and departures from the scene (where the integral describes integration over time between t=0 and the present):

$$\text{Seroprevalence} = \frac{\int\text{arriving seropositives} + \int\text{seroconversions} - \int\text{departing seropositives}}{\left(\begin{array}{l}\text{Number IDUs at } t=0 + \int\text{arriving seropositives}\\ + \int\text{seroconversions} - \int\text{departing seropositives}\\ + \int\text{arriving seronegatives} - \int\text{seroconversions}\\ - \int\text{departing seronegatives}\end{array}\right)} \qquad [4]$$

$$= \frac{\int\text{seroconversions} + \int\text{arriving seropositives} - \int\text{departing seropositives}}{\left(\begin{array}{l}\text{Number IDUs at } t=0 + \int\text{arriving seropositives}\\ - \int\text{departing seropositives} + \int\text{arriving seronegatives}\\ - \int\text{departing seronegatives}\end{array}\right)}$$

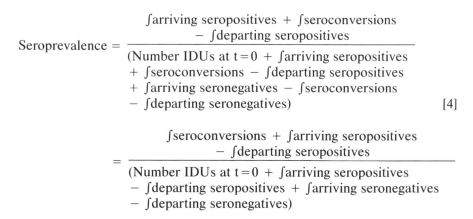

In this equation, each of the terms within the integrals is a function of time, and the shape of these functions is by no means predetermined.[1] They can be nonlinear or, indeed, discontinuous functions. (The equations to estimate which behavioral risk factors are associated with seropositivity are much more complex. Behaviors vary over time, so the functions used to describe behaviors must be time-dependent.)

[1]In addition, it should be noted that definitions of "drug injector" may vary, particularly in terms of how many times one must inject within what time period to be considered an injector.

TABLE 1. *Major forms of arrival and departure of drug injectors from the scene*

- Departures
  - Death
    - AIDS[a]
    - "Non-AIDS" HIV[b]-related fatal diseases
    - HIV-related suicides
    - Overdoses
    - Homicides
    - Other deaths
  - Voluntary geographical movement
  - Involuntary geographical movement out of scene
    - Incarceration
    - Hospitalization, including residential drug treatment
    - Gentrification, urban renewal, neighborhood burn-out
    - Flight from police or others
  - In cohort studies
    - Refusal to be re-interviewed
    - Inability of researchers to re-locate subjects
- Arrivals[c]
  - New injectors
  - Voluntary geographical movement
  - Semivoluntary geographical movement
    - Return from incarceration
    - Flight into the scene

[a]AIDS, acquired immunodeficiency.
[b]HIV, human immunodeficiency virus.
[c]In addition, there may be "non-arrivals" if people avoid becoming drug injectors.

IMPLICATIONS OF THE MODEL RELATED TO HISTORICAL PATTERNS OF VIRAL SPREAD

Clearly, the seroprevalence rate is the outcome of a number of complicated social and epidemiologic processes. In an epidemic like that in New York City, where HIV infection among drug injectors dates back at least 15 years, these adjustments to the "naive" Equation 2 can be both quite extensive and quite complex. This means that attempts to understand the risk factors for infection using cross-sectional seroprevalence data require increasing care as the epidemic matures.

There are several ways in which the development of the epidemic influences Equation 4. Most obviously, in a long-term epidemic in a high-seroprevalence city, the terms for departures due to deaths will increasingly include large numbers of HIV-related deaths. Thus, in New York City, by 1986 (approximately 10 years into the epidemic among drug injectors), Stoneburner et al. (35) reported that there had been at least 1,803 acquired immunodeficiency syndrome (AIDS) deaths and at least as many "non-AIDS" yet HIV-related deaths among drug injectors. Since then, over 9,500 additional AIDS deaths have been reported among drug injectors in New York City (E. J. Fordyce, *personal communication,* 1992).

As a further complication, these deaths would not be expected to be a random selection of the infected drug injectors. Deaths due to AIDS or other HIV-related diseases or conditions will be overrepresented among those who were infected earlier and perhaps among those who have maintained high injection rate lifestyles (36). Thus, efforts to estimate risk factors for infection from seroprevalence should adjust for changes over time in the behavioral and sociodemographic characteristics of those who became infected at different times, including consideration of differential depletion of the population caused by death from disease progression as a function of time since infection and perhaps of behaviors since infection. In some cities, there might also have to be adjustments due to suicide after notification of HIV antibody test results.

In addition, there is some reason to think that the normal pattern of spread of HIV among drug injectors in a community means that the functions for seroconversion rates and for the risk factors for seroconversion are both functions of the seroprevalence rate. Table 2 shows that, among 10 cities with seroprevalence rates less than 12%, seroconversion rates increased with seroprevalence. On the other hand, the rate of seroconversion as a function of seroprevalence seems to level off later in the epidemic (see Table 3). Also, the leveling off of seroprevalence rates in many cities has a similar implication (2).

Tables 2 and 3 also indicate that risk factors for seroconversion may change over the course of the epidemic. At first, when seroprevalence is low, a key determinant of probability of seroconversion in intravenous drug users (IDU) may be whether or not they are located in "pockets of infection" (i.e., those groups of IDU who have the closest network connections to the first local drug injectors to become infected). Thus, in the ten cities in Table 2, black and Puerto Rican drug injectors are particularly likely to seroconvert. As the epidemic progresses, however, it appears that the virus becomes more widespread throughout the drug injector networks, and specific behavioral propensities become the factors more likely to determine seroconversion. Among the 4 cities with seroprevalence rates greater than 20% in Table 3, for example, renting used syringes (typically, in shooting galleries or other multiperson injection settings) and cocaine injection fre-

TABLE 2. *Risk factors for seroconversion in 10 cities with seroprevalence <12%*

	Cox regression	
	Risk ratio	95% CI[a]
City seroprevalence (per 1% increase)	1.27	1.10, 1.46
No prior drug abuse treatment	2.94	1.16, 7.43
Black[b]	2.77	1.08, 7.09
Puerto Rican[b]	13.17	1.58, 110.02

[a]CI, confidence interval.
[b]Reference group is other subjects, who are primarily white (non-Latino) and Mexican.

TABLE 3. *Risk factors for seroconversion in 4 cities with seroprevalence >20%*

	Cox regression	
	Risk ratio	95% CI[a]
Any renting used syringes in last 6 months	2.15	1.50, 3.07
Cocaine injections per day	1.20	1.01, 1.43

[a]CI, confidence interval.

quency are risk factors for seroconversion (but race/ethnicity variables are not). Seroprevalence studies will tend to reflect the local history of all of these processes—with an averaging function described more precisely by Equation 4—but in a locality with an older epidemic, some of the significant predictors of infection may reflect previously important risk factors rather than currently important ones. For example, in a city where black and white drug injectors have had relatively little contact, the following scenario might occur:

1. HIV enters first among black IDU.
2. HIV spreads rapidly among black IDU, barely entering white IDU networks. At this stage of the epidemic, both seroconversion and seroprevalence studies will show that being black is a risk factor.
3. Rate of seroconversion declines among black IDU to the same (low) level as among white IDU. A seroprevalence study will show black race/ethnicity as a risk factor at this stage, but a seroincidence study will find race/ethnicity unrelated to seroconversion.
4. The epidemic spreads to white IDU, who begin to seroconvert rapidly. At this stage, a seroprevalence study will still show blacks to be at higher risk, but a seroincidence study will show whites to be at higher risk.
5. White seroconversion levels off, perhaps to a seroprevalence rate slightly below that of blacks (due to still being a few years "behind" them). Here, seroprevalence studies might find a slight racial/ethnic effect, but seroincidence studies would not.
6. If the white epidemic lagged behind that among black IDU by several years, higher death rates among those (predominantly black) IDU who were infected earlier might lead to equalization or even inversion of relative seroprevalence rates among blacks and whites. Yet seroincidence studies during this period would continue to show no racial effect.

This pattern is already quite complex, but might be even harder to untangle if the different race/ethnicity groups started out with different levels of risk behaviors and if their behaviors changed at different rates during the course of the epidemic. Consider what would happen if black drug injectors—and those white drug injectors among whom HIV was most widespread—switched from drug injection to crack smoking as their primary way of taking drugs in Stage 4, in an attempt to prevent HIV from spreading so quickly. Under these circumstances, a seroprevalence study might conclude that crack smoking was the primary risk factor for HIV.

IMPLICATIONS OF THE MODEL RELATED TO CHANGES IN SCENES OVER TIME THAT ARE NOT DIRECTLY RELATED TO THE EPIDEMIC

There are many other ways that patterns of arrival and departure of drug injectors can lead to difficulties in interpreting seroprevalence and seroconversion risk factors. Basically, these arise if the seroprevalence rates of new arrivers or new departers change over time. Here, we will present a few examples:

1. Changes in in-migration patterns. Consider a city like San Francisco, in which seroprevalence has stabilized at about 15% among drug injectors. If there were to be a sudden influx of high-frequency needle sharers from a very low seroprevalence city, seroprevalence studies might even find needle sharing to have a protective effect. This same conclusion might arise through a different process (e.g., if a large number of seropositive drug injectors who had learned never to share moved into the city from New York with its 50% seroprevalence rate). A cohort study that recruited its subjects prior to the beginning of these migrations would shed no light upon these findings (which also might be easily missed by a seroprevalence study that did not specifically analyze migration).
2. Consider new injectors, who are *ipso facto* new arrivals to the scene. Typically, cities or countries vary over time in the extent to which new persons begin to inject drugs. In New York City, for example, there was a wave of new injectors in the late 1960s, followed by a lower rate of recruits over the years since then (37). The Netherlands saw a wave of new heroin injection beginning in the 1970s (38), and Glasgow saw such a wave begin in the early 1980s and continue to increase through the rest of the decade (39). In a 14-city international study sponsored by the World Health Organization, the New York wave stands out in that the average years of injection and average age of New York subjects are considerably higher than those in the other 13 cities (M. Carballo, *personal communication*).

   In seroprevalence studies, it is commonly found that newer injectors are less likely to be infected than longer-term injectors. This is undoubtedly due at least in part to newer injectors having had less opportunity of exposure due to having shared injection equipment less, but which may also be due in part to differences in the likelihood of their networks including infected persons (21,40,41).

   More detailed understanding of findings about new injectors involves considerations of patterns of viral spread, and thus the histories and social epidemiologies of local epidemics. Thus, seroincidence studies have found a different relationship between years of injection and seroconversion rates. Ciaffi et al. (42) found that seroconversion in northern Italian cities (with high seroprevalence rates and relatively low seroincidence rates of 4.0 per 100 person-years at risk) was significantly greater among new injectors than among longer-term injectors. Our current data on New York City drug injectors indicate a similar pattern. Data from the studies reported on in Tables 2 and 3, on the other hand, show a more complex picture. Among the lower seroprevalence cities (with less than 12% seropositive), seroincidence rates are low (<1 per 100 person-years at risk) and are not related to the length of time a drug injector has been injecting. Among four cities that have both high seroprevalence (>20%, <50%) and high seroconversion (7.9 per 100 person-years at risk) rates, subjects who have been injecting for more than 7 years have an incidence rate of 9.55 per 100 person-years at risk, as compared to 3.57 per 100 person-years at risk for newer injectors ($p < 0.06$).

We suggest that these seemingly confusing results may be explained as follows:

a. In cities with high seroprevalence and low seroincidence—those with "mature" epidemics—the long-term injectors are less likely to seroconvert because of saturation effects. That is, those long-term injectors most vulnerable to infection have already become infected; for example, the seronegative may be those who either have fewer risk behaviors or who are in networks that are somewhat isolated from infected networks. New injectors in these cities are thus more likely to seroconvert than longer-term ones. Even though they may be somewhat protected if their networks consist mainly of other new injectors, the overall high seroprevalence rate makes their (perhaps occasional) risk behaviors in the presence of longer-term injectors highly dangerous.
b. In cities with both high seroprevalence and high seroincidence—that is, those where the epidemic is widespread but has not yet stabilized—this limited protection of new injectors caused by their network composition may tend to hold their seroconversion rates below those of longer-term injectors.
c. In cities with less developed epidemics, where both seroprevalence and seroconversion are low, the pockets of infection in which HIV is spreading do not seem to be based on years of injection.

Yet another possible complication may arise while studying new injectors. In most situations, we would expect them to have relatively low seroprevalence—roughly equal to that of the great majority of persons in their age group. Another pattern might occur, however, if a group of homosexual or bisexual men should start to inject drugs after they already have substantial seroprevalence due to sex with other men. (Homosexual/bisexual male drug injectors have been suggested as a bridge group that enabled HIV to be transmitted from homosexual/bisexual male noninjectors into wider drug-injecting circles in both New York City [1] and Rio de Janeiro [43]. However, no evidence has yet been found of a situation in which a large group of gay or bisexual men started to inject after HIV had become widespread among them.) Another situation in which significant numbers of new drug injectors might be seropositive might arise in localities in which large numbers of sexual partners of drug injectors begin to inject.

In general, then, understanding the history of drug-injection scenes will be necessary when interpreting seroprevalence or seroconversion data. Other examples can readily be provided. Patterns of policing that differentially incarcerate a particular subset of drug injectors may mean that the remaining subjects provide an unrepresentative picture of overall seroprevalence, or can even affect patterns of loss to follow-up in a cohort study in ways that may affect estimates of seroconversion rates or of risk factors.

RESEARCH IMPLICATIONS FOR LOCALITIES WITH OLDER EPIDEMICS

Seroprevalence studies may be particularly difficult to interpret in localities where the virus has been present for a considerable time. In such places, the long history of risk behaviors by drug injectors, the changing distribution of the virus among different networks over time, and the patterns of arrival and departure from the scene create a situation where data about current risk behaviors may provide misleading clues about how people have gotten infected. Nonetheless, seroprevalence studies can still discover "new" risk factors even in a city with as long a history of the epidemic as New York. We will conclude with an example of such a finding and of some of the issues raised by the preceding discussion for how this should be assessed and tested.

Jose et al. (44) recently reported that "backloading"[2] is a risk factor for HIV seropositivity: that is, that persons who report that they have shared drugs by having them dispensed from another person's syringe into their own syringe within the last 2 years are more likely to be infected than those who report that they have not done this. So far, this relationship seems to hold in cross-sectional multivariate analyses, although we do not have sufficient data to test whether backloading is a predictor of seroconversion at the current time. Of particular importance, backloading is also a risk factor among the subset of new injectors, whose personal history of risk behavior is of shorter duration and thus somewhat less likely to be obscured by complications stemming from historical dimensions of the epidemic. Nonetheless, we lack adequate historical and comparative data to ascertain whether backloading has been a detectable risk factor at all stages of the epidemic. The only other data that have been presented on the relationship of back-

[2]The terms "backloading" and "frontloading" have become virtually interchangeable names for syringe-mediated drug sharing.

loading to HIV were from Baltimore, a city with a lower seroprevalence rate (24%) than New York's and with a stable seroconversion rate of approximately 4 per 100 person-years at risk (31,45). In the Baltimore study (46), backloading was not related to seroprevalence among subjects who did not share syringes, whereas this relationship was significant among both syringe-sharing and non-syringe–sharing subsets in the New York data (44). It is not clear at this time whether these different findings are due to differences in methodology, to differences in drug scenes or behaviors between the two cities, or to inter-urban differences in stage of the epidemic.

In conclusion, the overall implication of this paper is that neither seroprevalence nor seroincidence studies by themselves can show the entire picture. In isolation, either can sometimes be misleading. Fortunately, the combined results of both kinds of studies should usually allow us to minimize these misinterpretations and, perhaps, to achieve a synthesis that more closely approximates the actual dynamics of the epidemic. Moreover, if sufficient and reliable data can be obtained about behaviors, seroprevalence, and seroconversion over an extended number of years, these may provide an even deeper level of understanding.

In addition, ethnographic and historical data about drug scenes are invaluable in studying how and why an HIV epidemic spreads and in interpreting findings about risk factors. These should include data about migration patterns, relationships between heterosexual, bisexual, and homosexual drug injectors, and changes in drugs used and in the settings where they are used. Thus, as a final point, one lesson that we have learned during the course of our research into the HIV epidemic among drug injectors is that research on this topic requires a combination of a variety of types of data and analyses. Understanding how and why HIV spreads comes from the total picture developed through a series of different kinds of studies, rather than through any one study or approach in isolation.

ACKNOWLEDGMENTS

The research in this paper was supported by National Institute on Drug Abuse grants DA05283 and DA06723. The views expressed in this paper do not necessarily reflect the positions of the granting agency or of the institutions by which the authors are employed.

We would also like to acknowledge the editorial assistance of Tom Ward of National Development and Research Institutes, Inc.

REFERENCES

1. Des Jarlais DC, Friedman SR, Novick D, et al. HIV-1 infection among intravenous drug users in Manhattan. *JAMA* 1989;261(7):1008–1012.
2. Friedman SR, Des Jarlais DC. HIV among drug injectors: the epidemic and the response. *AIDS Care* 1991;3(3):239–250.

3. Boxaca M, Libonatti O, Muzzio E, et al. HIV-1 prevalence and the role of other infectious diseases in a group of drug users in Argentina [abstract 3141]. Presented at the Sixth International Conference on AIDS, San Francisco, California, 1991.
4. Caussy D, Weiss SH, Blattner WA, et al. Exposure factors for HIV-1 infection among heterosexual drug abusers in New Jersey treatment programs. *AIDS Res Human Retroviruses* 1990;6:1459–1467.
5. Chaisson RE, Baccheti P, Osmond D, et al. Cocaine use and HIV infection in intravenous drug users in San Francisco. *JAMA* 1989;261(4):561–565.
6. Choopanya K, Vanichseni S, Plangsringarm K, et al. Risk factors and HIV seropositivity among injecting drug users in Bangkok. *AIDS* 1991;5(12):1509–1513.
7. D'Aquila RT, Peterson LR, Williams AB, Williams AE. Race/ethnicity as a risk factor for HIV-1 infection among Connecticut intravenous drug users. *AIDS* 1989;2:503–513.
8. De Rossi A, Bortolotti F, Cadrobbi P, Chieco-Bianchi L. Trends of HTLV-1 and HIV infection in drug addicts. *Eur J Cancer Clin Oncol* 1988;24(2):279–280.
9. Fay O, Taborda M, Fernandez A, et al. HIV seroprevalence among different communities in Argentina after four years of surveillance [abstract 3263]. Presented at the Seventh International Conference on AIDS, Florence, Italy, 1991.
10. Friedman SR, Rosenblum A, Goldsmith D, et al. Risk factors for HIV-1 infection among street-recruited intravenous drug users in New York City [abstract 12]. Presented at the Fifth International Conference on AIDS, Montreal, Canada, 1989.
11. Koblin BA, McCusker J, Lewis BF, Sullivan JL. Racial/ethnic differences in HIV-1 seroprevalence and risky behaviors among intravenous drug users in a multisite study. *Am Epidemiol* 1990;132:837–846.
12. Loimer N, Presslich O, Hollerer E, et al. Monitoring HIV-1 infection prevalence among intravenous drug users in Vienna 1986–1990. *AIDS Care* 1990;2:281–286.
13. Marmor M, Des Jarlais DC, Cohen H, et al. Risk factors for infection with human immunodeficiency virus among intravenous drug abusers in New York City. *AIDS* 1987;1(1):39–44.
14. Muga R, Tor J, Llibre J, et al. Risk factors for HIV-1 infection in parenteral drug users. *AIDS* 1990;4:259–260.
15. Nguyen S, Reardon J, Wilson MJ, et al. HIV-1 infection among female injection drug users (IDU) in the San Francisco Bay area, California 1989–1991 [abstract 1553]. Presented at the Eighth International Conference on AIDS, Amsterdam, The Netherlands, 1992.
16. Page JB, Smith PC, Kane N. Shooting galleries, their proprietors, and implications for prevention of AIDS. *Drugs and Society* 1990;5:69–85.
17. Sasse H, Salmaso S, Conti S, et al. Risk behaviors for HIV-1 infection in Italian drug users: report from a multicenter study. *J AIDS* 1989;2:486–496.
18. Schoenbaum EE, Hartel D, Selwyn PA, et al. Risk factors for human immunodeficiency virus infection in intravenous drug users. *N Engl J Med* 1989;321(13):874–879.
19. Telles PR, Bastos FI, Lima ES, et al. HIV-1 epidemiology among IDUs in Rio de Janeiro, Brazil [abstract 4265]. Presented at the Eighth International Conference on AIDS, Amsterdam, The Netherlands, 1992.
20. van den Hoek JAR, Coutinho A, van Haastrecht HJA, et al. Prevalence and risk factors of HIV infections among drug users and drug-using prostitutes in Amsterdam. *AIDS* 1988;2:55–60.
21. Vlahov D, Munoz A, Anthony JC, et al. Association of drug injection patterns with antibody to human immunodeficiency virus type 1 among intravenous drug users in Baltimore, Maryland. *Am J Epidemiol* 1990;132(5):847–856.
22. Williams ML. HIV seroprevalence among male IVDUs in Houston, Texas. *Am J Public Health* 1990;80:1507–1509.
23. Anthony JC, Vlahov D, Nelson KE, et al. New evidence on intravenous cocaine use and the risk of infection with human immunodeficiency virus type 1. *Am J Epidemiol* 1991;134:1175–1189.
24. Des Jarlais DC, Friedman SR, Marmor M, et al. Development of AIDS, HIV seroconversion, and potential co-factors for T4 cell loss in a cohort of intravenous drug users. *AIDS* 1987;1(2):105–112.
25. Des Jarlais DC, Choopanya K, Vanichseni S, et al. AIDS risk reduction and HIV seroconversion among injecting drug users in Bangkok [in press].

26. Friedman SR, Des Jarlais DC, Deren S, et al. HIV seroconversion among street-recruited drug injectors: a preliminary analysis. *Proceedings of the 54th Annual Meeting of the College on Problems of Drug Dependence*. Rockville, MD: NIDA Monograph [in press].
27. Friedman SR, Jose B, Deren S, et al. Preliminary analysis of HIV seroconversions among drug injectors in 13 cities. *Proceedings of the Third Annual Research Conference of the National AIDS Demonstration Research Project*. Rockville, MD: NIDA Monograph [in press].
28. Klein CW. HIV seroconversion and risk behaviors: analysis by gender. Presented at the 119th Annual Meeting of the American Public Health Association, Atlanta, Georgia, 1991.
29. Metzger DS, Woody GE, Watkins KE, et al. Risk behaviors and seroconversion among intravenous drug users in and out of treatment [abstract 3320]. Presented at the Seventh International Conference on AIDS, Florence, Italy, 1991.
30. Moss AR, Bachetti P, Osmond D, et al. Seroconversion for HIV in intravenous drug users in San Francisco [abstract 11]. Presented at the Fifth International Conference on AIDS, Montreal, Canada, 1989.
31. Nelson KE, Vlahov D, Munoz A, et al. Incident HIV-1 infections in a cohort of intravenous drug users (IVDUs) [abstract 4698]. Presented at the Eighth International Conference on AIDS, Amsterdam, The Netherlands, 1992.
32. Nicolosi A, Leite MLC, Musicco M, et al. Parenteral and sexual transmission of human immunodeficiency virus in intravenous drug users: a study of seroconversion. *Am J Epidemiol* 1992;135:225–233.
33. Solomon L, Astemborski J, Warren D, et al. Differences in risk factors for seroconversion among female and male IVDUs [abstract 3050]. Presented at the Seventh International Conference on AIDS, Florence, Italy, 1991.
34. van Ameijden EJC, van den Hoek A, Coutinho RA. Risk factors for HIV seroconversion in injecting drug users in Amsterdam, the Netherlands [abstract 104]. Presented at the Seventh International Conference on AIDS, Florence, Italy, 1991.
35. Stoneburner RL, Des Jarlais DC, Benezra D, et al. A larger spectrum of severe HIV-I-related disease in intravenous drug users in New York City. *Science* 1988;242:916–919.
36. Galli M, Des Jarlais DC. Evolution of causes of death in IVDU in Milan and New York. Presented at the Conference on Models and Methods of Epidemiologic Research on HIV Infection, Capri, Italy, 1992.
37. Des Jarlais DC, Uppal G. Heroin activity in New York City, 1970–1978. *Am J Drug Alcohol Abuse* 1981;7(3&4):335–346.
38. van de Wijngaart GV. *Competing perspectives on drug use: The Dutch experience*. Amsterdam, The Netherlands: Swets & Zeitlinger B.V.; 1991.
39. McKeganey N, Barnard M. *AIDS, drugs and sexual risk: lives in the balance*. Buckingham, UK: Open University Press; 1992.
40. Friedman SR, Neaigus A, Jose B, et al. Social structures and processes that affect HIV spread among drug injectors. Presented at the 119th Annual Meeting of the American Public Health Association, Atlanta, Georgia, 1991.
41. Friedman SR, Des Jarlais DC, Neaigus A, et al. AIDS and the new drug injector. *Nature* 1989;339:333–334.
42. Ciaffi L, Nicolosi A, Correa Leite ML, et al. Incidence of HIV infection in intravenous drug users from Milan and Northern Italy, 1987–91 [abstract 1552]. Presented at the Eighth International Conference on AIDS, Amsterdam, The Netherlands, 1992.
43. Lima ES, Telles PR, Bastos FI, et al. Homosexual and bisexual male drug injectors as a potential bridge for HIV to reach other drug injectors in Rio de Janeiro [abstract 4258]. Presented at the Eighth International Conference on AIDS, Amsterdam, The Netherlands, 1992.
44. Jose B, Friedman SR, Neaigus A, et al. "Frontloading" is associated with HIV infection among drug injectors in New York City [abstract 1551]. Presented at the Eighth International Conference on AIDS, Amsterdam, The Netherlands, 1992.
45. Proletti F, Vlahov D, Alexander S, et al. Corellates of HTLV-II/HIV-1 seroprevalence and incidence of HTLV-II infection among intravenous drug users [abstract 4392]. Presented at the Eighth International Conference on AIDS, Amsterdam, The Netherlands, 1992.

46. Samuels JF, Vlahov JC, Solomon L, Celentano DD. The practice of "frontloading" among intravenous drug users: association with HIV-antibody. *AIDS* 1991;5(3):343.

DISCUSSION

Dr. Halloran: I agree that it is important to include the temporal aspect because, although a lot of things are the same as in chronic diseases, the temporal changes are so much more dramatic. Gonorrhea is an example. In a closed population, if men are cured more quickly than women, women would probably have a higher seroprevalence and men would have a higher incidence. If you did a seroprevalence study only in a sexually transmitted diseases clinic, you'd say that the men were the problem. There are a lot of other examples like that. To make any sense, what we need is to have a picture of what is going on in our population. If we jump from prevalence to odds ratios in our equations, we don't know what parameter we're estimating—the cumulative incidence or the hazard ratio? And what are we doing with the odds ratio anyway? There are a lot of steps that are then used for attributable risk, and we end up with this mish-mash. I think the points you were making are fundamental for the whole discussion here.

Dr. Biggar: I have a question concerning the stratification versus the multivariate analysis that you did with respect to backloading. I wonder whether you are not picking up some of the errors in people's self-reported sharing whereas, if you stratified it with sharing and no sharing, it may be less of a problem. Is that a possibility?

Dr. Friedman: I'm not sure that I understand what you mean by stratifying.

Dr. Biggar: In the Baltimore study, you said they stratified according to sharing or no sharing.

Dr. Friedman: We did that.

Dr. Biggar: But you also said that you did it in multivariate analysis, which I thought referred to the degree of sharing rather than the degree of backloading.

Dr. Friedman: We did different things. One of them was to stratify according to whether they said they shared or not. Within both of those categories, backloading was a significant predictor.

Dr. Vlahov: One of the earlier comments concerned looking at behaviors over time. One of the things we did in our study was take a 10-year retrospective history. We ended up collapsing the data because it became very complicated to look at it all. Originally, we looked at 7 different injection patterns and divided the 10-year history into 4 calendar periods, which makes a total of 2,401 possible drug injecting combinations for the 2,921 individuals. What we found was that there were 753 different patterns and that there were only 8 groups of patterns that had at least 50 people, indicating that there is tremendous variability in injection patterns over time in this population. So, some of the preconceived notions about drug users and what we would perhaps like to think about in terms of following one or two or three different standard patterns just weren't borne out by the data.

My second point is that, subsequent to your presentation in Amsterdam, we went back and looked at our seroconverters who reported not sharing needles in the 6 and 12 months prior to their first seropositive visit. Two percent of them reported what we're calling frontloading at this meeting. So, again, we didn't go for controls to look at developing odds ratios for that.

Dr. Friedman: It's a fascinating question of why the two studies are different because, when we compared methods, our first reaction was to say, "Ha! We know how to do this research, and David doesn't." But, anyone who knows David Vlahov will know how absurd that statement is. So we talked to David, checked his publications, and so on and found that he'd done pretty much the same as we had, which is not surprising because, to some extent, we had copied our methods from him. This makes us think that something is going on that is different in the two cities, and we're going to have to find a way of figuring out what that is.

Dr. Des Jarlais: One overall comment. Despite all of the complexity that you've illustrated very well with respect to seroprevalence and seroincidence studies, I think that there is still tremendous worldwide consistency in terms of the factors for seroprevalence and seroincidence, even including frontloading and backloading. Where inconsistency exists, this often relates to sexual behavior: whether male with male sex, or crack use and the supposedly greater sexual activity associated with crack use, is an important factor. With all of this complexity, we're still getting remarkably consistent results in terms of drug injection behavior and both seroincidence and seroprevalence. Where we're getting the least consistency is in relation to the importance of the sexual behavior of intravenous drug users.

Dr. Rezza: You sometimes find inconsistent results comparing cross-sectional and incidence studies. An example is the association between the duration of drug use and HIV infection. Adopting a cross-sectional approach that uses prevalent cases of HIV infection, you can find that a long duration of drug use is associated with HIV infection because of the cumulative effect. If you use incidence cases, you can find that a short duration of drug injection is associated with HIV infection because those who start to inject are sometimes more likely to seroconvert than long-term seronegative drug injectors. So, if you can, it's better to compare incidence and prevalent data before getting to definite conclusions.

Dr. Friedman: On that, we have been trying to figure out what happens as new injectors begin to inject because that's clearly a very important issue for intervention purposes. By analogy, from the perspective of stopping heterosexual or gay epidemics, we also have to consider the new sexually active people. One of the differences we are finding is that although seroprevalent studies are absolutely consistent in finding that new injectors are less infected (because there is obviously a serious pattern with long-term injectors of more potential exposure), there are also differences in seroconversion between different cities. Trying to tease out this difference may give us some clues as to how some of the networks are structured, how they vary over time, and how we can plan social interventions. Some of the implications of the kinds of research I'm doing imply prevention interventions that do not involve individual patients coming to the doctor for treatment, although this is also necessary if our aim is to stop seroconversions.

Dr. Vermund: In one of your earlier slides, you said that in high prevalent zones (in one seroincidence study you did, it was 7.89 per 100 person-years) cocaine use was a strong predictor. This works in a couple of ways: one is the injection of cocaine, the other is the sex for crack exchange that the Montefiore Medical Center group found to be especially prominent in their older drug users. There was almost a transition of predictors. In earlier seroconverters, it was the drug injection patterns and gallery sharing that were most highly predictive. Later in the epidemic, sexual variables were more predictive. This may be highly plausible through the saturation of highest risk sharers and with ongoing sexual risk in a person where high-risk sharing hasn't occurred. But as far as sexual risk is concerned, the obvious research challenge is teasing these factors out. Since the theme of this afternoon is issues in confounding, I wanted to hear some of your thoughts on how you tease out the difference between these highly colinear needle sharing and sexual variables.

Dr. Friedman: First of all, let me say I was referring to cocaine injection, not cocaine use. So it was not the crack phenomenon, it was what Dick Chaisson, Andrew Moss, and their team originally identified.

We've been trying to find some sexual predictors of seroconversion in this data set. When you don't find anything, it is, of course, always possible that your measures are poor, and that is a real possibility. But whichever way we look, we haven't been able to find anything. The only potential sexual variable we've found is for the total sample. Among the women who seroconverted, the predictors were city seroprevalence and having engaged in woman-with-woman sex. This is unlikely to be due to sexual transmission from woman-to-woman because if that were going on, the case data would be absolutely unmistakable; there would be thousands of cases among non-injector lesbians.

At this stage, we have two hypotheses. One is that the women in question were injecting with gay injecting men who, in some cities, are more likely to be infected than other injecting men, because many of these cities have a low seroprevalence among drug injectors.

The second hypothesis is that, rather than injecting with gay men, they are having sex with gay men. Either of those could be right. But, even if we had this kind of data, the number of cases involved is probably too small to allow this study to demonstrate it. Thirty percent of the seroconverting women said that they had had sex with another woman in the previous 6 months, and there might have been some others who underreported (we have reason to think that there is underreporting of woman–woman sex among drug users). When I say 30%, understand that that's 3 out of 10, which limits our ability to do statistical analyses. All we can do is offer the information and say: "Look, there's something going on; several other cross-sectional studies have similar kinds of findings. We have to get on top of this and we'd be glad to help anyone get such a study together." But that's just another conundrum.

HIV Epidemiology: Models and Methods, edited by Alfredo Nicolosi. Raven Press, Ltd., New York © 1994.

12

Methodological Issues in the Measurement of Sexual Behavior and Interpretation of the HIV Epidemic

*Anne M. Johnson and †Jane Wadsworth

**Academic Department of Genito Urinary Medicine, University College, London Medical School, London W1N 8AA, and the †Academic Department of Public Health, St. Mary's Hospital Medical School, London, W2 1NY United Kingdom*

The measurement of sexual behavior is an essential component of many studies that attempt to elucidate the epidemiology of human immunodeficiency virus (HIV) infection. Quantification of sexual exposure has been crucial to understanding the etiology of acquired immunodeficiency syndrome (AIDS) in case-control studies, in cohort studies examining HIV seroconversion and disease progression, in partner studies examining risk practices for transmission, and in sexual behavior surveys (1–6). Methods for estimating the magnitude of the epidemic frequently rely on population estimates of behavior. These include mathematical models, methods that attempt to link HIV seroprevalence measures to estimates of the proportion of the population involved in different risk behaviors, and indirect methods that attempt to derive the true number infected from knowledge of the number of *known* seropositives and from the proportion of individuals with particular risk behaviors who are known to have been tested for HIV (7). More recently, consideration has been given to measuring patterns of sexual mixing in order to ascertain differential spread of HIV in different populations (8).

CASE-CONTROL AND COHORT STUDIES

The earliest epidemiological studies of AIDS depended on measuring patterns of sexual behavior in cases and controls and indicated that the likely cause of AIDS was a sexually acquired organism. Following the identification of HIV, cross-sectional studies were able to demonstrate that the probability of HIV infection increased markedly with increasing numbers of reported sexual partners (3). Such a pattern is typical of many sexually acquired organisms and in a situation of a new condition of unknown etiology, relatively simple analyses can rapidly elucidate fundamental aspects of an epidemic. However, as research has advanced, investigators have attempted to tease out the relative efficiency of different sexual practices for HIV transmission (and not the numbers of sexual partnerships alone) that may be altered by behavioral intervention, as well as biological factors amenable to treatment (e.g., other sexually transmitted diseases [STD]).

CONFOUNDING

One of the difficulties in examining risk factors that may increase or decrease the likelihood of HIV infection is that the relationship may be distorted by confounding. For example, many cross-sectional studies have found an association between history of other STD and HIV infection. It is postulated that STD may enhance the transmissibility of HIV infection by either increasing infectivity of the HIV-positive individual or increasing susceptibility of the exposed contact. This relationship is confounded by the fact that STD and HIV infection have similar sexual risk behaviors. This problem can theoretically be overcome by controlling for sexual behavior in the analysis (e.g., by stratification on the basis of number of sexual partners). Mertens et al. (9) cogently illustrate this relationship, indicating that an apparently increased relative risk may be measured in a cross-sectional study, where none exists, simply because those with HIV and those with STD both have many sexual partners. However, unravelling such a relationship demands both that the confounder can be measured sufficiently accurately and that it is a reliable predictor of STD and HIV infection in the population studied. Mertens et al. (9) also demonstrate that misclassification of the level of sexual activity in a stratified analysis may lead to overestimation or underestimation of the true relative risk associated with the presence of other STD. This problem of residual confounding remains extremely difficult to overcome in cross-sectional studies.

A further difficulty arises because number of sexual partners or a history of drug injection is used as a proxy measure of exposure to an HIV-infected individual. Very frequently, because all sexual partners are not traced, the true exposure to HIV infection cannot be measured. For example, Halsey et al. (10) concluded that there was an "independent" association between smoking and HIV infection in a logistic regression analysis in a study of Haitian women. It was assumed that sexual behavior had been adequately controlled by dichotomizing the study population into those with or without three or more lifetime sexual partners. In this situation, the relationship may remain confounded by the inability to accurately measure exposure through sexual intercourse to an HIV-positive person (11).

PARTNERS STUDIES

The problem of exposure to an HIV-positive person is overcome in heterosexual partner studies because contacts are only selected who have known exposure to an HIV-infected individual (see Chapter 7). However, problems in assessing the relationship between behavior and probability of infection remain. These include the inability to measure the true duration of exposure and potential bias between positive and negative contacts in reporting sexual behaviors after a diagnosis has been made. There is the possibility of interviewer bias and underreporting of particular behaviors in seronegative partners because those who are positive may be more zealously investigated for other risk behaviors in addition to heterosexual contact. Finally, it is necessary to consider the potential bias of preferentially assuming that risks such as transient homosexual contact or drug injection are the source of infection rather than heterosexual contact itself, which may result in underestimation of transmission risk.

MEASURING SEXUAL BEHAVIOR IN GENERAL POPULATION SAMPLES

Many mathematical models of the transmission of HIV and other STD depend largely on relatively simple deterministic models. In these, the case reproduction rate (Ro) is dependent on the probability of transmission of infection, the mean and variance of rate of partner acquisition, and the duration of infectiousness (12,13). Rate of partner acquisition is a key variable here, but how accurately can we measure this in human populations? While models are now being developed that take account of assortative and disassortative mixing, even in the simplest cases, is it possible to accurately measure "rate of sexual partner change" in the population?

It demands that in a given population of interest, we can measure the mean and the variance of distribution of new sexual partners per unit time. In reality, this is a difficult item to measure and most sexual behavior surveys in practice measure the disacquisition rather than the acquisition of partners, focusing not on new partners but on the total number of partners in a given time interval.

A further application of general population surveys is to estimate the proportion of the population who engage in different kinds of activities. These have been used to estimate the number of people infected when linked with the estimated seroprevalence (14,15). For example, the population is subdivided into estimates of number of homosexual men, injecting drug users, hemophiliacs, and heterosexuals with different characteristics. The difficulty here is the lack of information on the size of these different populations, how they should be best defined on the basis of behavioral characteristics, and how they relate to populations under surveillance through unlinked anonymous prevalence monitoring (16). Data from representative population samples are clearly required for such approaches to understanding the epidemiology of HIV.

The study of human sexual behavior is one to which modern survey methodology has only recently been applied (2,17). The sample must be both adequately representative of the population of interest and of sufficient size to provide robust estimates of rare behaviors. Important design issues include the selection of an appropriate sampling frame and adequate sample size. In the analysis, estimates of sampling errors, assessment of response rate, response bias, and the use of weighting strategies are essential to derive reliable population-based estimates. Too little attention has perhaps been paid to detailed evaluation of measurement instruments assessing the reliability and validity of question formats. It is essential to consider carefully definitions of key variables and to ensure comprehensibility of questions (18). Comparability between different surveys must be made with great care and must consider precise question formats for key variables before conclusions can be drawn about variability in behaviors or differential spread of HIV in populations. Interviewers require careful training in standardized interview techniques in order to minimize the effects of their personalities and experience on response rate and response bias. Respondents may be influenced by recall bias, by situational influences such as the level of privacy when the interview is undertaken, and by the degree of willingness to report censured behaviors.

Numerous different sampling strategies have been used in sexual behavior surveys (17,19–21). Quota samples are generally employed by market research companies, using age, sex, and social classes as controls, but neither response rate nor response bias can be measured from these (22). Random sampling strategies include the use of electoral or other population registers that allow direct selection of individuals, but their ability to select a representative sample depends upon the completeness of such registers. The use of households, which is employed in the British survey, has proved a useful method, but both this approach and the use of telephone numbers to select households results in oversampling of individuals who live in single-person households. It is therefore necessary to weight the final dataset for household size in order to achieve population estimates of behavior.

Some groups have oversampled certain populations, such as urban populations, or have attempted to oversample those with particular risk behaviors by the use of filter questions. The latter method has been employed in the French national study, but depends crucially on the effectiveness of the filter question in identifying those at particular risk, such as men who have sex with men.

Representativeness of a sample can be assessed by the usual methods available to social researchers, such as response rate, characteristics of nonresponders, and the comparisons of the demographic characteristics of the sample with the national census (2,21).

Further work is needed on the comparisons of the validity of results achieved from different forms of interview (e.g., face-to-face, self-completion, and telephone interviews). Question design experiments can indicate otherwise unrecognized flaws in question design. Such split-run experiments on question design and ordering were carried out in the British survey and crucial differences in the prevalence of key variables were found to be dependent on particular question formats, which often resulted from wording that was ambiguous to respondents. The use of internal consistency checks enabled questions that were badly worded or misunderstood to be discarded, while qualitative work helped to guide the form of language used (18). For same-sex experience, a very wide range of estimates can be derived dependent on whether it includes any transient experience defined by the respondent as sexual (all inclusive), to a partnership defined in strict anatomical terms in a structured questionnaire, in a defined time period (2).

WHAT IS A SEXUAL PARTNER?

Measurement of the number of sexual partners over a given time period is often a key measure used, not only for the purposes of controlling for confounding by sexual behavior in biological studies, but also as a key parameter in many mathematical models. Different surveys have adopted different definitions. For example, in the British random survey, for the purposes of analysis, a heterosexual partner is defined as "someone of the opposite sex with whom the respondent has had vaginal or anal intercourse, or oro-genital contact." In a volunteer sample of gay men in the United Kingdom, Project Sigma uses the following terminology: "a sexual partner is any person with whom you have had sexual contact, where the aim was orgasm for one or both of you" whereas they re-define a penetrative sexual partner as "someone with whom the respondent has had anal or vaginal intercourse" (23). By making this distinction between sexual partners and penetrative sexual partners, they demonstrate that estimates of key parameters such as the mean and the median number of partners are remarkably reduced by considering only penetrative sexual partners, which are partnerships in which transmission could potentially occur. Furthermore, in almost all behavioral surveys, there is very substantial variability in behavior. The distribution of numbers of partners is extremely skewed, thus the mean is an unstable summary statistic heavily influenced by those in the top 5% of the distribution. It differs markedly from the median, and the variance is very large. This is particularly true for lifetime partners reported. This is likely to provide the most inaccurate estimate, measuring different time periods for different individuals and being the most subject to recall bias. For this reason, the 5-year estimate may be one of the most useful comparisons between groups and populations, allowing not only sufficient representation of variability in numbers of partners, but also less subject to recall difficulties.

Thus, in assessing the measurement error in sexual behavior research, it is essential that good qualitative research in the design of measurement instruments is undertaken and that question design experiments are carried out. Once the data are available, internal consistency checks may be useful by repeating data items in different formats. Comparisons can also be made with independent datasets, such as STD statistics or abortion statistics. Statistical checks can be used, such as male/female comparisons. For example, provided a random sample is selected from a closed population, the mean number of partners over relatively short time periods should be similar for men and women, as should the frequency of sexual acts.

In Great Britain, men and women were very consistent in the reporting of frequency of vaginal intercourse and of socially censured practices such as anal intercourse (2). Estimates of the proportion reporting a visit to an STD clinic in the feasibility study were at least consistent with data available from national statistics, although with wide confidence limits.

Despite these remarkable consistencies between men and women, one of the inconsistencies in nearly all studies of sexual behavior is the differential reporting of numbers of sexual partners between men and women, with men consistently reporting more partners than women (17,24). Why should this be the case? One possibility is the instability of the mean. The mean is strongly influenced by those who have reported large numbers of partners and who may be the most likely to be inaccurate in their reporting. The second possibility is mixing outside the sampled population, such as commercial sex or partners abroad. Next is the influence of differential age mixing and the tendency of older men to mix with younger women, who themselves report higher rates of partner change than do their older compatriots (25). This has some influence on the difference, but does not overcome it and this is an area for the modelers to consider further. Memory error and social acceptability bias are clearly very real problems in this kind of data, but the consistency of this result in different groups raises questions of whether this relationship should be expected to always hold true, or whether the sampling strategies that select individuals and not partnerships may have a part to play in this discrepancy.

This leads to the question of development of methodologies, which ask not only how many partners, but also who mixes with whom. Some models have attempted to differentiate between different activity classes and to make assumptions about patterns of mixing (8). One of the key issues is the extent to which assortative mixing or disassortative mixing occurs. In assortative mixing situations, mixing occurs only within particular activity groups, such that those with many partners mix only with those with similar patterns of behavior. Under conditions of disassortative mixing, there is effective mixing between high activity classes and low activity classes, a phenomenon that happens particularly in societies where many partnerships occur within the sex industry and clients of prostitutes mix with their lower activity regular partners. There are also important differences between heterosexual populations in which men can mix only with women, and homosexual populations in which all men can mix with one another, and for a given population size a greater number of partnerships is possible.

Measurement of sexual behavior is a key problem in epidemiological studies of HIV that has received relatively little attention. Standardized methods of measurement need to be more widely employed using well validated measures. This is pertinent both to clinical studies and to large-scale population surveys. If the differential spread of HIV in different societies is to be better understood and the component attributable to behavior and that attributable to biological and other influences defined, it is essential that attempts are made to standardize and improve existing methods of measurement.

REFERENCES

1. Johnson AM. Social and behavioural aspects of the HIV epidemic: a review. *J R Stat Soc A* 1988;151:99–114.
2. Wellings K, Field J, Wadsworth J, et al. Sexual lifestyles under scrutiny. *Nature* 1990; 348:276–278.
3. Winkelstein W, Lyman DM, Padian N, et al. Sexual practices and risk of infection by the human immunodeficiency virus. *JAMA* 1987;257:321–325.
4. Johnson AM, Laga M. Heterosexual transmission of HIV. *AIDS* 1988;2:S49–S56.
5. Padian N, Marquis L, Francis DP, et al. Male-to-female transmission of human immunodeficiency virus. *JAMA* 1987;258:788–790.
6. European Study Group on Heterosexual Transmission of AIDS. Comparison of female to male and male to female transmission of HIV in 563 stable couples. *Br Med J [Clin Res]* 1992;304:809–813.
7. Report of a working group. AIDS in England and Wales to end 1993: projections using data to end September 1989. *CDR* 1990;1–12.
8. Potts M, Anderson R, Boily M-C. Slowing the spread of human immunodeficiency virus in developing countries. *Lancet* 1991;338:608–612.
9. Mertens TE, Hayes RJ, Smith PG. Epidemiological methods to study the interaction between HIV infection and other sexually transmitted diseases. *AIDS* 1990;4:57–65.
10. Halsey NA, Coberly JS, Holt E, et al. Sexual behaviour, smoking and HIV-1 infection in Haitian women. *JAMA* 1992;267:2062–2066.
11. Davey Smith G, Phillips AN. Confounding in epidemiological studies: why "independent" effects may not be all they seem. *Br Med J* 1992;305:757–759.
12. May RM, Anderson RM. Transmission dynamics of HIV infection. *Nature* 1987; 326:137–142.
13. Hethcote HW, Yorke JA. Gonorrhoea: transmission dynamics and control. Lecture notes. *Biomathematics* 1984;56:1–105.
14. Report of a working group. *Short term prediction of HIV infection and AIDS in England and Wales*. London: HMSO; 1989.
15. Centers for Disease Control. Human immunodeficiency virus infection in the United States: a review of current knowledge. *MMWR* 1987;36:1–48.
16. PHLS AIDS Centre, PHLSVRL, Academic Department of Genito-Urinary Medicine, and collaborators. The unlinked anonymous HIV prevalence monitoring programme in England and Wales: preliminary results. *CDR* 1991;1:R69–R76.
17. Wadsworth J, Johnson AM. Measuring sexual behaviour. *J R Stat Soc A* 1991;154:367–370.

18. Spencer L, Faulkner A, Keegan J. *Talking about sex*. London: SCPR; 1988.
19. ASCF Principal Investigators and Their Associates. Analysis of sexual behaviour in France (ACSF): a comparison between two modes of investigation: telephone survey and face-to-face survey. *AIDS* 1992;6:315–323.
20. Carballo M, Cleland J, Carael M, Albrecht G. A cross national survey of patterns of sexual behaviour. *J Sex Res* 1989;26:287–299.
21. Melbye M, Biggar RJ. Interactions between persons at risk for AIDS and the general population in Denmark. *Am J Epidemiol* 1992;135:593–602.
22. Department of Health and Social Security and Welsh Office. *AIDS: monitoring response to the public education campaign: February 1986–February 1987* London, HMSO; 1987.
23. Hunt AJ, Davies PM, Weatherburn P, Coxon AP, McManus TJ. Sexual partners, penetrative sexual partners and HIV risk. *AIDS* 1991;5:723–728.
24. Centers for Disease Control. Number of sex partners and potential risk of exposure to human immunodeficiency virus. *MMWR* 1988;37:565–568.
25. Johnson AM, Wadsworth J, Field J, Wellings K, Anderson RM. Surveying sexual lifestyles (Letter). *Nature* 1990;343:109.

DISCUSSION

Dr. Detels: I might add two anecdotes regarding studies that we have done in homosexual men. In 1981, when it was not clear what the modes of transmission were, I did a cross-sectional study of gay students at the University of California at Los Angeles and asked them about the number of partners they had. Two years later, when it had become quite apparent that anal intercourse was a risk factor in the gay community, I convinced the same group of men to form a cohort. At the second interview, their cumulative number of lifetime partners had actually declined. Obviously, knowing that this was not a wise practice had influenced their answers considerably.

The other experience came when we were at the beginning of the Multi-center AIDS Cohort Study (MACS), and we were arguing vigorously about whether to have an interviewer-administered or a self-administered questionnaire. One of the reasons why I wanted a self-administered questionnaire was that I saw an example of the same questionnaire that had been administered to a group of homosexual men by three interviewers: one was a very attractive gay gentleman, one a not very attractive gay gentleman, and one a woman. You can guess which one had the highest number of sexual partners reported!

Dr. Padian: In your list of the things to be careful about, there was one point I think that particularly needs to be emphasized. Sam has mentioned the time dependence of independent variables, but there is also the time dependence of dependent variables. Of course, the best way to cover this is to follow the same person as they go through their sexual history, but then you run the risk of all of the problems associated with cohorts and people telling you what you want to hear. This is another issue that makes it difficult to use chronic disease methodology when dealing with this and other infectious diseases.

Dr. Friedman: One of the things that always strikes me when we talk about modelling processes is that people usually go for parameters primarily derived on the basis of concepts of frequencies of behaviors or numbers of partners. We've now had one or two hundred years of sociology and other disciplines and we've developed other categorizations of societies, such as race, ethnic groups, social classes, intravenous drug users, and so on. These represent socially cohesive network patterns and may help to define the spread of epidemics from within pockets of infection in a way that is more socially than model defined. Do you have any comment on that?

Dr. Johnson: I'm afraid I'm not a modeler, although I've worked with many people who are. But models have helped me to think about the epidemic itself and not just the kinds of things that may drive it. Particularly, in relation to these deterministic models, it seems to me that the modelers themselves would call them "What if . . ." thought experiments. They try to come up with parameters that are likely to be keys in determining an STD epidemic, and then try to look at how different scenarios might alter the course of the epidemic. Although such models are seen as being highly quantitative, much of what they say seems to me to be qualitative. Of course, they don't necessarily mimic real life and, in fact, they're a gross oversimplification of it. But, it seems to me that some of the stochastic or more complex models might tell us more. We're always told that the modelers are ahead of the data collectors. And it's true that once you've collected the data, the models seem to have moved on as well.

Dr. Friedman: One of the things that a congress like this should do is increase the extent to which some of the substantive findings of some risk factor studies (such as seroconversion, seroprevalence, and so on) get into the models. That might be useful to both groups of researchers.

Dr. Musicco: One of the things that we found in our cross-sectional study on heterosexual transmission was that awareness of a partner's seropositivity was one of the strongest protective factors. This was not explained by condom use, anal sex, oral sex, or any kind of conventionally investigated sexual behavior. What seems to me to be relevant (and, in part, this can also be applied to the data on intravenous drug use) is that we are probably not really measuring the behavior that affects transmission. I cannot believe that the short or long duration of intravenous drug use is enough by itself, it needs to be coupled with a particular behavior (maybe a risk factor). And, unless we suppose the higher susceptibility of particular racial groups, it seems that race is just an indicator of some behavior that we have not investigated. The unexpected behavior of back and frontloading (which is relevant for transmission) is another good example. In sexual transmission, we need more refined ways of investigating behavior, including nonconventional behaviors.

HIV Epidemiology: Models and Methods,
edited by Alfredo Nicolosi. Raven Press, Ltd.,
New York © 1994.

13

The Logic in Ecological*

Mervyn Susser

Gertrude H. Sergievsky Center, Columbia University Faculty of Medicine, New York, New York 10032

The prime justification of the ecological approach in epidemiology is to study health in an environmental context. The aim is ambitious, no less than to understand the effect of context on the health of persons and groups through selection, distribution, interaction, adaptation, and other responses. Neither nutrition, nor sexuality, nor cognition, nor violence, nor epidemic spread can be accurately or fully explained by counts of individual attributes. Pairings, families, peer groups, schools, communities, cultures, and laws are all contexts that alter outcomes, and often they do so in ways inaccessible to studies solely of individuals.

In 1939, however, E. L. Thorndike warned of the problem involved in making inferences about individuals from studies of groups (1). In 1950, W. S. Robinson warned of this again (2). It was left to H. C. Selvin to label the ecological fallacy in 1950 (3). The naming of names often influences attitudes and thought. In epidemiology particularly, the fallacy has brought the ecological approach into disrepute. This work will in some ways be one of rehabilitation. Its concern is with the utility of the approach in its own right and not as a substitute for more respectable ones. In epidemiology, much attention has been given to abuses (4–6), the barest minimum to uses (7,8).

The fallacy is an issue of analysis and inference. One needs to clarify the logic of analysis before going on to the logic of design and practice. As an analytic issue, ecological questions reduce to the technical if not simple matter of taking groups and not individuals as the unit of study. Its essence lies in the distinctions between levels of organization (9–11). Individual units at one level are assembled into groups; these groups become the units of the next level. Each level acquires collective properties that are more than the sum of the properties of its individual members.

---

*The copyright for this paper, in press with the *American Journal of Public Health*, is held by the American Public Health Association, which gives permission for its publication, in part, as Proceedings of the International Workshop on Methods and Models in HIV Epidemiology, held by the National Research Council of Italy on Capri, September 4–7, 1992.

The problems special to ecological analysis arise in extrapolating upward or downward from one level to another (10–13), and these are not unique to the population sciences. They arise in the ascent from gene to protein molecule, from molecule to cell, from cell to tissue or organ, from organ to person, as well as from person to group and, be it noted, in the reverse on descent.

The task is to unravel the phenomena that emerge when persons, the individual units of the usual analytic currency of epidemiology, are assembled into larger units. These phenomena require, in addition to all those familiar dimensions involved in the analysis of individuals, study of the effects of the group dimension itself on the manifestations under observation. Individual level analysis cannot capture this sometimes crucial dimension. Hence, two broad kinds of variables enter the calculation: everyday variables common to individual and grouped units; and special variables peculiar to groups.

VARIABLES IN COMMON

Three general kinds of variable are shared by individual and group analysis:

1. Independent: individual, x; group, X.
2. Dependent: individual, y; group, Y.
3. Associated: individual, a; group, A.

Association is with either the independent variable, the dependent variable, or both. Thus, A along with a may be antecedent conditions, intervening variables, moderator variables, potential confounders, etc.

VARIABLES PECULIAR TO GROUPS

Two analytic dimensions (here termed integral and contextual) are unique to group analysis, as explained below. In the analysis of group phenomena, both integral and contextual variables can serve as independent, associated, or, if mutable, dependent variables, but it is their role as independent or associated variables that complicates ecological studies.

Integral Variable (*I*)

Such a variable affects all or virtually all members of a group (13). The variable reflects an antecedent condition that varies between groups but not appreciably within groups. It may be discrete and dichotomous (e.g., an intervention or a disaster), scaled and polytomous (e.g., social disorganization or intensity of newborn care), or continuous (e.g., altitude or latitude). When groups as the analytic unit are assembled in a manner that renders them uniform with regard to I, meaningful analysis with individuals as the unit is precluded.

Contextual Variable (C = Median, Mean, or Proportion Within Groups of an Attribute (c) of Individual Group Members)

A contextual variable, derived from a measured attribute of individuals within each group, characterizes the group and not the individual (14–16). Thus, individuals are known to be infected or not, information that collectively affords the group prevalence rate as a measure of context. The grouped variable C will always be the appropriate characterization for measuring group effects (adjusted as necessary when groups are compared). For individuals, C will be effective when its contribution to variation in the individual dependent variable y is over and above that of the ungrouped individual level variable c. The association of C with the grouped dependent variable Y incorporates the individual as well as the group effects of the variable on y.

For instance, during a communicable disease epidemic, the independent variable x characterizes individual exposure to microorganisms, and X exposure across the population. A person will have an immune state, c, that governs susceptibility and the individual likelihood of being infected, y; a group will have a threshold value for herd immunity, C, which is in turn governed by the proportion of susceptibles. C modifies the probability of contact with infection (i.e., x). Thus, C alters the individual likelihood of infection, y, as well as the population likelihood of spread and hence incidence and prevalence (i.e., Y).

For convenience, we exemplify with a linear regression model. In many instances, categorical multivariable models better reflect the data (5). Here, c is an individual predictor of y, measured by the position of the individual on the slope $x \rightarrow y$. C is a contextual predictor of y, also measured by the position of the individual on the slope $x \rightarrow y$. C/c allows for simultaneous effects at the individual and grouped level, that is, the interaction of individual and contextual predictors of the position of the individual on the slope $x \rightarrow y$. All of the above are incorporated in the group relations $X \rightarrow Y$.

Another relation that can obtrude on measured associations is an analogous contextual effect of grouped dependent variables on outcome, aptly described as "contagion." This effect is governed not by independent (X) or associated (A) variables, but by the dependent variables (Y and y), Y/y being the predictor. In Ronald Ross' theory of happenings (17), the "dependent happenings" recently resurrected by Halloran and Struchiner (18) serve well to describe this fundamental dynamic of communicable disease. For instance, the prevalence of any transmissible infection in a defined group at any moment governs the probability of transmission to an individual in the group. Koopman's synthetic model of the transmission of HIV infection provides a cogent reminder that in the face of group effects, individual measures of risk (odds ratios) may serve poorly. Where prevalence is low, the odds of infection with high-risk behavior compared with low-risk behavior rise as prevalence rises; where prevalence is high, the risks with low-risk behavior increase, and the odds ratio of high to low risks decline (19). The dependent happenings of contagion render the individual measure unstable, since it changes as contagion (i.e., context) changes. The obvious moral is that epidemic spread cannot be captured by analysis at the individual level. To gauge risks of transmission, the supraindividual context is a key element. This includes the transactions between individuals, and in turn the social and cultural dynamics that rule them.

Figure 1 is a simple path model that illustrates the relations engendered by sets of the individual and group variables described. Within groups, the presence of associated variables multiplies the number of pathways (x_i,a_i,y_i) among individuals assembled in more than one group. The presence of *A* at group level further exaggerates the number of relationships. The more variables, the more complex the analysis and for that reason alone the more liability to mismeasurement, bias, and confounding. Interactions are likely to be more intrusive if not more detectable, covariation or colinearity compounded and difficult to disentangle, and confounding ever present and unapparent. These are problems of scale and not unique to group variables.

Between groups, however, pathways special to groups are added; these multiply relations within groups still further. Integral and contextual dimensions, when in the form of associated variables, are bearers of bias and confounding in individual but not in group analysis. With human immunodeficiency virus (HIV) infection, for instance, integral variables like geography (e.g., Africa and the United States) and contextual variables (e.g., parental

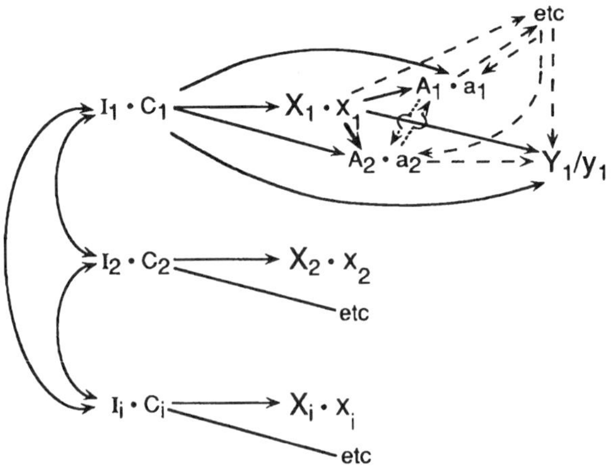

FIG. 1. Scheme of paths between individual and grouped variables in i groups. Solid lines represent definite relationships between variables that must be accounted for. Broken lines represent potentially influential relations within each group. Letters designate variables: *I*, integral, *C*, contextual, *X*, grouped independent, *x*, individual independent, *Y*, grouped dependent, *y*, individual dependent, *A*, grouped associated, *a*, individual associated.

drug use or, as noted, HIV prevalence) act powerfully on risks of transmission. The possibilities of imprudent inference from extrapolating between levels are patent but avoidable.

COMBINATIONS OF INDIVIDUAL AND GROUP UNITS

We now turn to the arrangement of variables in ecological studies. A fourfold table of independent and dependent variables at individual and group levels separates studies that do and do not mix levels (Table 1). Where extrapolation must occur is made evident.

Unmixed Studies

Unmixed studies (a and d below) involve variables on the same level. In the absence of the requisite data, extrapolation can arise only if one level is used to infer to the other. Unmixed group studies present few special problems except for those of scale and hence in the complexity of confounding, control, and interpretation. Unmixed individual studies present the familiar problems of epidemiology except for neglect of group effects when subjects are assembled from more than one group.

The problems of complexity in themselves are neither insignificant nor simple. They arise from the multifarious ways in which individuals can be assembled into groups (7–9). The nature of the problem is illustrated in Fig. 2 (20). In this model of associations at the individual and group level, the same regression slope between groups *(XY)* for each of two groups (B_e) conceals quite different slopes for individuals *(xy)* within groups (B_i).

The advantage does not always lie with the simpler individual analysis. The instance of epidemic infection and the relation $X \rightarrow Y$, with *X* an integral ecological effect, has been well illustrated for severe dengue fever in Mexico. Temperature during the rainy season was by far the most powerful factor in transmission (21). The mosquito *Aedes aegypti* is the vector of dengue. That the detection of larvae around households, a contextual variable, added to the risk lends validity to the ecological analysis, *XY*. Mosquitoes are an obligatory condition for transmitting dengue, but this relationship could not be demonstrated at the individual level, *xy*.

TABLE 1. *Combinations of independent (X,x) and dependent (Y,y) variables in ecological studies*

Dependent variable	Independent variable: Ecological	Independent variable: Individual
Ecological	a. XY	b. xY
Individual	c. Xy	d. xy

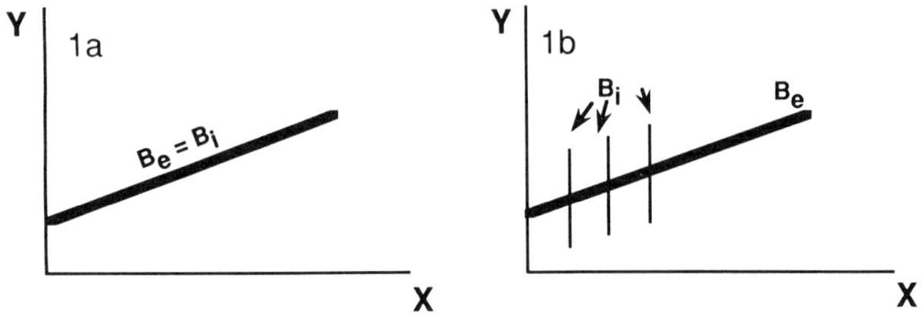

FIG. 2. Example of possible relations (expressed as regression coefficients) *within* a number of groups (B_i) and *between* groups (B_e) in the form of regression slopes between two variables at individual (*xy*) and group (*XY*) levels. Adapted from Lincoln and Zeitz (20).

Mixed Studies

Mixed studies (b and c in Table 1) do present special problems. These stem from the choices to be made about levels of variables for analysis and from the potential intrusion of integral and contextual effects. In mixed studies, some degree of extrapolation is inherent. The relation *xY,* with *Y* a contextual effect, is illustrated by vaccinated persons, *x,* who influence the spread and the prevalence of infection, *Y. Xy* appeared above as in the influence of the proportion vaccinated on the probability of individual infection.

The distinction between levels is not always sharp. Aside from the hybrid forms in the fourfold table above, blurring can be a matter of degree. Only nice distinctions between measures of independent or dependent variables may exist. For instance, a true individual risk can be derived from observing the timing of an outcome (single or repeated) in relation to repetitive exposures in one person (e.g., exercise and cardiac ischemia, or life stress and epileptic seizures). To measure individual risk by the convention of cumulative incidence in a cohort, however, is for a purist a step toward grouping; to do so using period incidence or incidence density as a measure is a still larger step.

RELATIONSHIPS AMONG VARIABLES

Four basic relationships of independent (*x* or *X*) and dependent (*y* or *Y*) variables inhere in an assembly of data that contains measures of the character of both groups and the individual members who comprise them (22). Previous writers have expressed these relations in terms of correlations and regression coefficients. For convenience, I use only regression coefficients as the more robust (23,24). Correlations add more problems of instability when, as is common, they vary across groups according to the distributions of the variables within each group.

The coefficients refer to the following:

1. Between the total assembly of individuals ignoring groups, B_t.
2. Between groups (ecological, with groups the unit), B_e.
3. Between individuals within each or any given group, B_i.
4. Weighted average of the group-specific coefficients for individuals within groups, B_w.

If effects special to groups or grouping are absent, then $B_t = B_w = B_e$. Conversely, contextual and integral variables will produce an "aggregation effect" and cause B_t and B_e to differ (properly an "aggregation bias" only if individuals are the sole concern). If grouping brings confounding and interaction with it, B_t and B_w will differ, a "specification effect" (again a bias only if individuals are the sole concern).

A logical estimate of relations among the whole assembly of individuals is the weighted average group-specific coefficient, B_w (22). When available, it is also likely to be a logical estimate for groups, in that it facilitates adjustment for group characteristics. B_t is in fact a weighted average of B_w and B_e and must lie between them. In theory, given random assembly of both groups and group membership, the order of magnitude of the two group coefficients cannot be predicted (22). In practice, commonly B_e is larger than B_t for two reasons: naturally formed human groups tend to have a greater degree of homogeneity and covariance than occurs randomly; and, by design, competent research eliminates as much extraneous variation as possible.

THE ECOLOGICAL FALLACY

At this juncture, the bugbear of the ecological fallacy can be defined. The nub is simply the assumption that an association at one level of organization can be inferred from that at another level. In terms of regression analysis, it is the assumption that a between-group coefficient will be equal to the weighted average within-group coefficient (i.e., $B_e = B_w$).

The fallacy stems from "crosslevel" bias (25,26). This bias reflects one or both of the two kinds of group effect, aggregation (or "atomistic," with extrapolation downward) (27) and specification errors. Aggregation bias (integral or contextual) is special to groups; specification bias is usually, if not invariably, aggravated by grouping (4,15), but, of course, also occurs with individuals as units. An appendix to this chapter gives mathematical expression to these biases.

Besides the sources of bias discussed above, in the form of special group effects and macrolevel confounding or interactions, special problems reside in measurement (5). We have illustrated how a variable measured as an attribute of individuals (e.g., infection, or immunity, or social class, or education) takes on added meaning as an attribute of groups when it signifies context. But other results can follow. Suppression of associations may result from the transfer of variables across levels in **either direction.** Loss of specificity results when a mean or proportion masks the variation between individuals. Conversely, an inadequate individual measure can suppress associations present at the group level. In individuals, measures of blood pressure or urinary sodium or dietary intake are notoriously unreliable, and in groups distinctly less so (28,29).

CONCLUSION

In this explication, my aim has been to clarify the nature, the utility, and the problems of studies that use grouped data as the unit of analysis, whether of necessity or by preference, and to treat ecological studies not merely as a resort of second-class research or a sandbox for methodologists. Such studies, I have tried to show, have their own obligations and legitimacies.

Many of those familiar with the relevant research areas will concede that some ecological studies have produced knowledge that has stood uncontested for many years. Nonetheless, hazards reside in ecological studies, and still more in extrapolation across aggregate and individual levels. Protective rules are needed.

While certain features are special, the elements, first, are those of epidemiological research regardless of level: accurate measures of the independent variable, of the dependent variable, and of associated variables, supported by multiple indices; the strongest design within the constraints of possibility; a sufficiency of numbers to ensure adequate statistical power; and rigorous analysis that does not neglect elaboration as a mode of *a priori* hypothesis testing (30–32). Among these elements, weak measures of exposure, weak design, and an insufficiency of grouped units are the besetting sins of ecological studies.

Six rules special to grouping are useful:

1. Ensure a sufficiency of groups for testing hypotheses with groups as units.
2. Take account of integral and contextual effects.
3. Prefer small groups, which have fewer interrelations and hence simpler and more manageable properties than large ones. But weigh the disadvantage with rare outcomes that small numbers within groups may sacrifice the stability of outcome measures.
4. To elicit maximum association in hypothesis-testing research, aim for similarity (homogeneity) between groups in all respects other than the independent and dependent study variables.
5. In hypothesis-testing research, again, aim by contrast for the greatest difference (heterogeneity) between groups on the independent variable. In other words, assemble the groups around X. A corollary is that if a study

is designed around Y^{24} on the case-control analogy, then the design should aim for the greatest differences between groups in Y.

6. Finally, if perforce the number of groups is limited, try to alleviate lack of power to test hypotheses by increasing the number of strata or antecedent conditions *a priori,* in the simplest cases by stratifying on demographic variables. The success of comparisons across conditions will be governed by the usual considerations of power, namely, the number of groups, the frequency or standard deviation of the outcome, and the size of the differences in outcome between groups.

REFERENCES

1. Thorndike EL. On the fallacy of imputing the correlations found for groups to the individuals or smaller groups composing them. *Am J Psychol* 1939;52:122–124.
2. Robinson WS. Ecological correlations and the behavior of individuals. *Am Sociol Rev* 1950;15:351–357.
3. Selvin HC. Durkheim's suicide and problems of empirical research. *Am J Sociol* 1958;63:607–619.
4. Brenner H, Savitz DA, Jockel K-H, Greenland S. Effects of nondifferential exposure misclassification in ecologic studies. *Am J Epidemiol* 1993;135:85–95.
5. Greenland S, Morgenstern H. Ecological bias, confounding, and effect modification. *Int J Epidemiol* 1989;18:269–274.
6. Greenland S. Divergent biases in ecological and individual-level studies. *Stat Med* 1992;11:1209–1223.
7. Susser M. *Causal thinking in the health sciences: concepts and strategies in the health sciences*. New York: Oxford University Press; 1973.
8. Morgenstern H. Uses of ecological analysis in epidemiologic research. *Am J Public Health* 1982;72:1336–1344.
9. Menzel H. Comment on Robinson's ecological correlations and the behavior of individuals. *Am Sociol Rev* 1950;15:674.
10. Goodman L. Ecological regressions and behavior of individuals. *Am Sociol Rev* 1953;18:663–664.
11. Blalock HM. Causal inference in non-experimental research. Chapel Hill: University of North Carolina Press; 1964.
12. Lazarsfeld PF, Menzel H. On the relation between individual and collective properties. In: Etzioni A, ed. *Complex organizations: a sociological reader.* Glencoe, IL: Free Press; 1961:422–440.
13. Selvin HC, Hagstrom WO. The empirical classification of formal groups. *Am Sociol Rev* 1963;28:399–411.
14. Barton AH. Allen Barton's comments on Hauser's "context and consex." *Am J Sociol* 1970;76:514.
15. Hammond JL. Two sources of error in ecological correlations. *Am Sociol Rev* 1973;38:764–777.
16. Farkas G. Specification, residuals, and contextual effects. *Sociol Methods Res* 1974;2:333–363.
17. Ross R. *The prevention of malaria*. 2nd ed. London: John Murray; 1911.
18. Halloran EM, Struchiner CJ. Study designs for dependent happenings. *Epidemiology* 1991;2:331–338.
19. Koopman JS, Longini IM, Jacquez JA, et al. Assessing risk factors for transmission of infection. *Am J Epidemiol* 1991;133:1199–1209.
20. Lincoln JR, Zeitz G. Organizational properties from aggregate data: separating individual from structural effects. *Am Sociol Rev* 1980;45:391–408.

21. Koopman JS, Prevots DR, Vaca Marin MA, et al. Determinants and predictors of dengue infection in Mexico. *Am J Epidemiol* 1991;133:1168–1178.
22. Piantadosi S, Byar DP, Green SB. The ecological fallacy. *Am J Epidemiol* 1988;127:893–903.
23. Duncan OD, Davis B. An alternative to ecological correlation. *Am Sociol Rev* 1953;18:665–666.
24. Goodman LA. Some alternatives to ecological correlation. *Am J Sociol* 1959;64:610–625.
25. Hannan MT, Burstein L. Estimation from grouped observations. *Am Sociol Rev* 1974;39:374–392.
26. Firebaugh G. A rule for inferring individual-level relationships from aggregate data. *Am Sociol Rev* 1978;43:557–572.
27. Riley MW. *Sociological research.* vol. 1. Merton RK, ed. New York: Harcourt, Brace, Jovanovich; 1963;700–718.
28. Frost CD, Law MR, Wald NJ. II. Analysis of observational data within populations. *Br Med J [Clin Res]* 1991;302:815–818.
29. Rush D, Kristal AR. Methodologic studies during pregnancy: the reliability of the 24 hour dietary recall. *Am J Clin Nutr* 1982;35(Suppl 5):1259–1268.
30. Susser M. What is a cause and how do we know one? A grammar for pragmatic epidemiology. *Am J Epidemiol* 1991;133:635–648.
31. Maclure M. Multivariate refutation of aetiological hypotheses in non-experimental epidemiology. *Int J Epidemiol* 1990;19:782–787.
32. Greenland S, Robins J. Ecologic studies: biases, misconceptions, and counterexamples. *Am J Epidemiol* 1992;136.

APPENDIX ON ECOLOGIC REGRESSION COEFFICIENTS

Bruce Levin

This appendix gives mathematical expression to the changes in regression coefficients that can arise when group level data are used instead of individual level data. To reduce the discussion to its elements, we consider three variables only: individual level exposure x, individual outcome y, and a grouping variable, G, which serves to identify the distinct group to which an individual belongs. G usually specifies a finite number of discrete groups, but need not do so: we allow groups to be defined by levels of a quantitative variable. To abstract from sampling variability, we shall assume large samples within groups, and use the convenient notation of mathematical expectation.

Consider a model that specifies a linear relation at the individual level between x and y given membership in group G:

$$E(y|x,G) = \alpha + \beta x + f(G), \qquad [1]$$

where the left side of (1) denotes the conditional mean of y given x and G. Model (1) is additive with respect to the effects of x and G, so that $\beta = \beta_w$ is the within-group regression coefficient of interest, constant across all groups. We specify the group effect $f(G)$ as an entirely arbitrary function to allow for various possibilities. Thus, if there are k distinct groups, a conventional form for the group effect would be

$$f(G) = \gamma_1 I[G=1] + \cdots + \gamma_{k-1} I[G=k-1],$$

where $I[G=i]$ is a zero-one indicator for membership in group i, and γ_i is the difference in mean response y between group i and reference group k, given fixed exposure x. Alternatively, if groups are defined by levels of a quantitative variable (denoted by G as well), then $f(G)$ could assume the linear form $f(G) = \delta G$ or any other appropriate function of G.

The group effect $f(G)$ is straightforward to observe with individual level data. When we move to group level variables $X = E(x|G)$ and $Y = E(y|G)$ by taking averages within groups, model (1) implies that

$$E(y|G) = \alpha + \beta E(x|G) + f(G),$$

or simply

$$Y = \alpha + \beta X + f(G). \qquad [2]$$

In ecologic analysis, the group effects $f(G)$ are generally unavailable, entering (2) as perturbations of the linear relation between group variables X and Y. Unlike ordinary error terms in regression models, however, $f(G)$ may be correlated with X, leading to a different regression equation. Moreover, $f(G)$ may not even be linearly related to X. To investigate these circumstances a bit further, we suppose the relation between X and Y appears approximately linear, so that for ecologic analysis one will obtain the best linear predictor of Y given X based on the observed pairs (X, Y). The best linear predictor of Y given X, $BLP(Y|X)$, is that linear function of X that minimizes the mean squared error $E\{Y - L(X)\}^2$ among all linear functions $L(X)$, where the expectation is taken with respect to the distribution of (X, Y) across groups.[1] We distinguish here between $BLP(Y|X)$ and the true regression of Y on X, $E(Y|X)$, because the latter may not be a linear function of X.[2] The coefficients of $BLP(Y|X) = a + bX$ are given by $a = EY - bEX$ and $b = \mathrm{Cov}(X, Y)/\mathrm{Var}(X)$, which agree with the familiar formulas for regression theory in which $E(Y|X)$ is assumed to be linear.

Given (2), it is easy to show that the best linear predictor of Y given X is $BLP(Y|X) = (\alpha + c) + (\beta + d)X$, where c and d are the coefficients of the best

---

[1]Here and below, expectations, variances, and covariances of group level variables across groups are written EX, $\mathrm{Var}(X)$, $\mathrm{Cov}(X, Y)$, etc. In calculating these quantities, groups are often weighted proportional to their size. For example, with k discrete groups of size n_i ($i = 1, \ldots, k$), $EX = \Sigma_i n_i X_i / \Sigma_i n_i$. For continuous groups, the moments are weighted by the probability density function of G.

[2]What characterizes the best linear predictor is that the residuals $Y - BLP(Y|X)$ have mean zero and are uncorrelated with X. These are weaker conditions than the usual requirement in linear regression that the error term have zero conditional expectation given X.

linear predictor of $f(G)$ given X, $BLP(f(G)|X) = c + dX$, with $c = Ef(G) - dEX$ and $d = \mathrm{Cov}(f(G),X)/\mathrm{Var}(X)$. The ecologic coefficient of X is thus $\beta_e = \beta + d$, and we see that $\beta_e = \beta_w$ if and only if $d = 0$. This occurs when either (i) $f(G)$ is identically zero, or (ii) the group effect $f(G)$ is uncorrelated with X. Condition (i) occurs when there are no group effects on individual outcome y in model (1) given individual exposure x, i.e., when outcome is conditionally independent of group membership given exposure, even if G is highly correlated with X. For example, if $E(y|x) = \alpha + \beta x$ in model (1) and G is defined by grouping of individuals in subintervals of x, the ecologic coefficient of X agrees with β. Condition (ii) would occur, e.g., if groups were constructed as random samples, and thus uncorrelated with X. Of course, one recognizes conditions (i) and (ii) as conditions sufficient to ensure that G is not confounding between x and y in the linear model (1). In cases where neither (i) nor (ii) obtain, coefficients β_e and β_w generally differ.

If we elaborate on model (1) to allow β to depend on group, say $\beta = \beta(G)$, then the shift in the ecologic coefficient of X contains an additional component. Let $\delta(G)$ denote the effect modification of group G on exposure: $\delta(G) = \beta(G) - \beta_w$, where β_w is the weighted average of within-group slopes.[3] Then the ecologic coefficient is $\beta_e = \beta_w + d$, where the shift is now $d = \mathrm{Cov}(\{\delta(G)X\} + f(G),X)/\mathrm{Var}(X)$. The additional component $\mathrm{Cov}(\delta(G)X,X)/\mathrm{Var}(X)$ will not generally equal zero unless the group effect modifications $\delta(G)$ are uncorrelated with both X and X^2.

DISCUSSION

Dr. Padian: Where you're clearly using an individual as the unit of analysis for both the independent and dependent variables, you're not doing an ecological study at all but you still have the effect of contextual variables. If you're doing a study of cancer, for example, it apparently doesn't matter how many people have it, but in reality, it does matter.

Dr. Susser: That's entirely true. I don't think you can ignore the contextual effect even in individual studies. You can analyze an individual situation or an individual group, but you can't generalize this analysis to other groups unless you take contextual variables into account.

Dr. Padian: Even the weight of the independent variables for any particular individual depends on the context.

Dr. Susser: Absolutely. I'm a great believer in context.

Dr. Moss: You said that most of the ecological studies you can think of failed. Can you give us some examples?

---

[3]The weights are proportional to $\mathrm{Var}(x|G)$: $\beta_w = E\{\beta(G)\mathrm{Var}(x|G)\}/E\{\mathrm{Var}(x|G)\}$. The linear combination of β_w and β_e mentioned in the text which produces the slope β_t of the best linear predictor of y given x ignoring G is $\beta_t = V\beta_w + (1 - V)\beta_e$, where $V = E\{\mathrm{Var}(x|G)\}$ / $[E\{\mathrm{Var}(x|G)\} + \mathrm{Var}(X)]$ gives the proportion of total variance in x accounted for by the average within group variance.

Dr. Susser: The Guatemala study of nutritional supplementation in four villages: high protein in two and low protein in two. There were not enough groups, and so they simply resorted to melding the whole lot, forgetting about the intervention and taking it as high supplement/low supplement for whoever happened to volunteer. They threw away the intervention model, the experimental design.

That's just one, but there was also a very interesting Rockefeller study in Egypt in about 1950 (I can't remember who did it). They tried to look at the effects of sanitation, nutrition, and DDT as three separate interventions in six villages. This was very interesting because we didn't know anything about such villages; but they got no result.

Although it's vulnerable in some of its design features, there's the recent exemplary study by Alfred Sommer and his colleagues on long-acting vitamin A supplementation in children in 450 Indonesian villages—one long-acting shot of vitamin A, one follow-up 1 year later, and how many died in the randomized treated and untreated villages.

Dr. Halloran: I wrote a paper in which Ronald Ross discussed dependent happenings. We described the dependent happening problem in a series of four different study designs and discussed the groundwork for some infectious disease contexts, and the third of these was an ecological study. There are situations in infectious diseases where, if you take a preintervention baseline as your study comparison, the comparisons of the effects are so dramatic that you can really see the difference. For example, if you compare measles immunization in the U.S. before and after intervention, it's quite clear that the vaccine has had an effect. The same thing is true for the schistosomiasis program in Brazil, where the prevalence of enlarged liver goes from about 80% to 20%. There's a good chance that that had to do with the intervention program. There's also the Garki malaria project in Nigeria, which involved different villages and preintervention and postintervention comparisons, although you can't always be sure that the change is attributable to what you have. And you can have real problems when you have an n of one or two.

Dr. Susser: I have a paper being reviewed at the moment in which I discuss a lot of design examples of different kinds to illustrate what I've called salience and different levels of salience.

Dr. Friedman: When we think of doing randomized assignments of communities to various kinds of acquired immunodeficiency syndrome (AIDS) interventions (e.g., needle exchanges or education on condoms to schools in different U.S. communities), we run into problems of contamination and control. These obviously have to be added to your list, but do you have any comments or suggestions to make?

Dr. Susser: You're right that they belong in my list. I think they're a genuine problem where people change their behavior regardless of whether they are being intervened—in the Stanford Heart Programme studies, for instance, and even in the Mister Fit studies. It's a design issue, and I think you can only use your wits.

In Uganda, the British Medical Research Council people are doing an interesting study in an attempt to control sexually transmitted diseases, and in turn, to control the spread of HIV (at least that's the hypothesis). This involves the ethical problem as to whether you can withhold treatment from some people. I think this is an insoluble problem at the individual level, but not at the group level, and certainly not in Uganda, where people are not being treated anyway. It's perfectly acceptable to introduce your intervention in communities selected at random from the total number of groups, and to do it successively to the limits of your resources. You can do it in that situation because they're spread randomly. You may not be able to do it in the U.S., although I think sometimes even there . . .

Unidentified: But then you get contamination from one community to another.

Dr. Susser: Only if they are close to one another. If you select your communities randomly across a whole country, you're not faced with the same problem. Of course, you need resources.

Dr. Vlahov: In some situations, randomization may not be possible. Do you have any comments on the possibility of using a natural experimental situation?

Dr. Susser: If you've got a natural experimental situation, exploit it. In the paper I was talking about, I describe a few ecological examples. But you've got to be lucky because you need to have a setting where you have some antecedent measures, and this doesn't often happen in the Third World.

However, we have recently had an example when children studied before the Bangladesh flood were measured again 6 months after it. No differences could be shown between individual children in terms of the amount of danger they were exposed to (e.g., the depth of the flood waters) or in terms of how many people they had seen die. However, the behavior of the group was obviously affected and there was a vast increase in bedwetting over 6 months. Here, I agree with the very bright suggestion that we're dealing with the integral variable of terror, which is not directly measurable by individual measures of physical danger. In this case, ecological analysis actually demonstrated what couldn't be seen at an individual level.

We used a natural (or rather, an unnatural and savage) experiment during the well-demarcated 6-month period of famine in Holland at the end of World War II. In that situation, we looked for the effects of prenatal exposure to famine on the outcome of subsequent development in young men. It had to be an ecological analysis, but we did have measures of the rations and all of the data were there.

We can talk at length about exploiting situations for ecological analyses. Ever since William Farr or John Grant, we have been using ecological analysis for descriptive purposes when we look at mortality in populations. In Britain, we've got 30 quinquennia of mortality data that are very precise for descriptive purposes, but the exposures are very badly measured for analytical purposes.

HIV Epidemiology: Models and Methods, edited by Alfredo Nicolosi. Raven Press, Ltd., New York © 1994.

14

Obstacles in the Pursuit of an AIDS Vaccine

Alan M. Schultz

Vaccine Research and Development Branch, Division of AIDS, BRDP, NIAID, NIH, Bethesda, Maryland 20892

Vaccines have long been an essential weapon in the worldwide fight against morbidity and mortality caused by infectious disease. When they are successful, they provide a low-cost and effective barrier, protecting entire populations against epidemic spread of infectious agents. A vaccine against acquired immunodeficiency syndrome (AIDS) is thus desperately needed to combat the worldwide epidemic facing us. Epidemiologists have been tracking its spread and identifying its contributing risk factors; they are also establishing the baseline studies in human populations that will permit subsequent efficacy testing of candidate vaccines against human immunodeficiency virus (HIV). Thus, it is reasonable to ask what are the most promising vaccine candidates and when are these trials likely to begin. The answers are complex and, unfortunately, not entirely satisfying. This chapter attempts to provide an overview of the significant scientific unknowns that stymie definite predictions about progress in this important area, and briefly reviews the status of the efforts, especially in the United States, to develop and test vaccines against AIDS.

In concept, creating a successful vaccine is a straightforward activity, once the causative agent is known. The vaccines need to induce an immune response(s) that is strong enough to repel natural exposure to the agent, broad enough to deal with variants of the agent that may circulate in the population, and that lasts long enough to provide lifelong immunity.

The classic steps in vaccine development are summarized in Table 1. Once the causative agent is known and can be grown in culture, rational vaccine development can begin. By examining patients recovering from the infection, important clues to the most significant immune responses and sensitive targets in the causative agent can be established. Various preparations of vaccines from the infectious agent, created most simply by inactivating or attenuating it, can then be tested for their ability to induce those responses.

TABLE 1. *Classic vaccine development*

1) Identify causative agent
2) Develop large-scale *in vitro* growth
3) Examine recovered patients, to correlate an immune response with recovery
4) Develop vaccines that induce that response
5) Establish the number of serotypes
6) Do challenge studies in humans

   OR

   preclinical vaccine trials in animals
7) Phase I/II safety and immunogenicity
8) Monitor phase III trials through established infectious disease surveillance

Then the potential issue of multiple variants or serotypes of the agent can be addressed to determine whether a monovalent vaccine will be adequate or, alternatively, if a polyvalent vaccine against multiple strains must be developed. Finally, initial indications of efficacy can be obtained if an adequate animal model exists, or even by vaccination and challenge studies in humans if the disease is not life-threatening or has good treatments available, as in the case of adenovirus or measles. Safety and immunogenicity studies on a small scale are a necessary preamble to larger trials. Phase III trials, to establish their degree of efficacy, are least expensive if the time between exposure and onset of clinical signs is short, and if there is already an existing surveillance for the disease.

A fundamental problem complicating AIDS vaccine development is lack of knowledge about what immune response(s) will be protective. In other diseases, people who have recovered from the infection can be examined to see what strong immune responses to the agent they have that may correlate with recovery. Accelerating these particular responses by vaccination is then likely to prevent disease. Spontaneous recovery from HIV infection is exceedingly rare, and there is no known population that clearly has suppressed HIV and can be said to have "recovered" from the infection. Thus, there are few unequivocal clues about protective immunity. In fact, until the string of successful primate vaccination and protection experiments in 1989 through 1991 (1–5), there was a significant opinion that a vaccine for HIV was a theoretical impossibility.

It is hoped we will be able to learn what the correlate(s) of protection is through a variety of approaches. Study of long-term survivors of HIV infection may offer some help, but there is the chicken–egg paradox. Does high neutralizing antibody produce long-term survivors, or does it develop because they *are* long-term survivors, keeping HIV and its variation in check by other mechanisms? As an alternative, those individuals who can be studied during the acute phase of HIV infection may show what immune responses have checked the initial infection. Longer-term study may then show common characteristics of the initial response that correlates with longer-term survival. Another human study population is a small group of so-called "exposed but uninfected" individuals who are at high risk for HIV but show no antibodies while having T-cell responses, when assessed by very sensitive techniques. Are these T-cell responses "protecting" them from HIV infection so they never need to develop antibody? Or have they simply not been exposed to an adequate dose of virus? Further longitudinal study of more subjects may give the answer.

Infants born to HIV-positive mothers are another group where hypotheses about protective immune responses may be tested. Since the majority of such infants do not become infected, have they: (a) received passive antibody from their mother and thus been protected?; (b) produced their own T-cell responses as a consequence of *in utero* exposure and resisted the virus?; (c) been the beneficiary of a mother's immune responses that reduce *her* virus load and thus minimize exposure of the infant?; or (d) been the beneficiaries of a placental barrier that nonspecifically can resist HIV transmission? Studies of virus load, difference in the HIV isolates from mother and infant, T-cell responses in the newborn, and neutralization of both the mother's and infant's HIV by maternal serum are actively underway. And finally, therapeutic use of vaccines in infected individuals, if shown to slow disease progression, may provide information about a response that can effectively combat HIV even in the presence of an established infection.

However, in the absence of a clear pathway to the evaluation of what immune responses will be protective, *a priori* approaches have been relied on. The initial paradigm for HIV vaccine design was an assumption that protection could only be obtained by preventing the very first infectious event upon exposure. Vaccines normally prepare the recipient to rapidly respond to the infecting agent after exposure, so that the infection does not further progress and is cleared before the onset of pathologic sequelae. Thus, vaccines protect against disease and not infection. Because anti-HIV responses ultimately fail in infected people, it was felt that "sterilizing immunity" was the only hope. This was only conceivable by inducing and maintaining high levels of neutralizing antibody, and the first vaccines concentrated on the envelope gene. Chimpanzee experiments have shown that neutralizing antibody, when passively administered and if present at high enough levels (6–9), can by itself prevent infection. This establishes the strength of a particular response needed for protective immunity. It may be possible to achieve this, at least in the short term, by active immunization. Sera from baboons receiving gp120 vaccines has protected reconstituted SCID/hu mice from HIV challenge. The challenge to vaccine development based on this paradigm is to maintain that level for long periods of time. The question of cross-protection has not yet been addressed in experiments of this type.

Other paradigms are now evolving. In a cellular immunity equivalent to the passive antibody transfer experiments, SCID/hu mice reconstituted with α-HIV cytotoxic T-cell (CTL) clones isolated from infected humans have been protected from *in vivo* challenge with HIV (10). Thus, in this model cellular immunity alone can protect from the establishment of infection. Cytotoxic cells eliminate host cells that have become infected. To the extent that SCID/hu mice mimic the human situation, it is encouraging that recovery from HIV infection is possible. In macaque experiments, a number of vaccines have not provided "sterilizing immunity," especially when the challenge SIV has been produced in macaque cells. Nonetheless, several groups have shown that vaccinated monkeys are still alive and healthy, though SIV-positive, 1 year or more after challenge whereas naive control monkeys from the same experiment have died with simian AIDS. Though the mechanism of this is not at all clear, it indicates that vaccination has slowed disease progression. If combinations of responses can be effective, then lower levels of both neutralization and cellular responses can be effective in concert with each other, and the likelihood of eventual success for an HIV vaccine is increased.

It is important to remember that vaccines are used to protect populations, and that interrupting transmission is the goal. A vaccine can cause an HIV-exposed person to fail to pass the virus on by three mechanisms: (a) the vaccine prevents any HIV infection at all ("sterilizing immunity"); (b) a local infection results but HIV never becomes established, though HIV genome may still reside inactively in some cells; or (c) the individual becomes infected, but vaccination-induced immunity keeps the levels of HIV so low that transmission is unlikely. Even a vaccine that suppresses HIV for long periods of time but eventually fails to protect the individual from HIV re-emergence and death is still "successful" to the extent that it minimizes the number of people effectively exposed to HIV.

A paradigm that allows for recovery from a localized HIV infection suggests that additional HIV gene products that do not contribute to "sterilizing immunity" may nonetheless be important components of a vaccine. It is now considered possible that an HIV vaccine may work like other successful vaccines, by using neutralizing antibody to minimize re-infection plus cytotoxic cells to kill HIV-infected cells. An advantage of CTL is the fact that frequently their target sequences are in conserved regions of the viral genome.

Vaccines that induce strong responses must also be able to repel a variety of HIV variants that are circulating in the population at risk. The sequence variation of HIV, especially the envelope gene, is extreme. Nonetheless, computer analysis suggests that HIV exists in five or six large families, or clades (11) (Figure 1). The immunological significance of these groupings is now beginning to be explored in detail. HIV from some geographic areas, such as North America, are limited to one clade while other areas, such as Zaire and Thailand, have viruses from more than one clade. Cross-neutralization between HIV isolates, based on the principal neutralizing domain in

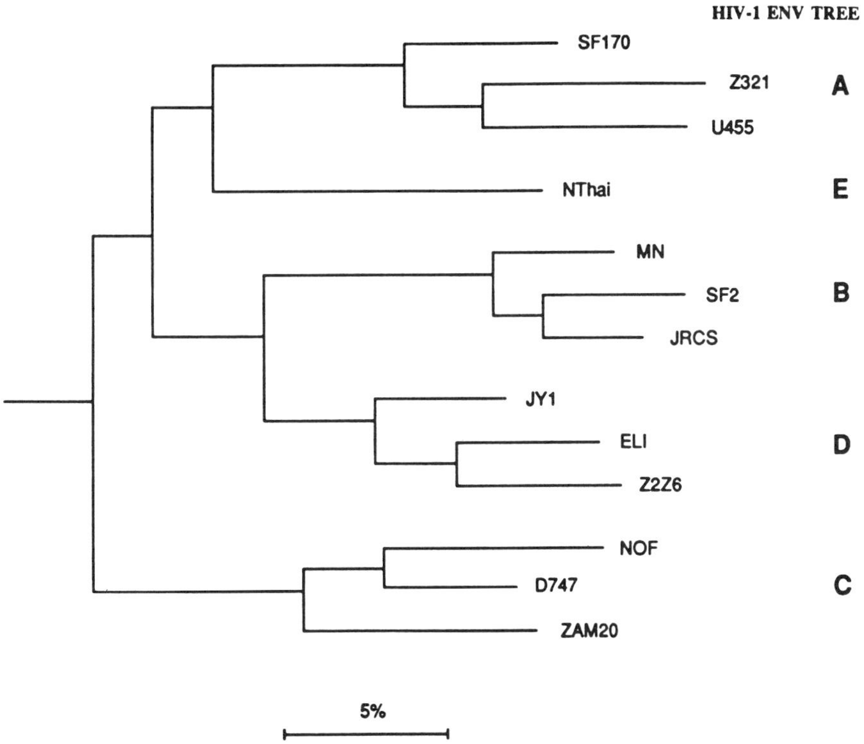

FIG. 1. Families (clades) of human immunodeficiency virus type 1.

the V3 region, is very limited even within one clade (12). However, antibodies directed to conformational determinants of the envelope are more cross-reactive (13). This geographical localization is most likely a temporary condition reflecting founder effects in various regions. In central Africa, where HIV has been prevalent the longest, several clades are found. It is only a matter of time before HIV mixtures are diverse everywhere.

PRIMATE STUDIES

Primates can be used in a strictly empiric sense to model human immune responses to vaccines and the likelihood of success in efficacy tests, and independently to supply the correlate of immune protection information that is missing from human studies. Unfortunately, the available models are less than ideal in both respects. If "sterilizing immunity" is the vaccine paradigm, then chimpanzees are adequate; alternatively, if recovery from infection is the vaccine paradigm, then the failure of HIV to cause disease in chimpanzees can be a concern. The reverse situation occurs with SIV in macaques, where the disease course of simian AIDS closely mimics the human condition. But SIV is not HIV, and for *env*-gene based vaccines specifically, the fact that SIV gp120 does not exhibit a linear epitope principal neutralizing domain like the V3 loop region of HIV gp120 severely impairs a test of "sterilizing immunity." This is probably the reason why subunit vaccines have been successful in chimpanzees with HIV-based subunits, but total failures in macaques with SIV subunit vaccines.

As far as understanding the mechanism of protection (the elusive "correlate") is concerned, neutralizing antibody seems to be it for the chimpanzees, whether induced by a gp120 (14) or a gp160 vaccine (15). However, these vaccines have been tested under extremely limited conditions. It should be appreciated that virtually all chimpanzee challenge studies have been done with a single HIV_{LAI} challenge stock, and that duration of protection and cross-challenge with other HIV isolates have not been tested yet. Thus, the "sterilizing immunity" paradigm works, but its relevance to real-world vaccine conditions is not clear. Since CTL have never been detected even in HIV-infected chimps, the ability to test other vaccine paradigms in this model may be limited. And it is well-appreciated that the expense of chimpanzees minimizes their use.

In the SIV/macaque model, a variety of SIV isolates are available that differ in biological and immunological properties, and CTL activity has now been reliably measured in both infected and vaccinated macaques. Thus, real-world conditions can be tested in this model, and holding facilities and animal supply are sufficient to do numerous experiments. The shortcomings of this model for *env*-based vaccines have already been mentioned. On the other hand, neutralizing antibodies directed primarily against the V3 domain may not be sufficiently cross-reactive to give protection under real-world conditions. That is to say, the failure of subunit vaccines to protect macaques from SIV challenge may be giving us the "real" answer. At this stage, a unitary path has not emerged from the primate studies, and it is difficult to propose any particular primate studies as gatekeepers for the progression of HIV vaccine candidates into human evaluations.

What can we hope to learn in the short-term from primate studies? The curious hybrid SHIV, with an HIV envelope on an SIV core (16–18), may solve some of the problems of both models if it fulfills its promise. At the present time, it can only test for the "sterilizing immunity" paradigm. An extremely important observation has been the strong protection induced in the SIV/macaque model by a live attenuated SIV vaccine (19). Protection here is certainly strong and lasts for a few years at least; breadth of protection will be evaluated soon in a series of expanded studies. Investigating the mechanism of protection of this very effective vaccine may be its most important contribution.

HUMAN STUDIES

Safety and immunogenicity of vaccines is established in phase I human trials as a necessary prelude to expanded study in phase II and beyond. Subunit proteins, synthetic peptides, and live, recombinant vaccinia expressing the HIV *env* gene have been tested so far in uninfected seronegative volunteers (20–25). In NIAID-sponsored trials, six varieties of envelope subunit have been tested, in addition to the HIVAC-1e vaccinia vector alone or in combination with a boost with insect cell gp160 (Table 2). All vaccines have been safe and well-tolerated. Immunization schedules have varied around the concept of two closely spaced inoculations (weeks apart), followed by a boost about 6 months later and, in some cases, an additional boost at 1 year. Doses have ranged, according to the protocol and vaccine product, from 15 to 1280 μg per dose.

Immunogenicity is presently being tested by measuring binding antibody titers to the HIV envelope and to a synthetic peptide from the V3 principal neutralizing domain. Vaccination-induced antibodies with biological activity are defined by homologous neutralization of the vaccine strain of HIV and by fusion inhibition antibody. If there is measurable homologous neutralization (LAI, MN, or SF2, depending on the vaccine), then cross-neutralization for non-vaccine strains of HIV is done. We are beginning now to test for antibodies that block the interactions of gp120 with CD4. This is a relatively low cost assay that may correlate with cross-neutralization.

This analysis suffers from the problems already described in the preclinical development of vaccines. What is the relevant immune response? Despite indications that some of these subunit vaccines induce CTL in mice, the only vaccine that has produced reproducible CTL in our volunteers is the HIVAC-1e/gp160 "prime-boost" combination. These have not been seen in all volunteers, and are short-lived. It is worth pointing out, however, that

TABLE 2. *Vaccines in phase I seronegative trial*

Subunit envelope proteins			Number of volunteers
gp 160	LAI	(insect cell)	46
gp 160	LAI	(mammalian cell)	70
gp 120 + novel adjuvant	SF2	(yeast)	18
			30
gp 120	LAI	(mammalian cell)	20
gp 120 + novel adjuvant	SF2	(mammalian cell)	24
			16
gp 120	MN	(mammalian cell)	48
Live vector			
env-gene	LAI	(HIVAC-1e)	41
Prime/boost			
HIVAC-1e plus gp 160		(insect cell)	33

CTL are harvested from the spleen in mice, since the tiny volume of blood makes it impractical to sample that for CTL. In humans, of course, CTL are sought from blood samples. The time of residence in the blood before homing to internal sites is not known. For other viral diseases, the most effective CTL are directed toward *core* proteins of the causative virus, and all vaccines tested so far by the NIAID are limited to the envelope gene of HIV. At this time, we cannot convincingly rank vaccines by their ability to induce CTL.

All of the subunit protein candidate vaccines in NIAID-sponsored trials have been tested at more than one dose. The serological responses after the first two inoculations have been very modest. The best antibody levels have been obtained after the third and fourth inoculations at a given dose, and have been proportional to the dose. Data are only now being accumulated on the persistence of these serological responses, as the trials of the highest doses of most of the products in Table 2 have begun within the last year; thus, 6-month and 12-month data are only now coming in. All of the products eventually induce neutralizing antibody against the vaccine strain of HIV at the highest doses of the particular vaccine. For the gp120 products, the induced levels of neutralization of the vaccine strain begin to approach the titers found in HIV-infected patients against the vaccine strain. However, the cross-neutralization against other laboratory HIV strains is somewhat lower.

Immunological analysis continues to concentrate on reliably measuring CTL responses and testing for neutralization of field isolates of HIV. The NIAID has embarked on a program of obtaining HIV from recent seroconversions, from the U.S. and from developing nations where vaccine trials are likely to occur. The development of domestic sites and Preparation for AIDS Vaccine Efficacy (PAVE) sites will be described in the accompanying chapter by Dr. Vermund. We also are receiving isolates from the long-term Multi-center AIDS Cohort Study (MACS), which has recently had dozens of seroconversions. We have had a ~50% success rate in culturing these isolates, and they are expanded in human PBL. These will prove valuable in the testing of volunteer sera, as decisions about initiating efficacy trials draw nearer.

Meanwhile, phase I trials are being initiated with newer types of products. "Second generation" subunit products are being evaluated by moving into adjuvants other than alum. Comparative adjuvant trials based on gp120 subunits will have begun by the summer of 1993. It is hoped that improved adjuvants can increase the strength of the immunological response, leading to increased breadth and duration of the serological response, and perhaps even to a more easily detected CTL-type response. A novel synthetic peptide vaccine trial begins in the spring of 1993, based on an octameric presentation of peptides that may be particularly immunogenic (26). And the NIAID will be following up a trial begun in France of an avipox vector that is immunogenic despite lack of replication in mammalian cells (27). This may provide the benefits of live virus immunization while avoiding most the concerns occasioned by the use of such vectors. Activity with these and other vaccines is necessary to keep the pipeline open to follow up on any efficacy trial results with current products. New approaches must be ready, either for use alone as better vaccines or in combination with existing ones.

Thorny problems remain before initiation of efficacy trials. This chapter has repeatedly emphasized the uncertainty about what immune responses will provide protection, and that uncertainty permeates all planning about prioritizing vaccines for entry into such trials and the time frame for beginning them. One problem that can be addressed as a general preamble to efficacy trial preparedness is the immune responses in target populations. Our phase I trials have largely been in very healthy, low-risk volunteers. Phase III trials will occur in developing world groups or in high-risk gay men, populations frequenting sexually transmitted disease (STD) clinics, and intravenous drug abusers. To address whether these populations also will respond as have the phase I volunteers, NIAID has recently begun phase II trials in those domestic populations. In this context, phase II refers not so much to number of volunteers as to a difference in the test population with respect to ethnic origin and health status. Results from such trials will be essential before beginning concrete plans for efficacy trials, which will involve thousands of volunteers.

The recurring theme of this chapter has been strength, duration, and breadth of protection, and the difficulty of defining and measuring it. There are a variety of scenarios for the future, depending on which turns out to be the biggest problem. Everyone involved in AIDS vaccine development hopes that initial efficacy trials will provide data that we have a vaccine of some utility, or at least point the way to improving the second generation of vaccines. If analysis of the trial indicates that there is some protection, but only against a group of HIV variants most like the vaccine strain, then lack of breadth of protection and HIV heterogeneity is the problem. This is actually good news, and solutions will most likely be approached by a complex polyvalent vaccine approach. If the vaccines show initial promise, but then protection decreases as the trial progresses, then duration of protection is the problem. We may have to rely on live vectors as vaccines, more frequent boosts, or hope that novel adjuvants can solve the problem. Finally, this chapter has not even mentioned sexual transmission of HIV and the fact that protection from transmission across mucosal surfaces may be a special problem for AIDS vaccines.

REFERENCES

1. Desrosiers RC, Wyand MS, Kodama T, et al. Vaccine protection against simian immunodeficiency virus infection. *Proc Natl Acad Sci U S A* 1989;86:6353–6357.
2. Murphey-Corb M, Martin LN, Davison-Fairburn B, et al. A formalin-inactivated whole SIV vaccine confers protection in macaques. *Science* 1989;246:1293–1297.

3. Carlson JR, McGraw TP, Keddie E, et al. Vaccine protection of rhesus macaques against simian immunodeficiency virus infection. *AIDS Res Hum Retroviruses* 1990;6:1239–1246.
4. Stott EJ, Chan WL, Mills KH, et al. Preliminary report: protection of cynomolgus macaques against simian immunodeficiency virus by fixed infected-cell vaccine. *Lancet* 1990;336:1538–1541.
5. Putkonen P, Thorstensson R, Walther L, et al. Vaccine protection against HIV-2 infection in cynomolgus monkeys. *AIDS Res Hum Retroviruses* 1991;7:271–277.
6. Emini EA, Schlief WA, Murthy KK, et al. Passive immunization with a monoclonal antibody directed to the HIV-1 gp120 principal neutralizing domain confers protection against HIV-1 challenge in chimpanzees [abstract 65]. VII International Conference on AIDS, Florence, Italy, 1991.
7. Emini EA, Schlief WA, Nunberg JH, et al. Prevention of HIV-1 infection in chimpanzees by gp120 V3 domain-specific monoclonal antibody. *Nature* 1992;355:728–730.
8. Prince AM, Horowitz B, Shulman RW, et al. Apparent prevention of HIV infection by HIV immunoglobulin given prior to low-dose HIV challenge. In: Brown F, Chanock R, Ginsberg H, Lerner R, eds. *Vaccines '90*. Cold Spring Harbor, NY: Cold Spring Harbor Laboratory; 1990:347–351.
9. Prince AM, Reesink H, Pascual D, et al. Prevention of infection by passive immunization with HIV immunoglobulin. *AIDS Res Hum Retroviruses* 1991;7:971–973.
10. Richard Koup, *personal communication.*
11. Myers G, Korber B, Berzofsky J, et al, eds. *Human retroviruses and AIDS: a compilation and analysis of nucleic acid and amino acid sequences.* Los Alamos, NM: Los Alamos National Laboratory; 1992.
12. Berman PW, Natthews TJ, Riddle L, et al. Neutralization of multiple laboratory and clinical isolates of human immunodeficiency virus type 1 (HIV-1) by antisera raised against gp120 from the MN isolate of HIV-1. *J Virol* 1992;66:4464–4469.
13. Haigwood NL, Nara PL, Brooks E, et al. Native but not denatured recombinant human immunodeficiency virus type 1 gp120 generates broad-spectrum neutralizing antibody in baboons. *J Virol* 1992;66:172–182.
14. Berman PW, Gregory TJ, Riddle L, et al. Protection of chimpanzees from infection by HIV-1 after vaccination with recombinant glycoprotein gp120 but not gp160. *Nature* 1990;345:622–625.
15. Girard M, Kieny MP, Pinter A, et al. Immunization of chimpanzees confers protection against challenge with human immunodeficiency virus. *Proc Natl Acad Sci U S A* 1991;88:542–546.
16. Shibata R, Kawamura M, Sakai H, et al. Generation of a chimeric human and simian immunodeficiency virus infectious to monkey peripheral blood mononuclear cells. *J Virol* 1991;65:3514–3520.
17. Li J, Lord CI, Haseltine W, et al. Infection of cynomolgus monkeys with a chimeric HIV-1/SIVmac virus that expresses the HIV-1 envelope glycoproteins. *J AIDS* 1992;5:639–646.
18. Sakuragi S, Shibata R, Mukai R, et al. Infection of macaque monkeys with a chimeric human and simian immunodeficiency virus. *J Gen Virol* 1992;73:2983–2987.
19. Daniel MD, Kirschhoff F, Czajak SC, et al. Protective effects of a live attenuated SIV vaccine with a deletion in the nef gene. *Science* 1992;258:1938–1941.
20. Dolin R, Graham B, Greenberg S, et al. Safety and immunogenicity of an HIV-1 recombinant gp160 candidate vaccine in humans. Ann Intern Med 1991;114:119–127.
21. Wintsch J, Chaignat C-L, Braun DG, et al. Safety and immunogenicity of a genetically engineered human immunodeficiency virus vaccine. *J Infect Dis* 1991;163:219–225.
22. Goldstein AC, Naylor PH, Sarin PS, et al. Progress in the development of a p17 based HIV vaccine: immunogenicity of HGP-30 in humans. *AIDS Res Hum Retroviruses* 1991;7:2–3.
23. Zagury D, Bernard J, Cheynier R, et al. A group specific anamnestic immune reaction against HIV-1 induced by a candidate vaccine against AIDS. *Nature* 1988;332:728–731.
24. Cooney EL, Collier AC, Greenberg PD, et al. Safety of and immunological response to a recombinant vaccinia virus vaccine expressing HIV envelope glycoprotein. *Lancet* 1991;337:567–572.

25. Graham BS, Belshe RB, Clements ML, et al. Vaccination of vaccinia-naive adults with HIV-1 gp160 recombinant vaccinia (HIVAC-1e) in a blinded, controlled, randomized clinical trial. *J Infect Dis* 1992;116:244–252.
26. Wang C-Y, Looney DJ, Li ML, et al. Long-term high-titer neutralizing antibody induced by octameric synthetic HIV-1 antigen. *Science* 1991;254:285–288.
27. Taylor J, Trimarchi C, Weinberg R, et al. Efficacy studies on a canary-pox-rabies recombinant virus. *Vaccine* 1988;6:497–503.

HIV Epidemiology: Models and Methods,
edited by Alfredo Nicolosi. Raven Press, Ltd.,
New York 1994.

15

The Efficacy of HIV Vaccines

Methodological Issues in Preparing for Clinical Trials

Sten H. Vermund

Vaccine Trials and Epidemiology Branch, Division of AIDS, National Institute of Allergy and Infectious Diseases, Bethesda, Maryland 20892

Human immunodeficiency virus (HIV) was discovered in 1983 and has been demonstrated to be the cause of the acquired immunodeficiency syndrome (AIDS) (1,2). In the brief time period 1977 to 1992, AIDS has become a major cause of death among adults in their most economically and reproductively active years. Losses have left a trail of tragedy not merely in the framework of family and friendship, but also on the global economic scale (3,4). Entire occupations, villages, and urban centers have been devastated by the HIV epidemic, which even today is increasing in incidence in Latin America, Africa, and Asia (5). In industrialized settings such as the U.S., relatively stable HIV incidence rates and prevalence (6) mask the contrasting trends reflecting the impact of chemotherapy and chemoprophylaxis of HIV-infected persons (7) and the growing AIDS problem among selected high-risk populations, including ethnic minorities and women (8). An especially poignant reminder of the ongoing torment left in the wake of this new plague is the living testimony of survivors, including the parents of dead children, the partners and spouses of dead loved ones (9), and the rising toll of children orphaned by HIV-infected parents (10,11).

The public health armamentarium for HIV epidemic prevention and control currently rests on securing changes in human behavior for reduction in illicit drug injection and needle sharing (12), protection of the blood supply, reduction in the number of unprotected sexual encounters and the number of sexual partners (13), expanded diagnosis and treatment of other sexually transmitted diseases (STD) (13), optimal prenatal care for pregnant HIV-infected women, and improved availability and compliance with antiviral chemotherapies that reduce seminal viral burden and probably reduce infectiousness (14). In impoverished developing nations, condoms, screening and treatment for sexually transmitted infections, antiviral chemotherapies, and HIV-seronegative blood and blood product supplies remain largely unavailable and unaffordable (15). Behavior changes in the field of human sexuality are possible, but may require intense intervention that may not be practical or affordable in all risk settings (16). In my view, an affordable, available HIV vaccine remains the single most important long-term prevention research goal (17–19), even as we must seek to expand HIV/STD education, condom marketing, STD control, prevention and treatment of injection drug use (IDU), and the development of an effective female-controlled virucide or microbicide (20–22).

A RATIONALE FOR HIV VACCINE EFFICACY TRIALS

Accepting the premise that HIV vaccines are a critically needed adjunct to behavior change, improved barrier contraceptives and microbicides, and a safe blood supply, one can still argue that HIV efficacy trials are premature. I agree at this time (September 1992). Yet, more than a dozen candidate HIV vaccines are currently in the U.S. Phase I trials investigate vaccine safety and immunogenicity in a small number (<50) of low-risk, HIV-seronegative volunteers. All vaccines have proven to be completely safe in the trials so far (23). Reactogenicity is mild and comparable to that seen with currently licensed vaccine products for other viral or for bacterial infectious agents (23). Some evidence of immunogenicity, as measured by binding antibody, neutralizing antibody, and cytotoxic T-lymphocytes (CTL), has been demonstrated for a variety of vaccines, though duration and magnitude of immune responses are not as great as those seen in natural infection. A Phase II study of safety, immunogenicity, and dosage schedule of two gp120 envelope subunit products in more than 200 higher risk volunteers began in early 1993. If one or more candidate(s) should be judged suitable, Phase III trials of vaccine efficacy in thousands of subjects could commence as early as 1994 or 1995. Planning for this eventuality is the subject of this presentation.

METHODOLOGIC ISSUES

While numerous issues could be presented regarding challenges in the design and conduct of large vaccine trials, I wish to present seven topics of special concern:

1. Vaccines must be selected using reasonable criteria, including safety, demonstration of an immunologic effector mechanism, and suitability of a given candidate vaccine for a given HIV strain circulating at the proposed trial site.

2. Maximum efforts must be made to apply current knowledge and use available epidemiologic cohort specimens and information to identify a natural correlate of protective immunity.
3. Efficacy trials must be designed to investigate both a primary endpoint (i.e., infection with HIV-1) and secondary endpoints (e.g., immunological and virologic status postinfection and early clinical events).
4. Behavioral research will need to be nested within trial preparations and in the trials themselves for compelling reasons that have no previous parallels in vaccine research history.
5. Route of viral exposure must be assessed in trials, and STD status and the impact of STD treatment on HIV seroincidence should be carefully considered within trials.
6. Site selection, plans for population identification and recruitment, and sample size estimates must be developed to maximize the efficiency and ultimate success of the study.
7. A host of ethical, social, and political issues must be addressed before, during, and after vaccines trials commence.

Vaccine Selection

Those vaccines selected for large field trials must satisfy concerns of many interested parties: potential trial volunteers and community advocates, vaccine developers and manufacturers, clinical trial investigators, international and local organizations with oversight responsibilities (e.g., the World Health Organization [WHO] and Institutional Review Boards), regulatory bodies (e.g., the Food and Drug Administration and the national Ministries of Health), and the funding and coordination agency (e.g., the National Institutes of Health [NIH] or European governmental research bodies).

To effectively forge consensus, criteria for vaccine selection have been developed by a working group convened by the Director of the National Institute of Allergy and Infectious Diseases (NIAID) in 1991 and again in 1992. Optimal criteria for vaccine selection present an idealized goal, while core criteria are meant to provide guidelines for identifying the time point at which the product would be worth testing in an efficacy trial (Table 1). These guidelines have been further refined by the NIAID in collaboration with academia, industry, other government agencies, and communities in 1993. The WHO is making similar judgments with its Vaccine Steering Committee for the Global Program on AIDS, focussed on trials that might go forward in WHO "target" countries: Brazil, Thailand, Uganda, and Rwanda (J. Esparza, *personal communication*).

The vaccine being taken into very large-scale efficacy trials must be safe, as judged by preclinical and clinical studies, including Phase I (small studies of safety and immunogenicity) and Phase II (larger studies of dosing and

TABLE 1. *Core and optimal guidelines for entry of HIV[a] vaccines into efficacy trials in uninfected volunteers*

What we realistically hope for	What would be ideal to see
1. Demonstrated safety in Phase I clinical trials	
2.* Demonstrated efficacy of a given vaccine construct in HIV-infected chimps or SIV-infected monkeys.	2.A Protects animals in challenge studies from HIV infection/disease induced by cell-associated as well as free virus.
3.* Elicits neutralizing antibody that is long-lasting and broadly reactive against heterologous isolates in Phase I clinical trials. A candidate vaccine would be more attractive if induction of long-term and broadly reactive cellular immunity were also seen.	3.A Protects against a broad spectrum of heterologous isolates. 3.B Protects against intravenous and mucosal challenge. 3.C Induces long-lasting immunity so that protection occurs when virus is administered months to years after immunization.
4.* Demonstrates immunological and/or genetic similarity to HIV isolates from the proposed efficacy trial site.	
	5.A Demonstrates induction of the likely correlates of immunity in Phase I clinical trials

Source: Modified from the Final Report of the NIAID Ad Hoc HIV Vaccine Advisory Panel, September 1992.
*It would be best if at least two of the three criteria with * would be met in addition to safety (#1) for a candidate vaccine to go into an efficacy trial.
[a]HIV, human immunodeficiency virus.

schedule, often in the same populations of higher HIV risk being considered for Phase III efficacy trials) studies. In the absence of knowledge of a correlate of protective immunity for HIV, some plausible immunological effector mechanism must be demonstrated, such as neutralizing antibody and/or CTL. The vaccine candidate should be judged for its suitability for use at a given trial site, ideally by demonstrating that vaccine-induced antibody is capable of neutralizing HIV-1 that is circulating in the geographic area of the proposed trial site. The duration of a given antibody response or other immunological effector mechanism must last as long as possible with adjuvants and antigens currently available or being developed. Thus, a candidate with a postboost antibody duration measured in weeks would, all other considerations being equal, be judged inferior to a candidate vaccine with an anamnestic antibody response that was measured in months or years. Whether CTL responses are needed to protect, particularly against cell-associated challenge, is unknown.

Site selection for a vaccine trial is intimately related to availability of a suitably engineered vaccine candidate. Industry is likely to have the greatest corporate interest in the MN family of HIV-1 strains, given their prominence in the areas that should have the strongest and most profitable vaccine markets in the future, namely, North America, Europe, and Australia. This introduces a special challenge for public and private sector advocates: provision of candidate vaccines for viral strains prevalent in impoverished regions of Sub-Saharan Africa, Latin America, and South Asia. Of course, a vaccine concept must be demonstrated to be *feasible* for these issues to be relevant. Hence, the early public health goal is to rapidly and ethically test promising candidate vaccines in communities that have a relevant circulating virus and are willing to participate in the vaccine trial.

Correlates of Protection

Before embarking on previous vaccine trials for other agents, a biological correlate of protective immunology has usually, but not always, been known. In the classic vaccine study of Edward Jenner in 1796, he noted that milk maids who had acquired cowpox in the course of their milking were spared full-blown smallpox; hence, the "correlate of protection" was prior infection with cowpox, suggesting its utility as a vaccine (24). In recounting the turn-of-the-century typhoid vaccine development by Sir Almroth Wright and others, Cockburn recalls that "properties of the serum of the inoculated [were compared] with serum from convalescent patients, and [it was] observed that the properties of the sera from the two sources were similar," (25) suggesting that this serum, if safe, might protect by the same immunologic mechanism by which nonlethal typhoid cases had recovered. For modern trials of polio by Francis and colleagues of the inactivated polio vaccine (Salk) in 1954 (26), and of hepatitis B by the New York Blood Center group (27) and the Centers for Disease Control multicenter study (28) in the late 1970s, high binding antibody titers were demonstrated to correlate with protection from disease in observational studies. The antibody response seen in natural infection could be reproduced by a safe vaccine product (three-dose course), suggesting likely vaccine trial success *prior* to the initiation of the trial. Disappointing malarial trial results were presaged by the absence of protection from the relevant antibody in conditions of natural infection (29).

For as yet unknown reasons, some persons who may be heavily exposed to HIV do not get infected. Furthermore, high neutralizing or binding antibody is not generally adequate to protect against eventual disease in the face of rapid viral mutation. Chimp studies, where high neutralizing antibodies have correlated with protection from challenge in somewhat ideal experimental circumstances, do suggest an important protective role for humoral immunity, though this may not be sufficient (30,31). In my opinion, discovery of a correlate of protection would be the single greatest advance in HIV immunology of relevance to vaccinology, having enormous impact on strategies for vaccine design and trial planning.

Trial Endpoint

It is not known whether the goal to prevent HIV infection is unrealistic or feasible (32,33). The suitable primary endpoint for measuring protection from infection is assessing the infection event itself in a placebo-controlled, double-blinded clinical vaccine trial. Vaccine-induced antibodies must be distinguished from wild virus-induced immune responses, preferably with field-appropriate technologies like epitope-specific enzyme-linked immunosorbent assay (ELISA) (34). However, no viral vaccines are known to protect against viral infection *per se* (35). Rather, infection is "permitted" in the vaccinated subject and success of immunization is judged by the prevention of disease. Given that such an outcome is of immeasurable significance in HIV/AIDS, as with other viral infections, efficacy trials must accommodate study of secondary endpoints with an assumption that the primary endpoint could prove disappointing. An example of a secondary endpoint includes CD4+ T-lymphocyte decline at the time of acute infection, which naturally averages about a 40% loss from baseline within 2 years after infection (36). Thus, blunting the loss of CD4+ cells during acute HIV infection might provide early suggestion of salutary vaccine impact. Measurement of viral burden postinfection, comparing vaccines and placebo recipients, should be evaluated for its utility as a secondary endpoint, preferably using a technique much less laborious and costly than quantitative viral culture such as quantitative RNA polymerase chain reaction (PCR) assessments (37). Whether viral surrogate markers are at all useful is an important subject for Phase II vaccine trials to address. Thus, the validity of early surrogate markers of disease, so important in antiviral drug and therapeutic vaccine trials, could be equally critical for prophylactic vaccine trials (38).

First generation HIV-1 vaccine candidates may or may not prevent infection; it is of critical importance to design vaccine studies to judge whether disease is modulated by assessing immunological, virological, and clinical parameters among infected recipients of vaccine or placebo. Nested studies may facilitate discovery of one or more correlates of protective immunity in subsets of subjects, even if the full trial is not deemed successful in proving efficacy of a given vaccine candidate. In this way, the testing of first generation vaccine candidates can contribute substantially to scientific progress, even if the optimal trial outcome is not achieved.

Behavioral Research

Few vaccine-preventable diseases are related to infection risk that can be modulated by human behavior. For example, measles, rubella, polio, mumps, *Haemophilus influenzae*, diphtheria, influenza, and tetanus are all ubiquitous in nature, capable of striking down prince or pauper and permitting little escape through prudent personal action. Hepatitis B is an exception to this, insofar as personal drug use or sexual behavior may change one's risk of exposure. If early HIV-1 vaccine candidates proved as highly efficacious as did the hepatitis B vaccines, then measuring risk behavior in HIV-1 vaccine trials might not be necessary to interpret the trial results. But if the HIV-1 vaccine candidates are less than optimally effective, behavior change within the context of the vaccine trial could have a major impact on the interpretability of the trial result. Several examples can be postulated.

A trial volunteer could seek HIV testing to find out whether his or her ELISA had converted to positive and whether the Western blot revealed new bands. We have termed this behavior "decoding," the unbinding of the volunteer through his or her seeking an HIV test. This has already occurred in Phase I trials sponsored by the NIAID (P. Fast, *personal communication*). If subjects who discover that they have received the vaccine are falsely reassured and they engage in high-risk behavior at a rate greater than that of the placebo recipients, then a less-than-optimal vaccine candidate (i.e., 50% to 60% efficacy) may be judged completely ineffective, as a consequence of *selective* high-risk behavior among decoded vaccinees. Work in progress to model this eventuality is underway both in our group (A. Sheon, *personal communication*) (39) and at Emory University (40).

A second eventuality might affect the feasibility of the trial. Volunteers could respond to the HIV-1 prevention education messages provided at the time of HIV-1 testing and trial enrollment. If incidence were to drop substantially among the trial subjects, then sample sizes and/or trial duration would have to increase to accommodate lower-than-expected incidence (Table 2) (41). Such an eventuality would be a positive event for a community; the vaccine researcher must be prepared with contingency plans to expand the study to ensure its scientific viability.

These two examples suggest the need to monitor risky behavior during the trial to assess whether risk is increasing or decreasing, selectively in one

TABLE 2. *Sample size calculations for a hypothetical two-arm placebo-controlled HIV[a] vaccine efficacy trial*

	Total sample size*			
	Annual HIV incidence rate			
Length of trial in years	1%	2%	3%	4%
2	13,700	6900	4600	3500
2.5	9600	4800	3200	2400
3	7400	3700	2500	1900

*For a two-arm trial with 90% power to detect 50% efficacy. Efficacy achieved gradually over a 6-month immunization period. Loss to follow-up is assumed to be 10% per year.

[a]HIV, human immunodeficiency virus.

Source: adapted from references 41 and 44 and Dr. Wasima Rida, personal communication.

arm of the study or overall in the volunteer population. Selection factors for entry into the study should be assessed to see whether lower risk subjects are coming into the trial. Compliance and study dropouts may be affected through understanding volunteer concerns and needs (42). Proper education as to the uncertainty of vaccine benefit and theoretical concerns of vaccine risk, such as enhancement of infection or disease progression, must be part of the enrollment and informed consent process to discourage a false sense of security among vaccinees.

Route of Exposure and STD Impact

It is conceivable that a vaccine product would work better against one route of virus inoculation than another. If a vaccine product induced systemic immunity but little or no mucosal immunity, the vaccine could conceivably protect a health worker from low-dose needle stick exposures or injecting drug users who had few sexual exposures and shared needles only occasionally, while failing to protect from mucosal exposure. (Hepatitis B is reassuring here, in that a systemically induced immune response still protects against disease from a mucosally mediated viral infection [43].) Or conversely, a given vaccine product may induce an immunological blockade adequate to ward off low-level exposures from sexual encounters, but would not protect from high-dose inocula such as those from IDU or contaminated blood and blood product transfusion. Hence, trials may have to be conducted with adequate recruitment among persons of varying risk exposures. Preparatory studies are being sponsored presently by the NIAID at 17 sites in 15 locales within 9 countries to assess the feasibility of large-scale (thousands of volunteers) vaccine efficacy studies (44).

Sexually transmitted infections bear special mention. It is known that genital ulcers are associated with HIV-1 risk, possibly due to the facilitation of contact between the HIV-1 and a CD4+ cell, and are more prevalent and accessible in disrupted mucosa, which may be friable and bleeding, than in epithelially intact mucosa (13,45,46). Could a given vaccine set up an immunological blockade adequate to protect from inocula exposed to an intact epithelial mucosal surface, but inadequate to protect from an exposure to inocula that infected more efficiently through a disrupted epithelial surface infected with a sexually transmitted infection? Nested studies of STD should be considered within HIV-1 vaccine trials to better evaluate the cofactors for protection or for failure of protection (47).

Perinatal transmission interruption by use of passive and/or active immunization will entail vaccination of mother and/or newborn. While some urge a more fundamental understanding of placental pathophysiology and viral tropism "before strategies to prevent maternal-fetal transmission of HIV can be developed," (48) I would argue for a parallel approach of empirical prevention research (to test key concepts such as utility of HIV-hyperimmune globulin [HIVIG]) at the same time that we engage in basic science and animal model work into cell biology, placental physiology, virology, and immunology of perinatal transmission. A vaccine with a less-than-optimal duration might still be quite efficacious in the perinatal setting where fetal protection may accrue even though the immune response induced by the vaccine wanes in just weeks to months.

Site Selection and Sample Size Calculations

The relevance of "matching" circulating virus and specific vaccine constructs may be a dominant factor in selecting sites to participate in selected vaccine trials. This is the first of several criteria for site selection that include genetic and serologic "match" of vaccine product to circulating virus; community and government support; ability to recruit and retain an adequate number of cooperative volunteers; costs; seroincidence in the study population suggesting a feasible trial, even after prevention counseling is provided; adequate laboratory and shipping capacity; adequate clinical evaluation facilities and expertise; ability to manage study data to meet U.S. Food and Drug Administration (and other suitable regulatory agencies outside the U.S.) auditing requirements; and ability to secure informed consent. Several thousand subjects are likely to be needed for a simple two-arm trial (Table 2). Testing multiple candidates or planning for stratum-specific analyses (e.g., by transmission risk status, STD status, or host genetics) would require yet higher sample sizes. Among high-risk populations of young homosexual men, injection drug users, professional sex workers, and others, HIV vaccine trials will, in my judgment, be among the greatest public health research challenges faced to date.

Ethical, Social, and Political Issues

Ethical and sociopolitical concerns are compelling topics that can only be briefly reviewed here. Ethical considerations must be considered well before trial initiation. Given the socially disenfranchised status of most persons at high HIV risk, subject exploitation must not occur or be perceived to be occurring within participating communities. Securing genuinely informed consent may be difficult in the context of poverty and illiteracy, as in some developing nations and in the inner cities of the industrialized world. Adolescents are at high risk in some environments (49,50) and are therefore suitable candidates for trial enrollment. This ushers in concerns that these youth not be manipulated or coerced, and that an appropriate parental role be established (51). Prisoners who have a history of illicit drug use or high-risk sex may be available for vaccination while incarcerated, and may revert to high-risk behavior upon their release from prison. They could benefit from vaccine trial enrollment, but the potential for their manipulation must be considered and minimized (52). Active drug users must be recruited only when they can understand the nature of the study. Persons at high risk may have special concerns to ensure that their trial participation does not "label" them for undesirable consequences of discrimination.

Examples of discrimination may include difficulties in securing employment or life and health insurance due to trial participation. This could come about from testing positive on an HIV screening test, or could even come about from participation in an efficacy trial, which will target persons "at risk" of HIV acquisition. The former concern has been addressed with considerable success by the NIAID-sponsored Phase I/II trials to date with provision of a vaccine trial participation identity card; a confirmatory toll-free telephone number, which a volunteer can provide to any skeptical prospective employer or insurance company; and an explicit agreement with a wide cross-section of the insurance industry not to equate seropositivity with infection in the vaccinee without first securing follow-up specialized testing (P. Fast and D. N. Lawrence, *personal communications*) (34,53). However, these protections have been applicable to only 800 vaccinees to date (1992) and are only relevant in the U.S. setting. When thousands of high-risk subjects are recruited, new agreements must be negotiated to maximize fair access to insurance for trial participants.

A concern for both consumer and manufacturer is the liability for any untoward effects of a given vaccine product. Within the research setting, no guarantees of safety can be made, and this must be made clear in the informed consent. (Products tested in the U.S. have proven safe so far). Upon licensure and broad distribution of a vaccine, however, industry is likely to require some risk-sharing for liability, to ensure profitability. An analogous circumstance nearly crippled U.S. production of childhood vaccination until the U.S. Congress passed legislation to control liability and accommodate its financial risk (54).

Political and social concerns are of paramount importance for the long-term success of vaccine trials. Trial volunteers may have many compelling social needs. These may include health care, housing, transportation, child care, treatment of addictions, and HIV education. Insofar as recruitment and retention depend on a subject's compliance, these issues *must* be considered for a trial to succeed. Community organizations, leaders, and advocates must participate in the process of trial planning if long-term community support is to be expected.

The trial funding agencies must be able to assure sustained support, if answers to vaccine efficacy are to be forthcoming. If first generation HIV vaccines are less-than-optimally successful or if they are unsuccessful, then funding for more promising vaccines may be difficult to secure if politicians do not have a sustained commitment to the goal of an effective and safe HIV-1 vaccine. Political support within governments and communities for vaccine trials may be stronger in some sites than in others. Recruitment and retention of trial subjects may not be feasible in some circumstances and in some populations. Political demagoguery could use the scientific uncertainties and suspicions of government-sponsored exploitation (55) to undermine even an ethical and important study. Finally, costs of this study may be so high as to be unaffordable in many locales.

In summary, the HIV/AIDS vaccine research effort is of compelling public health importance and preparations are in progress to test promising HIV-1 candidate vaccines in large-scale efficacy trials with volunteers at high risk of acquiring infection (30,44). The complexities of vaccine development (56), preclinical and Phase I/II human testing, and community-based Phase III efficacy trials will require a broad partnership of committed parties—scientists, communities, industry, governments, international health organizations, ethicists, advocates, and funding agencies—to achieve success.

REFERENCES

1. Barre-Sinoussi F, Chermann J-C, Rey F, et al. Isolation of a T-lymphotropic retrovirus from a patient at risk for acquired immune deficiency syndrome (AIDS). *Science* 1983;220:868–871.
2. Popovic M, Sarngadharan MG, Read E, Gallo RC. Detection, isolation, and continuous production of cytopathic retroviruses (HTLV-III) from patients with AIDS and pre-AIDS. *Science* 1984;224:497–500.
3. Anonymous. Global health care for HIV disease. *Lancet* 1990;336:1123.
4. Hellinger FJ. Updated forecasts of the costs of medical care for persons with AIDS: 1989–1993. *Public Health Rep* 1990;105:1–12.
5. Chin J, Sato PA, Mann JM. Projections of HIV infections and AIDS cases to the year 2000. *Bull WHO* 1990;68:1–11.
6. Vermund SH. Changing estimates of HIV-1 seroprevalence in the United States. *J NIH Res* 1991;3:77–81.
7. Rosenberg PS, Gail MH, Schrager LK, et al. National AIDS incidence trends and the extent of zidovudine therapy in selected demographic and transmission groups. *J AIDS* 1991;4:392–401.
8. Rosenberg PS, Levy ME, Brundage JF, et al. Population-based monitoring of an urban HIV/AIDS epidemic: magnitude and trends in the District of Columbia. *JAMA* 1992;268:495–503.
9. Monette P. *Borrowed time: an AIDS memoir.* New York: Avon Books; 1988.
10. Hunter SS. Orphans as a window on the AIDS epidemic in Sub-Saharan Africa: initial results and implications of a study in Uganda. *Soc Sci Med* 1990;31:681–690.
11. Michaels D, Levine C. Estimates of the number of motherless youth orphaned by AIDS in the United States. *JAMA* 1992;268:3456–3461.
12. Kaplan EH. Needle exchange or needless exchange? The state of the debate. *Infect Agents Dis* 1992;1:92–98.
13. Vermund SH, Sheon AR, Galbraith MA, et al. Transmission of the human immunodeficiency virus. In: Koff W, Wong-Staal F, Kennedy R, eds. *Annual review of AIDS research*. Vol. 1. New York: Marcel Dekker, Inc; 1991:81–135.
14. Anderson DJ, O'Brien TR, Politch JA, et al. Effects of disease stage and zidovudine therapy on the detection of human immunodeficiency virus type 1 in semen. *JAMA* 1992;267:2769–2774.
15. Mann JM. AIDS—the second decade: a global perspective. *J Infect Dis* 1992;165:245–250.

16. Rotheram-Borus MJ, Koopman C, Haignere C, Davies M. Reducing HIV sexual risk behaviors among runaway adolescents. *JAMA* 1991;266:1237–1241.
17. Karzon DT, Bolognesi DP, Koff WC. Development of a vaccine for the prevention of AIDS: a critical appraisal. *Vaccine* 1992;10:1039–1052.
18. Haynes BF. Scientific and social issues of human immunodeficiency virus vaccine development. *Science* 1993;260:1279–1286.
19. Koff WC, Hoth DF. Development and testing of AIDS vaccines. *Science* 1988;241:426–432.
20. Stein ZA. HIV prevention: the need for methods women can use. *Am J Public Health* 1990;80:460–462.
21. Elia CJ, Heise L. The development of microbicides: a new method of HIV prevention for women. Programs Division Working Paper No. 6. New York: The Population Council; 1993.
22. Kreiss J, Ngugi E, Holmes K, et al. Efficacy of Nonoxynol 9 contraceptive sponge use in preventing heterosexual acquisition of HIV in Nairobi prostitutes. *JAMA* 1992; 268:477–482.
23. Fast PE, Walker MC. Human trials of experimental AIDS vaccines. *AIDS* 1993;7(suppl 1):S147–S159.
24. Hopkins DR. *Princes and peasants: smallpox in history.* Chicago: The University of Chicago Press; 1983:77–81.
25. Cockburn WC. The early history of typhoid vaccination. *J R Army Med Corps* 1955;101:171–185.
26. Francis T Jr, Korn RF, Voight RB, et al. An evaluation of the 1954 poliomyelitis vaccine trials: summary report. *Am J Public Health* 1955;45:1–63.
27. Szmuness W, Stevens CE, Harley EJ, et al. Hepatitis B vaccine: demonstration of efficacy in a controlled clinical trial in a high-risk population in the United States. *N Engl J Med* 1980;303:833–841.
28. Francis DP, Hadler SC, Thompson SE, et al. The prevention of hepatitis B with vaccine: report of the Centers for Disease Control multi-center efficacy trial among homosexual men. *Ann Intern Med* 1982;97:362–366.
29. Hoffman SL, Oster CN, Plowe CV, et al. Naturally acquired antibodies to sporozoites do not prevent malaria: vaccine development implications. *Science* 1987;237:639–642.
30. Johnston M, Fast P, Schultz A, Hoth D. Progress toward development of a vaccine to prevent AIDS. *AIDS Res Hum Retroviruses* 1993;9(suppl 1):S115–S120.
31. Schultz AM, Hu S-L. Primate models for HIV vaccines. *AIDS* 1993;7(suppl 1):S161–S170.
32. Sabin AB. Improbability of effective vaccination against human immunodeficiency virus because of its intracellular transmission and rectal portal of entry. *Proc Natl Acad Sci U S A* 1992;89:8852–8855.
33. Ada G, Blanden B, Mullbacher A. HIV: to vaccinate or not to vaccinate? *Nature* 1992;359:572.
34. Hoff R, O'Shaughnessy MV, Schochetman G, et al. Monitoring immunogenicity and infection in HIV vaccine efficacy trials. *AIDS Res Hum Retroviruses* 1993;9(suppl 1):S69–S72.
35. Ada GL. The immunological principles of vaccination. *Lancet* 1990;335:523–526.
36. Stein DS, Korvick JA, Vermund SH. CD4+ lymphocyte cell enumeration for prediction of clinical course of human immunodeficiency virus disease: a review. *J Infect Dis* 1992;165:352–363.
37. Piatak M Jr, Saag MS, Yang LC, et al. High levels of HIV-1 in plasma during all stages of infection determined by competitive PCR. *Science* 1993;259:1749–1754.
38. Ellenberg SS. Surrogate end points in clinical trials. *Br Med J [Clin Res]* 1991;302:63–64.
39. Vermund SH, Hoff R, Lawrence DL, Fischer RD, Rida WN, Fast PE, Koff WC, Ungar BL, Hoth DF, Barker LF. HIV vaccine efficacy trial preparations. VIII International Conference on AIDS, Amsterdam, 1992, [abstract 4505, vol. 2]: C329.
40. Halloran ME, Longini IM Jr, Struchiner CJ, et al. Exposure efficacy and change in contact rates in evaluating HIV vaccines in the field (in press).
41. Dixon DO, Rida WN, Fast PE, Hoth DF. HIV vaccine trials: some design issues including sample size calculations. *J AIDS* 1993;6:485–496.

42. Vasquez R. A discussion of community concerns regarding HIV vaccines. *AIDS Res Hum Retroviruses* 1993;9(suppl 1):S23–S25.
43. Hilleman MR. Newer directions in vaccine development and utilization. *J Infect Dis* 1985;151:407–419.
44. Vermund SH, Fischer RD, Hoff R, et al. Preparing for HIV vaccine efficacy trials: partnerships and challenges. *AIDS Res Hum Retroviruses* 1993;9(suppl 1):S125–S130.
45. Cameron DW, Simonsen JN, D'Costa LJ, et al. Female to male transmission of human immunodeficiency virus type 1: risk factors for seroconversion in men. *Lancet* 1989;2:403–407.
46. Rodriguez EM, deMoya EA, Guerrero E, et al. HIV-1 and HTLV-I in sexually transmitted disease clinics in the Dominican Republic. *J AIDS* 1993;6:313–318.
47. Wasserheit JN. Epidemiological synergy: interrelationships between human immunodeficiency virus infection and other sexually transmitted diseases. *Sex Transm Dis* 1992;19:61–77.
48. Douglas GC, King BF. Maternal-fetal transmission of human immunodeficiency virus: a review of possible routes and cellular mechanisms of infection. *Clin Infect Dis* 1992;15:678–691.
49. Bowler S, Sheon AS, D'Angelo L, Vermund SH. HIV and AIDS among adolescents in the United States: increasing risk in the 1990s. *J Adolesc* 1992;15:345–371.
50. Wawer MJ, Serwadda D, Musgrave S, et al. Dynamics of spread of HIV-1 infection in a rural district of Uganda. *Br Med J* 1991;303:1303–1306.
51. English A. Expanding access to HIV services for adolescents: legal and ethical issues. In: DiClemente R, ed. *Adolescents and AIDS: a generation in jeopardy*. Newbury Park, CA: Sage Publications; 1992:262–283.
52. Dubler NN, Sidel VW. On research on HIV infection and AIDS in correctional institutions. *Milbank Q* 1989;67:171–207.
53. Stein RE. Insurance and liability issues in AIDS vaccine development. *AIDS Res Hum Retroviruses* 1993;9(suppl 1):S155–S157.
54. Clayton EW, Hickson GB. Compensation under the National Childhood Vaccine Injury Act. *J Pediatr* 1990;116:508–513.
55. Jones JH. *Bad blood*. New York: The Free Press; 1981.
56. Hilleman MR. Impediments, imponderables and alternatives in the attempt to develop an effective vaccine against AIDS. *Vaccine* 1992;10:1053–1058.

DISCUSSION FOR CHAPTERS 14 AND 15

Dr. Dianzani: This morning session is dedicated to vaccine trials, a subject that is very appropriate for an epidemiology meeting.

It took some time before we realized that, in order to design and plan a vaccine, we must also know something about the pathogenesis of the infection. In studying a new infection, you usually begin by considering its epidemiology (in order to learn how it is transmitted and spreads into the population); you then study the biology of the virus, the way it interacts with the host, and so on. Finally, you go into the aspects of molecular biology that enable you to refine this knowledge further.

As everybody knows, the general time course of the development of knowledge about AIDS did not follow the general rule because the molecular biology was already available. Consequently, we went straight from epidemiology to molecular biology, which probably explains why many of the early attempts to make an effective vaccine failed.

Having acknowledged this lack, a lot of work has been done on the pathogenesis of the infection, and we have now come to the point when we can design a vaccine in a more logical way, which is basically what our speakers today talked about.

Dr. Tsiatis: I'm interested in the possible problems that might occur if people find out that they're on vaccine and then change their behavior. This might show an effective vaccine to be ineffective.

Another possibility is to use a kind of intention to treat approach. If this were done in the community, it might reflect how people behave. If indeed something is only partially effective, maybe we should really test whether people change their behavior because they know a vaccine exists.

Dr. Vermund: In most vaccine studies, there are Phase I trials, which are largely concerned with efficacy and getting hints of immunogenicity; Phase II trials, which are much more focused on immunogenicity and getting a hint of efficacy; Phase III trials to see whether the candidate vaccine works; and Phase IV trials (which CDC, and not the NIH, have largely spearheaded in the U.S.), which are very much focused on the community-based effectiveness of a vaccine.

I would personally prefer to do so something closer to a human experiment on efficacy and then go to a Phase IV trial, because I think it would be a tragedy if we actually had an efficacious candidate vaccine, particularly in the context of counselling and testing, and we didn't know it.

Dr. Schultz: At the end of my talk, I was relatively pessimistic about our real preclinical knowledge concerning these vaccines; but, nevertheless, I was in favor of Phase III-type trials in order to get some clear answers. This idea is based on the premise that the worst thing that can happen in these trials is that the vaccine doesn't work. If a vaccine were not effective in a Phase IV trial, the net result would be that a lot more people would become infected because they had changed their behavior. In this case, the worst thing that happens is not simply that the vaccine didn't work.

Dr. Stein: I thought insufficient mention was made of perinatal infection. In these cases, we know the time of infection, who infected whom, that the duration of immunization from the mother can't be more than 9 months, and that there seem to be variations in the rate of transmission across the world—we would know the results sooner. As far as I'm aware, the chimpanzee/macaque explorations haven't considered perinatal transmission. Does SIV transmit? I don't know the answer, but it seems to me there's a lack of interest on the part of both epidemiologists and immunologists in this very important topic that seems to contain some principles that could be very interesting (apart from ethical and human considerations).

Dr. Schultz: I did indicate that the biggest failing of animal models is the modelling of transmission. In the first place, it's just too expensive to do chimpanzee transmissions. In the one case where we inadvertently did the experiment (a pregnant female who was not known to be pregnant was challenged with HIV), there was no transmission, but this was on an n of 1.

In the case of macaques, transmission through the mother has been so inefficient that people are now attempting to get high-efficiency transmission by introducing the virus into the amniotic fluid. You have to remember that Rhesus macaques are all seasonal breeders, and so you can't just do one experiment after another; you have to wait until the right time of the year. That's why there is a shortage of animal data. However, pediatric grants have been awarded to some people, and they are the ones who have given us some of these early data.

Concerning human trials, we come up against the indemnification and regulatory issues: the Food and Drug Administration (FDA) is demanding teratogenicity studies on these vaccines. One problem is that it may be the third, fourth, or fifth month before a pregnant, infected woman comes to your attention, and so how much time do you have even to start an immunization scheme?

If you deal with a cohort of infected women who continue to get pregnant despite counselling, you could then consider simply immunizing the whole cohort and looking for the breakthrough of pregnancy as your trial. There is clearly no ethical problem here because this represents a therapeutic vaccine modality for the mother; but there is evidence that vaccine treatment causes an initial slight increase in viremia, and does that put the child at greater risk? If the risk of transmission is low (say, 1 in 3 to the infant), that means that two-thirds of your study subjects are not at risk.

Speaking as a scientist, it's true that perinatal transmission represents the high rate of transmission you want to look at, but there are enormous problems involved. We're trying to address them, but we don't see the beginning of a perinatal trial in the next 6 to 12 months.

Dr. Dianzani: I might add that some preclinical assays are very discouraging from that point of view. For instance, if you take infected lymphocytes and apply them to cultured endothelial cells, the endothelial cells get infected through the direct transmission of the virus from the lymphocytes. If you remove the infected lymphocytes and replace them with new lymphocytes, those lymphocytes become infected through the endothelial cells. This is not prevented by antibodies, so we probably have to find some other strategy.

Dr. Des Jarlais: One comment on a purely scientific issue. The way people might react to receiving a vaccine by changing their behavior is an empirical question that can and should be studied prior to a Phase III trial. The biggest difficulty right now is a lack of adequate theory in terms of predicting how people might react. We need a theory that says: "Measure these variables as part of your counselling, testing, and vaccine administration, and that will then predict post-vaccine counselling behavior changes." And we also need a data theory to tell us what these variables are. Some competing theories do exist (disinhibition theory and so on), but we need to tie down the theoretical framework because, at the moment, we're in a phase of blind empiricism in predicting post-counselling and post-vaccine administration behavior. We need to get the empirical and theoretical work done before we go on to Phase III trials.

Second, I have a political comment. This epidemic does not exist in a political vacuum, particularly in the U.S. There, the people being asked to participate in vaccine trials suspect that HIV is a man-made virus that is being deliberately put into highly stigmatized groups. That's the political environment in which any U.S. perinatal trial will be conducted. If anything should go wrong, the political downside of "you have harmed babies of such and such a group" would be disastrous. We really need to think in terms of the downside risk for mounting a second or third trial, if anything should go wrong in the first. And people are likely to be least rational if something goes wrong with a perinatal vaccine.

Dr. Gail: Sample size calculations seem to be primarily dominated by considerations of low incidence or seroconversion rates. What would happen if you lost a little specificity in deciding whether someone was infected or not? This is something that might happen if, for example, you gave someone an envelope vaccine and had to relinquish or relax some of the criteria for diagnosing infection based on other antigens that the virus would present. I was a little shocked when I found that if your specificity only dropped to 99% (that is, you got 1% false positives), you'd almost double the required sample size. Any loss in specificity of endpoints would really hurt your sample size.

Dr. Vermund: Here we're considering problems with PCR, because we would use culture and PCR rather than a modified ELISA or Western blot positivity category for something like that. If culture were not feasible (say, in a developing country or where the positivity yield would plummet), PCR would be a reasonable alternative. A 1% loss in specificity in PCR is actually industry-standard and, even in the cleanest labs, a little bit of carry-over contamination can cause the 1%. So I think you're making an excellent point. It gives us a lot more incentive to do cultures as an endpoint.

Dr. Cameron: I'd like to make another point about sample size calculations based on seroconversion rates per annum in high-risk populations in developing countries. The annualized seroconversion rate in an STD clinic is based on a population that, at entry to that clinic, has already been exposed and is in the process of primary infection. At the first visit, the patient is seronegative. The following year's seropositivity reflects conversion subsequent to primary infection. This could lead to an overestimation of the target population in that setting.

Dr. Halloran: Some of my colleagues have been working on the problem of people changing their behavior and increasing their contacts. By separating the contact process from the susceptibility issue, you can formulate all of the possible parameters of evaluation as a function of the number of contacts people make, the probability of transmission per contact, and the effect of the vaccine on transmission probability. You can then create a parameter called behavioral efficacy, which is the increase in the number of contacts per time. If you do a small study in which you get a lot of good behavioral information and you know the number of partners who are infective, you can measure the difference in transmission probability with and without the vaccine.

The interesting thing is that there are two vaccine models that Smith, Rodriguez, and Fine developed in 1984, and that some of us are refining. One model reduces the probability of transmission upon contact, and that would be one efficacy measure. Another efficacy measure is that a proportion of your population has complete protection. (I think that was what Sten Vermund was saying: 60% efficacy means that 60% of the people are completely protected.)

These two models have consequences in terms of deciding whether to do a placebo trial or not, which also depends on which parameter you choose. This is a long and complicated issue, but we have calculated what the biases would be under certain circumstances. If you imagine a situation in which the vaccine affects everybody equally and reduces the probability of transmission, you have behavioral change; in this case, you have a negative bias in biological vaccine efficacy that could be adjusted for behavioral information.

But if you have a model 2 vaccine (which completely protects some people while others don't respond), the nonresponders who test themselves will think they belong to the placebo arm and so will not change their behavior. Only the responders will change their behavior. In this case, there's a parameter that will not change. If you then control for behavior, you will get what will look like increased efficacy because the parameter of interest is not the change in transmission probability, but the proportion of people who are completely protected. Under model 2, the people who are completely protected will change their behavior, the others won't. And, if anything, it's going to look as if the vaccine is protecting more people.

Given the vaccine model, it depends on the parameter you choose and you can calculate that out by using the correct equations and then estimating how far off you're going to be under the conditions of different numbers of people changing their behavior.

Dr. Vermund: Both scenarios sound biologically plausible and are definitely worth developing further.

Dr. Schultz: Can I make a comment that perhaps reflects the fact that people believe more in the data that they themselves can generate? We have been talking about the fact that a trial would be uninterpretable because of the impossibility of modelling behavioral changes.

But, as a biologist, I believe that the people who fail to be protected will be those who have been exposed to a virus rather far from the vaccine virus. To investigate that (and this also addresses the breakthrough problem of how to find out whether someone is merely responding to the vaccine or whether he has been infected), it's absolutely essential to isolate the virus from everyone in the trial who becomes infected. In the absence of any statistically significant measure of protection, if you find a missing window of viruses in vaccinated people (because that's the window of viruses closest to the vaccine), you've at least a biological measurement of this set of viruses while the other viruses are all over the place. Although the percentages stink in terms of a public health intervention (you would not want to recommend this vaccine for widespread use because its not very efficacious), you will have learned something very important and you will have made a first step.

Dr. Dianzani: It's probably even more complicated because, from a biological point of view, establishing the efficacy of a vaccine only using laboratory parameters is probably not enough. Let's imagine a vaccine that does not prevent infection but prolongs latency for 20 or 30 years; we'll never know whether it is effective unless we wait long enough.

Dr. Detels: First of all, I understand that isolation is only 90% accurate. That's another margin of error to consider and, as we both know very well, PCR has tremendous problems.

However, I would like to ask the virologist whether we really know at what level in the process of infection of the cell, and in the replication of the virus, that a vaccination is actually going to work. Is it going to work by preventing the virus from entering the cell, or is it possible that the virus may enter the cell but not complete infection? If it's the latter, I think that you're making some isolations, particularly if the vaccine group is being more promiscuous, since it's a question of the probability of the transient presence of virus and the frequency of exposure, and I think measurement of the outcome may be difficult.

Dr. Vermund: That's what I meant when I showed the vaccine outcome slide for scenario 2 (and possibly for scenario 3, which is permissive of acute infection). What I meant by blunting viral replication was the presence of some modified infection (an unnatural infection) that, although it may have been seen in some people, is not generally seen naturally. Or in scenario 3, viral location is largely permitted but chronic disease is delayed.

Dr. Schultz: Here is a case where there are some relevant animal data. You can't do these experiments in chimpanzees because they don't get sick; but all of the SIV under study do kill the animals. That's what I meant when I said at the beginning that we wouldn't talk about how a vaccine might work because, since we don't know what's necessary for protection, we look at things that might work and then try to induce those.

There is a spectrum of SIV: those that kill animals in 6 to 12 months and that have actually been manipulated by animal-to-animal passage to get that, and other SIV that take 2 to 3 years to kill the animals (those are the ones represented on the slide of different challenge viruses that I didn't go into in detail). If you immunize and then challenge animals with the more aggressive rapid viruses, you do prolong survival in many cases. The animals fail the challenge, they all get infected, and have high viremia; however, instead of dying in 6 to 12 months, they die in 2 to 3 years. That's good, but the virus level stays high. But if you look at the other biological variant of SIV (the one that takes 2 to 3 years to kill), the animals that have been vaccinated and are then challenged also give virus isolation positivity early on, but then go virus isolation negative in a period of 3 to 6 months (some of them even go PCR negative).

In terms of whether we are making progress with a vaccine and how far we still have to go, I tend to think that the less aggressive SIV in vaccinated monkeys suggests promise. HIV and other SIV that have been manipulated for the sake of convenience are not necessarily giving us bad news. But there are now clear data in the animal model that vaccines that fail do give prolonged life, even for aggressive SIV. Because they behave as if they are fully infected, the animals are presumably highly efficient transmitters, it's just that they stay alive longer. But there is other evidence that the endpoint of a successful vaccine could be PCR positivity and virus isolation negativity: stopping the epidemic and probably indefinitely prolonging the life of the vaccine recipient.

Dr. Vermund: Some of you will remember the paper by Anderson, Gupta, and May published in *Nature* about a year ago, where they modelled the international epidemic and tried to model the impact of treatment. I thought they had the monstrously wrong assumption that treatment had no effect on infectiousness. I thought it was a mistake not to run the model with the assumption that treatment did have an impact on infectiousness because, by not doing so, they had an almost Malthusian discussion section saying that if we treated more people, there would be a greater spread of the virus. I didn't like the paper, but I think it's much more legitimate as a concern for vaccine trials where it is conceivable that life could be prolonged as in the case of treatment, but that infectiousness would not necessarily diminish very much. We don't know which way it might go but, knowing virology/immunology, it is not implausible that one could have an infectious patient who lived longer and the population impact of that might very well be what Anderson, Gupta, and May postulated.

Dr. Dianzani: On the other hand, the macaque evidence suggests that the best vaccine is probably human cells.

Dr. Schultz: No, the data on low virulence SIV refer to vaccine priming and boosting that do not have that problem.

Dr. Dianzani: However, the European experience shows that if you vaccinate macaques with killed virus derived from human lymphoblastoid cells, you get consistent protection; but you don't get the same effect if you vaccinate the monkeys with virus grown in their own infected cells.

Dr. Schultz: Although it's true that the majority of the macaque trials have been done with a vaccine of the type you mention, a limited number of trials are not confounded by that variable because the vaccine has nothing to do with human antigens. Even though the challenge virus may have been grown in human cells, that is irrelevant to the protection induced by the vaccine.

Dr. Dianzani: I was not denying that possibility, I was just pointing out that you can vaccinate macaques with human cells. This is another possibility because probably some type of HLA antigen or something else is involved (perhaps something that has not yet been considered).

Dr. Vlahov: Intravenous drug users (IDU) seem to be singled out in terms of their willingness to cooperate with the needs of both epidemiological and clinical trial protocols. However, I would like to point out that it might be unfair to single out IDU in this case. I think that there is a growing body of evidence that, working with this population, you will see rates of cooperation that are similar to those of other populations.

My second comment is that you raised the issue of informed consent and talked about special populations (including IDU and prisoners). The point to come back to there is that the mechanical aspects of informed consent have been fully worked out in these populations for different types of vaccines, under different therapeutic protocols and in different situations; however, emphasis needs to be placed on the level of comprehension of these populations. Selection should be extended to other populations where comprehension may be a problem; people initially agree, but their motivations for participating in trials may be different.

The third issue is the interest that people might have in finding out what their vaccine status might be. Although this is of great theoretical concern, I'm not convinced that it will be a major issue in practice. Given my experience in working with these populations, I don't think the number of patients in clinical trials who will spend time or energy finding out their results will represent a major problem.

Finally, is any discussion concerning vaccine trials being conducted in Italy?

Dr. Dianzani: In Italy, there is a vaccine development program that is mainly carried out in collaboration with other European countries; that is, Italy is part of the European project and we lost a lot of macaques because of their response to human cells, although we are now starting again.

Furthermore, therapeutic vaccine trials are being planned in collaboration with commercial enterprises; for example, a reasonably large trial using GP160 is about to begin. So far, we have been much more deeply involved with advanced chemotherapy trials, but we are very interested in other opportunities that may arise and, as we are doing with the European community, we would be happy to participate in international projects.

Dr. Vella: Before we start any trials, we must be clear about the fact that no known vaccine protects against infection; we are looking for something that protects from disease, not infection. I would like to know whether Dr. Schultz thinks that we are likely to find something that protects against infection looking at the portal of entry? Have the challenges in animals been done by intravenous administration or by mucosal routes? I can imagine neutralizing antibodies that protect against infection if they are administered intravenously, but not from a non-local portal of entry.

Dr. Schultz: I said in my talk that the concept of sterilizing immunity (that is, preventing the first infective event) was not a meaningful way of planning the working of a vaccine. You can demonstrate that the transfer of huge amounts of antibody to chimpanzees seems to have worked in that way, but I think that one is going to have to be able to recover from some early infectious events. The result of a successful vaccine will be PCR-positive people who have been exposed, have replicated virus, and then have suppressed that virus very, very deeply by means of some immune mechanism so that it doesn't come back.

The animal challenges have largely been done intravenously. There have been vaginal challenges in monkeys, which require approximately 1000-fold more virus laid gently in the vaginal vault in order to do a purely mucosal challenge. Once again, we are facing the transmission issue. What are we modelling in the animals? How much is compromising the mucosal barrier part of transmission? Is that really the way people are exposed, or are there micro-tears and even frank lesions?

Encouraging results from the animal model include the fact that monkeys have been protected against rectal challenge with a whole activator vaccine; but, of course, the actual mechanism of protection may well involve human antigens (given that there is confounding by that variable). Nevertheless, the animals are not only protected against intravenous challenge, they are also protected against rectal challenge. So far, attempts at making vaginal challenges with the same vaccines have not been successful. It is as if the vaginal vault is more sensitive to infection than the cells lining the rectal cavity. This year, however, by using oral and tracheal immunizations, the first protection against vaginal challenge in monkeys has just been reported. That's an encouraging advance. Again, it's human-grown virus and human-grown challenge, so maybe the modality hasn't changed. But we have made an advance from the negative results obtained by doing intramuscular vaccinations and failing to get any vaginal protection. Now, using mucosal surface immunizations, we are getting protection against mucosal challenges. Incremental steps and advances are being made in terms of science, it's just that we do not know how far we have to go before expanding human studies.

Dr. Muñoz: I would like to have some information on the status and future plans for therapeutic vaccine studies, especially with reference to scenarios 5 and 6 that concern enhancing the infection and accelerating the disease process.

Dr. Vermund: That's a very big subject. Therapeutic vaccines have strong industry interest and tremendous interest in communities of HIV-infected people. We haven't highlighted it for this presentation because it wasn't our assigned topic and because it's not as tightly networked to epidemiology communities, although biostatisticians find the issues to be analogous to those in drug trials. As you can imagine, there is interest in the issue of surrogate markers, and there is now a raging debate as to whether trials can go forward with surrogate-marker endpoints as recently proposed to the FDA by the U.S. Army. We have a number of therapeutic trials being sponsored by the U.S. Government, by the Europeans, and by private companies. In academic centers, there must be at least 20 such trials, though some of them are modest Phase I studies.

Jonas Salk is in the middle of a controlled Phase II trial with the Immune-Response Corp. candidate that, as you probably know, is a whole-killed virus stripped of envelope. This is quite a nontraditional approach since most people think envelope is the most immunogenic part. Salk has chosen to inactivate the vaccine and make absolutely sure it's safe by stripping it of envelope and feeling that core antigens will be adequate. But Salk's actually developing a whole series of theories that antibody is not particularly relevant any more and has some very controversial points of view concerning the need for cell-mediated immunity for protection.

In a nutshell, I think there are enormous challenges in these therapeutic trials; we must beware of nontraditional approaches towards evaluation by taking immunological responders, segregating them, and analyzing them separately from the immunologic nonresponders. There are various post-hoc analyses that, if you read, say, the Redfield paper in the 1991 *New England Journal of Medicine,* I think some of us interested in clinical trial methodology would have some concerns about. There are some very interesting immunologic and surrogate marker data forthcoming. The first trial to be done as a full-scale Phase II trial is the Walter Reed/Redfield trial, and the code broken on that has been in 1993. That result will be explosive regardless of what it shows.

Dr. Friedman: On the question of behavior change, I think we should be thinking of it as a kind of Phase II study, with all of the theoretical development we can get into it. But when we talk about doing it as Phase III, we're talking about fairly serious large numbers in communities where people at risk have already reduced their risk a lot and have a pent-up wish they could relax their precautions; some of the community's members could go back to some dangerous behaviors. You could be talking about taking stabilized epidemics and potentially destabilizing them. Also, when you talk about Anderson and May's model, I agree with you that the way they dealt with it was not adequate, but the questions of behavior change are also relevant there. As we do these trials, and as we go into full-blown application of a vaccine to a community, we need to be sure that the behavior change parameters are correct. With a partially effective vaccine, people are going to increase their risk and increase infectiousness towards others. One very powerful method that we know from some of the stuff on counselling and testing outcomes among drug users is that simply by making them fully aware of their responsibilities towards others, we get a response, and it works.

Dr. Moss: This question is about people who are thinking about participating in possible Phase III trials. What are visible on the horizon are the envelope protein vaccines and if we're really going to do this in 1½ or 2 years from now, that's what we're looking at. What do we need to see over the next year that would make us believe that this is a good thing to do?

Dr. Schultz: I quickly went over the Phase I candidates that have chimpanzee data. I am awaiting with great interest the results of two chimpanzee trials that will certainly be accomplished by the time any final decisions concerning Phase III trials are made. These are the two mammalian GP120 products that have been giving the most promising results in our Phase I trials in terms of the ratio of neutralizing antibody married to binding antibody and also cross-neutralizing antibody, although the percentage of people responding is not high. And both Chiron and Genentech have immunized animals, so this will be the first test of this product to see if it shows the same kind of benefit that the Genentech product has shown.

Genentech is moving on now; its first chimpanzee experiment was with the IIIB-based product, which protected against IIIB challenge. They now have several chimpanzees immunized with the MN product (the same GP120 but now using the MN strain, which is entering a Phase I trial). Interestingly enough, it seems to give better immune responses to MN and other viruses than the IIIB product gave to IIIB and other viruses. Genentech have built in short-term homologous challenge. They are also using six animals—two to be challenged 2 weeks after the completion of the course with original MN; two to be challenged 2 weeks after the completion of the immunization with IIIB for the variation issue; and then two that were started sooner, so that at the time that they are challenged along with the other animals, it will have been several months since they received their last shot—to look at the decay of antibody and the duration of protection issue. The MN stock is not going to be available on the expected trajectory. But, SF2 and MN are close enough that I have been formally requested by Genentech to supply them with the SF2 challenge stock, which they will use.

I think that, within a year from now, these two crucial experiments will have been accomplished in chimpanzees on the two leading candidates for subunits. We can revisit the good news or the bad news or the intermediate news at that time.

Dr. Vermund: Can I just make the point that we are committed to *preparing* for vaccine efficacy trials; we are not committed to doing them if the candidates are not appropriate or if important details of the trials are not well worked out. We are not going to exploit an infrastructure inappropriately. We would like to have some degree of consensus within the scientific community that this is an appropriate thing to do. Having said that, we don't want to have a candidate that is suitable for testing, and not be ready to test it. So we are committed to setting up the infrastructure. Our goal is to have an infrastructure in place by the end of 1993. Should these infrastructures not be useful for a vaccine trial at any given time, they may very well be useful for other prevention trials. They might be very suitable environments for some of you to conduct other important trials, not necessarily vaccine trials.

Dr. Cameron: I'm familiar with the design of a Phase II controlled GP160 trial underway in Canada, and I would like to raise a design concern that I have. One of the primary outcome parameters of this therapeutic trial is immunologic modulation or response—a change in CD4 T-cell counts over time. The treatment arm is given GP160 with adjuvant, and the placebo arm is given an immunologically inert inoculation without adjuvant. I have a serious concern about the interpretation of clinical trials like this.

Second, the trial I'm referring to crosses over at a study endpoint, and will not, with subsequent follow-up, be able to test the hypothesis of subsequent disease acceleration even if there is transient response of primary outcome parameters, let alone durability of effect.

Dr. Des Jarlais: One of the things that didn't get emphasized much in the discussion, although it was briefly mentioned in the talks, was the whole idea of informed consent. For ethical vaccine trials, we really need to address this issue in much more detail than it's given in most of our studies. My own personal experience is that a lot of informed consents are simply lawyers writing a document to protect the Institution in case something should go wrong. I would also say that if informed consents are not understood by the subjects any better than they usually are by the Institutional Review Board, we're going to be in very big trouble for vaccine trials.

Dr. Dianzani: There is increasing evidence that, during acute infection, recovery coincides with the development of both humoral and cell-mediated immune response. This suggests that, also in this disease, the immune mechanisms and defenses do their job. I don't think the fact that some infection remains is peculiar to retroviruses, it is probably true for polio virus and it's certainly true for measles. The key issue here is to make the initial infection mild enough not to interest a large number of latent cells. If this is true, we have to consider that immune response is both antibody and cell mediated. The envelope proteins usually make neutralizing antibody, they don't last long, and they don't neutralize various variants. Cell-mediated immunity is usually activated against capsid proteins. In theory, neither protein alone should induce a protective stage. Why hasn't a combined vaccine been tried so far (maybe with recombinant proteins, but one envelope and the other P24 perhaps). This is probably a strategy that should be considered.

Dr. Schultz: The short and unsatisfactory answer to that question is that the technology for combining the two different products generally doesn't exist in the same company. That's the problem with being dependent on the pharmaceutical industry to make these vaccines. Even to do it separately, how many years of negotiations did it take to get the HIVAC Vaccinia followed by the MicroGeneSys GP160? Bristol-Myers wanted to make sure that if the vaccine trial went sour, it wasn't going to be their fault. MicroGeneSys had the same fear, saying that their vaccine wouldn't have been bad if it hadn't been primed with the vaccine that was given in the first place. These are not simple issues.

A more optimistic answer (I passed rather briefly over the issue of pseudo-virions) is whole inactivated virus. Why hasn't that been used? There are the four chimpanzee studies. The Immune Response Corporation didn't design it to be stripped of envelope, but when they found that it didn't have envelope, they turned that into an advantage and said that's really what they wanted after all. But IIIB is a particularly poor virus at retaining envelope through purification. Some other strains (MN, remarkably enough) tend to hold on to their envelope better. There are now companies that have been producing genetically inactivated virions that do not contain a genome. In our freezer, we have virions made by two different techniques and a proposal from another group to do whole virus inactivation. We will test these various products in some of the new primate HIV macaque models (chimeric viruses and so on, which I won't go into). That way we can do a 20-animal experiment with 4 different products and then confirm any positive result in chimpanzees. This strategy is adopted knowing the $100,000 price tag of each chimpanzee experiment. Serving as a broker for the traditional products that the private sector considers as running the danger of being unsuccessful, we are doing what we can to take the most straightforward approach to vaccines.

Dr. Dianzani: In a sense, this reminds me of a recent experience I had when sailing with a friend of mine in his boat. The boat was a magnificent motor yacht, and the guy spent hours praising the quality of the motor while we were sailing. At a certain point, the sea got rough and we tried reaching the shore by sail in a rather unsafe way. I asked, "Why don't you switch the motor on?" "Because I don't have any fuel!"

But I really think that the vaccine program has made fantastic progress. We cannot yet say that we are around the corner, but at least we have arrived at the corner and, albeit with a periscope, we can see something.

HIV Epidemiology: Models and Methods, edited by Alfredo Nicolosi. Raven Press, Ltd., New York © 1994.

16

Concept and Estimation of Attributable Risks in HIV Epidemiologic Research

M. Elizabeth Halloran

Emory University School of Public Health, Atlanta, Georgia 30329

The concept of attributable risk was introduced by Levin in 1953 as a measure of the proportion of disease attributable to a given risk factor (1). Since then, attributable risk has been used extensively as a measure of the public health importance of an exposure. Nicolosi et al. (2) evaluated the relative role of parenteral and sexual transmission of human immunodeficiency virus (HIV) in seronegative drug users recruited from 25 drug dependence treatment centers in northern Italy. Between 1987 and 1989, 35 seroconversions occurred in 635 participants. The incidence rate ratios were 3.3 (95% confidence interval [CI], 1.4–7.5) for subjects aged <20 years, 2.4 (95% CI, 1.2–4.7) for <2 years of intravenous drug use, 2.2 (95% CI, 0.9–5.5) for syringe sharing, and 1.0 for subjects with an HIV-positive sexual partner. Nicolosi et al. performed a case-control analysis using multiple logistic regression and adjusting for sex, age, area, and prevalence. The analysis yielded odds ratios of 13.2 (95% CI, 3.1–56.8) for frequent syringe sharing and 4.0 (95% CI, 1.5–10.4) for sexual contacts with seropositive partners. The authors conclude that parenteral transmission is the most important route of infection with HIV among intravenous drug users, and sexual transmission plays a relevant, additive role.

Greenland and Robins (3,4) have shown that the attributable fraction is actually a family of causal parameters containing at least three distinct concepts. The excess fraction is the proportionate increase in number of infections produced by an exposure in a specified time interval. The etiologic fraction is the fraction of infections produced by a causal pathway in which the exposure has an effect. The hazard fraction at some time t is the fraction of the hazard rate that is due to the exposure. This family of parameters corresponds closely to the family of vaccine efficacy parameters that represent the prevented fraction in the exposed (5–9). Vaccine efficacy was discussed analogously to attributable fraction by Greenwood and Yule as early as 1915 (10).

In this paper, we review the family of concepts of attributable fraction and estimation of the excess fraction, including in the multivariate setting (11) with an application to HIV transmission in intravenous drug users. We emphasize the time-varying aspects of estimates of both the excess and the hazard fractions. This dependence on time makes causal interpretation of their values contingent on the duration of follow-up. We discuss the relationship to current research in concepts of vaccine efficacy and survival analysis, and show that the concept of excess fraction in the exposed has an added dimension under conditions of dependent happenings in infectious disease (12).

HIV TRANSMISSION IN INTRAVENOUS DRUG USERS

We construct a hypothetical study with some similarities to that of Nicolosi et al. (2) for this example. Suppose we begin at time $t = 0$ with a closed cohort of N seronegative intravenous drug users, and that at time t after the beginning of the observation period, $M(t)$ are infected. We assume that there are only two modes of transmission: (a) parenteral, through sharing syringes with HIV-infected people, and (b) sexual, through sexual contact with HIV-infected partners. Let $N_p(0)$ be the initial number of people in the cohort sharing syringes. Let $A_p(t) = N_p(0)(1 - S_p(t))$ be the number of infections in those exposed to infection by syringes by time t, where $S_p(t)$ is the survival function. Let $N_s(0)$, $A_s(t)$, and $S_s(t)$ be the corresponding quantities in those with HIV-positive partners.

There are four basic categories of exposure to infection in the cohort:

1. those who do not have sex, or at least do not have sex in any way that permits transmission, and also do not share syringes;
2. those who share syringes, but who do not have sex, or at least do not have sex in any way that permits transmission;
3. those who do not share syringes, but who have sex in some manner permitting transmission;
4. those who share syringes and also have sex in a manner permitting transmission.

People in category (a) will presumably have an infection incidence rate equal to 0. Let $P_+(t)$ and $P_-(t)$ be the proportions sharing and not sharing syringes at time t, respectively, and $S_+(t)$ and $S_-(t)$ be the proportions exposed and not exposed to sexual transmission, respectively. Then the cohort is divided into the four proportions: $P_-S_-(t)$ having no exposure to infection, $P_+S_-(t)$ and $P_-S_+(t)$ having exposure only to parenteral and sexual transmission, respectively, and $P_+S_+(t)$ having exposure to both types of transmission. The relative proportion of susceptibles in each category can change over time as people become infected.

Let $h_p(t)$ and $h_s(t)$ be the hazard rates, or incidence of infection from sharing syringes and sex, respectively. The hazard rate from syringes is a function of the transmission probability β from infective needle to susceptible, the frequency f of fixing, the probability r that a fix is done with a reused needle, and the probability $\theta_p(t)$ that the previous person using the needle was infective. The probability that the previous person using the syringe was infected can be estimated from prevalence of infection in the people sharing syringes under the assumption of random sharing of syringes.

The hazard of infection from sexual activity is a function of the transmission probability p between infective and susceptible, the number of sexual contacts per unit time c, and the prevalence of infection in the sex partner pool, $\theta_s(t)$. Each person i in the cohort could have individual hazards $h_{pi}(t)$ and $h_{si}(t)$. The transmission probability could be sex-specific. Also, the seroprevalence in the pool of sex partners could be sex-specific or could differ between areas. The overall hazard in men could differ from that in women. For simplicity, we begin by assuming that those who share syringes all do it at exactly the same rate and with the same pool of sharers, and that those who have any exposure to sexual transmission all have exactly the same exposure. We also assume that behavior is independent of time and that risk of infection from one route is independent of the risk of infection from the other. That is, the two routes of infection are independent competing risks in those who engage in both types of behavior.

The simplest multiplicative model yields the hazards of infection from each source as

$$h_p(t) = fr\beta\theta_p(t)$$

$$h_s(t) = cp\theta_s(t).$$

The overall hazard at the beginning of observation of the closed cohort will be

$$h(0) = S_+(0)cp\theta_s(0) + P_+(0)\beta fr\theta(0).$$

The proportion of the total population hazard due to syringes and sex at the beginning of the observation period, respectively, will be

$$\frac{S_+(0)cp\theta_s(0)}{S_+(0)cp\theta_s(0)+P_+(0)\beta fr\theta(0)}, \qquad \frac{P_+(0)\beta fr\theta(0)}{S_+(0)cp\theta_s(0)+P_+(0)\beta fr\theta(0)}.$$

The probability of a person j becoming infected by time t is

$$S_j(t) = 1 - \exp\left(-\int_0^t [h_p(t)x_{1j} + h_s(t)x_{2j}]dt\right), \qquad [1]$$

where x_{1j} and x_{2j} are indicator variables for whether the person is exposed to parenteral and sexual infection, respectively. The integral is the integrated hazard function $H_j(t)$ for person j in the time interval $(0,t)$.

There are nine factors that go into each of these. Any one of these nine factors can be affected by an intervention program. The transmission probabilities from sexual activity and from using an infective needle could be reduced by the use of condoms and bleach, respectively. Bleach will not affect the hazard of infection from sexual activity and condoms will not affect the hazard of infection from sharing syringes. If someone stops sharing needles, then the proportion $P_+(0)$ will differ. Having an HIV-positive partner is equivalent to a person choosing her or his partner from a pool of prevalence $\theta_s(t) = 1$.

By writing out these hazard functions, we have expressed one temporal level of the causal model. In the background there is a very dynamic system that we have not taken into account. We have not expressed the prevalence in the partner and syringe sharing pools as a function of incidence in the cohort under observation. The background prevalence could be increasing dramatically in the early stages of the epidemic. This might be influenced by an intervention program due to the dependent happenings (12,13) in infectious diseases. This is a further complicating factor in estimating the excess or hazard fraction that is touched upon briefly below.

ATTRIBUTABLE RISK: FAMILY OF CONCEPTS

We now examine the family of concepts of attributable risk on this example. Emphasis is on the difference between etiologic and excess fractions, the role of time in the definitions and estimates, the difference between the excess fraction and the hazard fraction, and the difference between the estimated causal effect in the exposed and in the entire cohort.

Excess Versus Etiologic Fraction

The excess fraction in the exposed is defined as the fraction of the infections in the exposed that would not have occurred by time t if the exposure had been removed. The etiologic fraction in the exposed are those infections in which the exposure played an etiologic role. To demonstrate the difference, we follow the development of Greenland and Robins (3). They consider a point exposure, while our example requires ongoing exposure to infection.

We focus on the sharing of syringes as the exposure. We identify three types of infected persons with the exposure of interest. Suppose that cumulative incidence is evaluated over a specified risk period or time interval $(0,t)$. Say the follow-up period was 4 years. Suppose we have a cohort of 1000 people, all of whom share needles and have seropositive sex partners. Then there are three types of infected people in this cohort.

Type 0: The exposure (sharing syringes) had no effect on the time of infection.
Type 1: The exposure (sharing syringes) made the time of infection earlier than it would have been in its absence. But had the exposure not occurred, the infection would still have occurred before *t*.
Type 2: Had the exposure (syringes) not occurred, the subject would not have become a case. In the absence of exposure, infection would have occurred after *t* or not at all. This would include infections in people using only syringes and not having sex with HIV-positive partners.

Type 0 infections are presumably from sexual contacts, while types 1 and 2 are from infection by syringe before elimination of the exposure to sharing syringes. The number of each type of infection at time *t* is $A_0(t)$, $A_1(t)$, and $A_2(t)$, respectively. Although we say that we can identify these three types of infection in principle, in practice we probably cannot distinguish whether a person became infected by sexual or parenteral transmission.

Type 0 infections are not attributable to sharing syringes or any aspect of transmission from syringes. Type 1 and 2 infections are both etiologic infections, in that sharing of syringes played a role in the infection. Type 1 infections are not excess infections, however, because they would have become infected by time *t* anyway. If we completely remove syringes as a source of infection, then some people become infected by sex who otherwise would have been infected by syringes. These are type 1 infections. If we consider the exposure to be the absence of a bleach program, where we assume that bleach reduces the transmission probability, then some of the infections from syringes might take place at a later time, but still before the time of analysis. These are also type 1 infections. Type 2 infections are the excess infections that would not have occurred by time *t* if the exposure to infection were completely removed, or if the hazard were reduced so that if infection still occurs, it will happen after the end of follow-up. If we lengthened our period of observation, some type 2 infections might become type 1 infections if the individual hazard rate from syringe sharing were not reduced to 0.

Consider now the cohort of 1000 people exposed to HIV through both sex and sharing syringes. Let the underlying constant hazard from both be h_s = 0.1 and h_p = 0.1 (Table 1). The number of infections from each route after 4 years of follow-up is 295, for a total of 590 infections. Thus, there are 295 etiologic infections from sharing syringes. The etiologic fraction in the exposed is 0.50. This fraction does not change from year to year in this example.

1. The excess fraction in the exposed decreases with time. In the first year, 100 of the 200 infections are through syringes. The excess fraction in the exposed after the first year is 0.50. If sharing of syringes were eliminated, the number of infections from sexual transmission alone would be 344 rather than 295. Although originally 295 of the infections after 4

TABLE 1. *Excess fraction of infections from sharing syringes in those who share syringes*

Year	Infections from Sex	Infections from Syringes	Susceptibles remaining	Infections from sex	Susceptibles remaining	$A_0(t)$	$A_1(t)$	$A_2(t)$	$EF_e(t)$
1	100	100	800	100	900	100	—	100	0.50
2	80	80	640	90	810	80	10	70	0.47
3	64	64	512	81	729	64	17	47	0.44
4	51	51	410	73	656	51	22	29	0.41
Total	295	295		344		295	49	246	

years were due to syringes, complete elimination of sharing syringes will not reduce the number of infections by 295. After 4 years of follow-up, the excess fraction of infections due to syringes in those sharing syringes has declined from 0.50 to (590–344)/590 = 0.41. Since everyone in this subpopulation is exposed to infection through the sexual route, eventually everyone will become infected, ignoring mortality. The excess fraction from those sharing syringes in those exposed to both sexual and syringe transmission will approach 0 if follow-up is long enough.

2. The etiologic fraction and the excess fraction are not necessarily equal. In this situation of assumed independent competing risks, when one entire pathway of infection is eliminated, there are more infections due to the other pathway because the amount of person-time at risk increases. The hazard rate due to sexual exposure, however, does not increase.
3. If the cohort were exposed to infection only by sharing syringes, the excess fraction due to syringes at all times would be equal to 1. If that route of transmission were to be eliminated, no one would get infected. In a group or subpopulation exposed to infection only by sexual transmission or not at all, the excess fraction from syringe sharing is at all times is equal to 0.

Estimation of the Excess Fraction

We cannot observe the same cohort sharing syringes and not sharing syringes. So to estimate the excess fraction, we need a comparison group that we assume to be comparable in every way except that they do not share syringes. Let $CI_1(t)$ and $C_0(t)$ be the cumulative incidence in the exposed and unexposed at time t, respectively. The excess fraction in the exposed is estimated by

$$EF_e(t) = \frac{CI_1(t) - CI_0(t)}{CI_1(t)}. \qquad [2]$$

In order to estimate this quantity, we have to have a group of people who are exposed to the exposure under study and an unexposed comparison group whom we assume are exchangeable.

A cohort of 1000 seronegative intravenous drug users could initially be distributed among the four exposure categories approximately as in Nicolosi et al. (2):

		share syringes		total
		no	yes	
sexual	no	560	240	800
exposure	yes	140	60	200
total		700	300	1000

In this distribution, the probability of sharing syringes is approximately independent of the probability of having an HIV-positive sex partner.

Nicolosi et al. (2) distinguished two categories of exposure to sexual infection somewhat differently from in our initial example. One category contains people with a proven seropositive partner, the other contains people with the serostatus of the partner apparently unknown. This does not preclude transmission in the second exposure category. Indeed, 9 of the 35 seroconversions observed in their study occurred in people who did not share syringes and did not have known HIV-positive partners. In this example, we consider the hazard of infection in the category with high sexual exposure to be $\lambda_h = 0.5$ and low sexual exposure to be $\lambda_l = 0.2$. The hazard of infection from sharing syringes is $\lambda_p = 0.1$.

If sexual exposure is equally distributed in the syringe sharers and the nonsyringe sharers, as in the first distribution given, we can estimate the excess fraction of infections in the exposed at time t by the relative difference in the number of infections in the exposed and the unexposed at time t. This is shown in Table 2. The excess fraction decreases over 4 years from 0.80 to 0.77.

We could also have a cohort of intravenous drug users in which people who share syringes have a higher probability of having HIV-positive sex partners than those who do not share syringes:

		share syringes		total
		no	yes	
sexual	no	550	150	700
exposure	yes	100	200	300
total		650	350	1000

If we do not take into account the difference in the distribution, then we will have an estimate of the excess fraction that is biased. Using this new distribution of the categories, and falsely assuming that the distribution of exposure to sexual transmission is the same in the syringe sharers as in the nonsyringe sharers, we would estimate the excess fraction of infections to be

TABLE 2. *Excess fraction of infections under independence and nonindependence of syringe sharing and sexual exposure*

		Nonindependence	
Year	Independence estimated $EF_e(t)$	Estimated $EF_e(t)$	Actual $EF_e(t)$
1	0.80	0.80	0.71
2	0.79	0.79	0.69
3	0.78	0.78	0.68
4	0.77	0.77	0.66

0.77 at the end of 4 years. The actual excess fraction in the exposed by the end of 4 years would be 0.66.

Care needs to be taken in choosing the comparison group. Suppose we want to estimate the excess fraction in the exposed of not using bleach. If the exposure is "sharing syringes and not using bleach," then the unexposed group is "sharing syringes and using bleach."

In summary,

1. All excess infections are etiologic infections. Etiologic infections are not necessarily excess infections.
2. In infectious diseases, the excess and etiologic fractions in the exposed can be equal, and they can both be equal to 1. Suppose the only route of transmission were parenteral. If this were eliminated, all infections would be eliminated. Thus, all infections that occur are etiologically related to sharing syringes, and would not occur if that exposure to infection were eliminated.
3. The excess fraction can be estimated easily. The biologically meaningful etiologic fraction is more difficult to identify. They should not be confused.
4. The excess fraction can decrease with time, and indeed can become 0. The time dependence needs to be taken into account when trying to interpret it as a causal parameter.

Hazard Fraction

The hazard fraction in the exposed at time t is the relative difference in the instantaneous probability of becoming infected under exposure and nonexposure:

$$HF_e(t) = \frac{h_1(t) - h_0(t)}{h_1(t)} = \frac{\rho(t) - 1}{\rho(t)}, \quad [3]$$

where $\rho(t) = h_1(t)/h_0(t)$. One advantage of the hazard fraction over the excess fraction is that it can be estimated in a dynamic cohort. Robins and Greenland (4) discuss estimability and estimation of the hazard fraction and its relationship to the excess fraction in detail. This discussion is also current in the vaccine efficacy literature (5,8,9,14). Since we cannot distinguish people who become infected from syringes from those infected through sexual contact in those who are exposed to both routes of infection, we can only estimate the hazard rates in those exposed to only one or the other routes. Then making the assumption of independent competing risks, we can compute the total number of infections from one route and from the other.

The four categories represent heterogeneities in the population. If the sizes of these categories are not taken into account, then the proportion of the incidence due to one or the other categories will be misinterpreted. If the hazard rate from sharing needles is greater than that from sexual exposure, then the proportion sharing needles will decrease more rapidly than the proportion with sexual exposure. Even if nothing else changes, and in the absence of an intervention program, the hazard fraction of HIV infection in the entire cohort due to sharing syringes will decrease with time due to effects related to frailty selection (15). Under equal distribution of sexual exposure in the syringe sharers and nonsharers, the overall incidence of infection changes:

$$h(0) = (.56)(.02) + (.12)(.05) + (.24)(.12) + (.08)(.15) = 0.06,$$
$$h(4) = (.65)(.02) + (.12)(.05) + (.18)(.12) + (.05)(.15) = 0.05.$$

Because of these frailty effects, Brunet et al. (5) have suggested that vaccine efficacy be defined based on the summary hazard ratio at the beginning of the observation period. This approach could also be applied to defining the hazard fraction.

EXCESS FRACTION ADJUSTED FOR MULTIPLE RISK FACTORS

Nicolosi et al. (2) estimate adjusted odds ratios using multiple logistic regression as if the cohort were a case-control study. The controls are those who did not become infected during the follow-up period. Assume there are k risk factors. Bruzzi et al. (11) provide a method to estimate the adjusted excess fraction at time t using multiple logistic regression based on the model:

$$\ln\left[\frac{p_j(t)}{1 - p_j(t)}\right] = \alpha + \sum_{i=1}^{k} \beta_i x_{ij}, \quad [4]$$

where $p_i(t)$ is the probability that the ith individual becomes infected by time t, and x_{ij} are the k covariate values for the subject j. The notation is partly from Kooperberg and Pettiti (16). The parameters α and β_i can be estimated by maximum likelihood.

The expected number of infections in the cohort is obtained by adding up the individual probabilities of becoming infected, given the covariates:

$$C(t) = \sum_j P(y_j = 1|x_j). \quad [5]$$

The adjusted excess fraction of infections in the cohort for any covariate in the model is estimated by computing the number of infections expected if no one had that covariate. If the covariate is dichotomous, then it is the number of infections $C_1(t)$ expected if $x_{1j} = 0$ for all j. If the covariate has different levels, it is the number expected when all with some level of interest were to take on another level of the covariate. We consider the dichotomous situation. Suppose that covariate 1 represents whether someone shares syringes or not. The number of infections expected in the time interval $(0,t)$ of follow-up in the absence of the covariate 1 is

$$C_1(t) = \sum_j \frac{\exp\left(\hat{\alpha} + \sum_{i=2}^{k}\hat{\beta}_i x_{ij}\right)}{1 = \exp\left(\hat{\alpha} + \sum_{i=2}^{k}\hat{\beta}_i x_{ij}\right)}. \quad [6]$$

The estimated adjusted excess fraction for the main effect of variable 1 is

$$\widehat{EF}_{p1}(t) = \frac{C(t) - C_1(t)}{C(t)}. \quad [7]$$

If the exposure under study were sharing syringes, then we could estimate in this way the adjusted excess fraction of cases in the cohort due to sharing syringes. Kooperberg and Petitti (16) provide a bootstrap method for standard errors and confidence intervals in an unmatched case-control study.

There are several important considerations when estimating the adjusted excess fraction using multiple logistic regression. First, we have emphasized that the probability of becoming infected increases as time progresses. Thus, the logit function $\ln[(p_i(t)/(1 - p_i(t)]$ is a function of time. As shown above, the probability of an individual j becoming infected by time t is a function of the person's hazard of infection from syringes and the hazard of infection from sexual activity. That is,

$$1 - p_j(t) = S_j(t) = \exp\left(-\int_0^t [h_p(t)x_{1j} + h_s(t)x_{2j}]dt\right). \quad [8]$$

Substitution of this expression for $p_j(t)$ into the multiple logistic equation demonstrates the relationship between the underlying survivor functions and the adjusted odds ratio estimators. Depending on the underlying biologic model, the estimated coefficients β_i may change with time. As shown above, the value of the excess fraction in the exposed as well as in the cohort could change with time.

Second, the logistic model provides only adjusted odds ratios. Odds ratios are estimators of parameters. Sometimes they are only approximate estimators under strict assumptions. One should always make explicit what parameter the odds ratios are supposed to be estimating. If we use the probability of infection at the end of follow-up, they are approximate estimators of the relative cumulative incidence. Just as in any other circumstance, if the analysis is done assuming that those who were not infected by time t are the controls, then the odds ratio is only a good estimate of the relative cumulative incidence if the cumulative incidence of infection is low.

Third, all covariates in the model should be considered in light of the model of incidence of infection and the assumed underlying dynamics of infection. Some of the other covariates have meaning only when the person shares syringes. For example, if covariate 4 represents using bleach or not, then if the data are good, we expect that anyone who does not share syringes would not be using bleach. The 2 × 2 table would look like:

		Share syringes	
		yes	no
Use bleach	yes	20	0
	no	80	100

Although we would possibly have obtained an estimate for β_4, all the covariate values would have to be set to 0 as well to estimate the adjusted excess fraction of the infections at time t. Thus, estimation of the excess fraction using this method requires examination of the meaningful relationship of the covariates.

Fourth, the joint distribution of the covariates values in the population should be made clear.

Fifth, in reporting a multiple logistic regression, the scoring procedure for each variable needs to be included.

Finally, just because the data are of a form that will fit into a multiple logistic regression analysis does not mean that these numbers will have direct causal interpretations in light of the underlying transmission system.

CONCLUSION

Estimation of the role of parenteral and sexual transmission of HIV is quite complex. It will be highly specific to the

- local proportion sharing syringes, $P_+(t)$,
- local proportion exposed to sexual transmission, $S_+(t)$,
- local prevalence of infection in the population sharing syringes, $\theta_p(t)$, and
- local prevalence of infection in the pool of sex partners, $\theta_s(t)$.

It will also depend on the distribution of individual risk factors, such as the number of sexual contacts, the frequency of shooting drugs, the probability of reusing a syringe, as well as the local transmission probabilities from HIV positives. The average infectiousness of HIV-infected people could even depend on the local stage of the epidemic, with very early infections and late stage infections presumably being more infectious.

Also, attributable risk is often used in cancer to try to delineate causes of effects. We see people dying of cancer and would like to know if smoking has an effect, and how much is the effect. In infectious diseases, we are very often interested in the effects of known causes. That is, we may know the cause is bleach or a vaccine, or an infectious agent. The causal pathway is easy to understand. But we want to know the efficacy of the cause in changing the rate of infection in the exposed, and, given the proportion of the population exposed to the exposure or intervention, the overall change in the number of infections.

The excess fraction as defined above does not take into account the possible indirect effects of an intervention in a population, and in certain ways is not applicable to infectious diseases at all. This is due to the violation of the stable unit treatment value under the conditions of dependent happenings. If we intervene in a group of intravenous drug users such that some of them do not become infected, then it is possible that some of the others who did not receive the intervention may be protected from infection because they no longer become exposed to infection. This is the indirect effect of the intervention. This is not measured in the estimation of the excess fraction as described above. The usual causal model that assumes outcomes are independent is violated in infectious diseases (17). Halloran and Struchiner (12) defined four types of study designs for evaluating direct, indirect, total, and overall effects of an intervention. The direct causal effect of an intervention in those receiving the intervention is defined as the difference in what the outcome would have been with and without the intervention, all other things being equal. In infectious diseases, it is difficult to assume that all other things are equal when there may be indirect effects.

The prevalence of infection in the partner pool and in those sharing syringes plays a crucial role in the hazard rate of infection. Under epidemic conditions, the prevalence of infection can change dramatically in either of the partner pools (18). Risk factors need to be defined clearly with respect to whether they represent

1. exposure to infection,
2. susceptibility, or
3. type of contact.

Intravenous drug users in the treatment centers may have a different prevalence of sharing syringes or having HIV-positive partners than the intravenous drug users in general. Thus, extrapolation of the estimated excess fraction or hazard fraction to the general intravenous drug user population for the purpose of making policy may lead to incorrect estimates.

In studying causal parameters, it must be kept in mind that there is no baseline spontaneous development of infection in the absence of exposure to infection. Exposure to infection is a necessary, but not sufficient, cause to become infected. If there are two different routes of becoming infected, then the assumptions related to competing risk, whether they are dependent or independent, need to be made explicit.

One should be very cautious when using any of the parameters in the family of attributable risk concepts. Perhaps none of these concepts is appropriate in particular settings. Transfer of concepts from chronic disease epidemiology to infectious diseases needs to be done with special attention to the underlying dynamics. The temporal trends can be much more dramatic, making some of the approximations in chronic disease epidemiology inappropriate. In particular, since the excess fractions in the exposed and in the population change with time, estimates of the temporal component must be carefully taken into account. Possibly a dynamic model would be more appropriate for studying what the effects of interventions would be (19).

ACKNOWLEDGMENT

M. E. Halloran was partially supported by NIAID grant 1-R01-AI32042-01.

REFERENCES

1. Levin ML. The occurrence of lung cancer in man. *Acta Unio Internationalis Contra Cancrum* 1953;9:531–541.
2. Nicolosi A, Leite MLC, Musicco S, Molinari A for the Northern Italian Seronegative Drug Addicts (NISDA) Study Lazzarin. Parenteral and sexual transmission of human immunodeficiency virus in intravenous drug users: a study of seroconversion. *Am J Epidemiol* 1992;135:225–233.
3. Greenland S, Robins JM. Conceptual problems in the definition and interpretation of attributable fraction. *Am J Epidemiol* 1988;128:1185–1197.
4. Robins JM, Greenland S. Estimability and estimation of excess and etiologic fraction. *Stat Med* 1989;8:845–859.
5. Brunet RC, Struchiner CJ, Halloran ME. On the distribution of vaccine protection under heterogeneous response. *Math Biosci* 1993;116:111–125.
6. Haber M, Longini IM, Halloran ME. Measures of the effects of vaccination in a randomly mixing population. *Int J Epidemiol* 1991;20:300–310.
7. Halloran ME, Haber MJ, Longini IM, Struchiner CJ. Direct and indirect effects in vaccine field efficacy and effectiveness. *Am J Epidemiol* 1991;133:323–331.
8. Rhodes PH, Halloran ME, Longini IM. Counting process models for differentiating exposure to infection and susceptibility [in press].
9. Smith PG, Rodrigues LC, Fine PEM. Assessment of the protective efficacy of vaccines against common diseases using case-control and cohort studies. *Int J Epidemiol* 1984;13(1):87–93.
10. Greenwood M, Yule UG. The statistics of anti-typhoid and anti-cholera inoculations, and the interpretation of such statistics in general. *Proc R Soc Med* 1915;8(part 2):113–194.
11. Bruzzi P, Green SB, Byar DP, et al. Estimating the population attributable risk for multiple risk factors using case-control data. *Am J Epidemiol* 1985;122:904–914.
12. Halloran ME, Struchiner CJ. Study designs for dependent happening. *Epidemiology* 1991;2:331–338.
13. Ross R. An application of the theory of probabilities to the study of *a priori* pathometry, Part 1. *Proc R Soc Series A* 1916;92:204–230.
14. Halloran ME, Haber MJ, Longini IM. Interpretation and estimation of vaccine efficacy under heterogeneity. *Am J Epidemiol* 1992;136:328–343.
15. Vaupel JW, Manton KG, Stallard E. The impact of heterogeneity in individual frailty on the dynamics of mortality. *Demography* 1979;16:439–454.
16. Kooperberg C, Pettiti DB. Using logistic regression to estimate the adjusted attributable

risk of low birthweight in an unmatched case-control study. *Epidemiology* 1991;2:363–369.
17. Halloran ME, Struchiner CJ, Robins JM. Violation of the stable unit treatment value assumption in vaccine evaluation. *Am J Epidemiol* 1992;136:993 (abst).
18. Koopman JS, Longini IM, Jacquez JA, et al. Assessing risk factors for transmission of infection. *Am J Epidemiol* 1991;133:1199–1209.
19. Halloran ME, Struchiner CJ. Prevention of AIDS in IV drug users and its consequences on the epidemic in an interacting heterosexual population. V. International Conference on AIDS, Montreal, Quebec, Canada, 1989.

DISCUSSION

Dr. Johnson: I get a bit lost with math, but I'm very interested in how much these models can help you think through a process. I wonder if we could discuss the use of the transmission probability beta, because it's a very fundamental parameter in all of these models. In some models, people talk about the transmission probability per partnership; in others, they talk about the probability of transmission per contact (which could be a needle stick with a positive person).

What most of us measure in partner studies is the transmission probability per partnership. Many people have said (I think erroneously) that the risk we are able to estimate is the risk of transmission per act of sexual intercourse with a positive person. But if 10 couples have sex with each other an average of 300 times over a period of 5 years and 1 person becomes infected, the transmission probability is 1 in 1500 or something, which is very low. But this is completely erroneous because you can only become infected once in that situation; it's more a question of becoming infected or not.

The only way you can measure transmission probability per contact is to look at the probability of infection in people who have sex once with an infected person. I would argue that the closest data we've seen to that is Bill Cameron's data, which give an estimate of 7% in the presence of sexually transmitted diseases (STD).

There are some real problems with models that confuse transmission probability per contact with transmission probability per partnership, and try to derive the first, per contact, parameter from long-term partner relationships. I feel we should all be very clear about this because of the very low beta values I've seen in some of the models, which will clearly give a crazy result. I don't think that any of us can go around saying that the risk of transmission per act of intercourse is 1 in 1000 or whatever. I don't think we know what it is.

Dr. Padian: I think there is such variation that it's really hard to come up with a number, but it's sometimes difficult to avoid when the media are pressing you.

Dr. Halloran: I know transmission probability is not a constant. In our modelling work, we have to look at several different things. I've used simple models in an attempt to make some concepts clear, but if you add distributions, you have to include them not only in the transmission probability, but also in the frequency of sharing. This is where you can look at using something like Gibbs sampling in the complex, in order to give an underlying structure to these unmeasurables, or some people use random effect models to look at distribution possibilities and so on.

But I think that we should start with the simplest, and then work our way up to the more complicated. If you are going to try to use something like incidence, or equivalent parameters such as attributable risk, you have to understand how it turns into transmission probability.

Dr. Padian: But what if the distribution range is from 0 to 1? If one possibility is that some people could become infected immediately, can you deal with distributions like that?

Dr. Halloran: Sure. That's where people use the binomial.

Dr. Musicco: I have three questions. You have clearly shown that attributable risk in the exposed is only a function of relative risk, so I don't see any particular advantage in using attributable risk. The real advantage comes when you talk about attributable risk in the population, because you can estimate the theoretical proportion of cases that you can prevent by removing certain risk factors with a particular kind of intervention. Unfortunately, we don't normally know the proportion of exposed subjects in the population: we don't know how many people have STD, we don't know how many drug addicts there are, we don't know the number of seropositives, and we rarely know the risk behaviors.

Second, reasoning as an epidemiologist, I think that when we try to refine our study designs in order to control confounding, we do exactly what you are suggesting. When we study the partners of seropositive men or women, we know that we are dealing with a population in which the probability of having sexual contact with a seropositive person is one, and we try to eliminate all of the variables that may interfere with our estimates.

Third, we consider that the probability of transmission is constant over time. This is an assumption that is not really supported by the data. Nancy Padian showed the log-linear relationship between the risk of becoming seropositive and the number of sexual contacts. I don't know whether model 1 can also include a change in transmission probability, but this is a real problem.

Dr. Halloran: The attributable fraction of any population is the attributable fraction exposed multiplied by the prevalence in the population of the given risk factor. This has different meanings and there are different ways of estimating it.

As to the question about whether you can include variabilities and changes over time in the model, if you start with the basic model and define what effects you think these risk factors may have, you can move to more complex methods of analysis where you get the beta values and other things coming out that you can't otherwise estimate. All of them can be time-bearing or made individual to the person, and you can make it as complicated as you want. Unless you start by relating what you think is happening in the system to what you are getting out at the other end in terms of these so-called odds ratios, you can't even begin making things more complex.

But none of this has any meaning unless it is related back to your underlying transmission model. Of course, you can make the model more complex, but you have to start building by thinking what's going on. There are only two possibilities: either whatever it is reduces the probability of transmission, or it removes it. You have to put your risk factors in that context.

Dr. Detels: If you're modelling what would happen if you had efficacy and trying to predict what the situation would be, my impression is that, because the transmission is heterogeneous in your population, you're trying to describe the different intensities of challenge. But as Nancy and Anne Johnson have said, I think that it's almost impossible to come up with all of them. Consequently, you end up with a series of statistics that are in any case a series of summaries.

Dr. Halloran: I haven't had a chance to work all of that out, but we have done a lot on heterogeneity, which is an area of intense research. I have begun to work on the different levels of effect that an intervention may have. We are also working on the problem that an intervention may have some sort of unmeasurable distribution of effect, as in the case of a vaccine or bleach program. Not only is the transmission probability distributed, but also the effect on the population. All I can say is that this is where we are. There are very advanced statistical methods for doing nonparametric maximum likelihood estimations where, even if you don't know how your vaccine effect is stratified, you can get estimates of the number of strata and what the effect might be.

HIV Epidemiology: Models and Methods,
edited by Alfredo Nicolosi. Raven Press, Ltd.,
New York © 1994.

17

Confounding, Multicollinearity, Measurement Errors, and Surrogate Markers and Their Relationship to Logistic Regression

Anastasios A. Tsiatis

*Department of Biostatistics, Harvard School of Public Health,
Boston, Massachusetts 02115*

THE LOGISTIC REGRESSION MODEL

The logistic regression model is a useful way of modelling the probability of response to a set of variables that are discrete or continuous. It is often used in epidemiological research to model the probability of disease to variables that may explain the etiology of the disease.

In a logistic regression model, it is the logit of the probability or (log odds) rather than the probability itself that is related to other variables, usually in a linear fashion. That is, if we denote by "p" the probability of disease, then the logit or log odds is defined as log $\{p/(1-p)\}$. The logistic regression model ordinarily assumes that the relationship of the probability of disease to other variables is as follows:

$$\log\{p/(1-p)\} = \alpha + \beta_1 X_1 + \cdots + \beta_k X_k,$$

where $X_1, \ldots, X_k$ denote the variables of interest, which can be continuous variables, discrete variables (coded as dummy indicators variables), or a combination of both. The logit of the probability is mathematically useful since a probability can only take on values between 0 and 1, whereas the logit can take on any value between $-\infty$ and ∞. This is important when using regression models as we do not have to put any restrictions on the possible values of the parameters $(\alpha, \beta_1, \ldots, \beta_k)$. There is also no loss in using the logit transformation since there is a one to one relationship between the logit and the probability. That is, if $l = \log\{p/(1-p)\}$, then

$$p = \exp(l)/\{1 + \exp(l)\}.$$

The logistic relationship is also convenient since the "β" coefficients in the model can be interpreted in terms of log odds ratio. This is important in epidemiological research since the odds ratio is invariant in a case-control design.

For example, in the simplest model where X denotes the indicator of exposure (i.e., $X=1$ if exposed, and 0 if unexposed), the value β in the logistic regression model

$$\log\{p/(1-p)\}=\alpha+\beta X,$$

corresponds to the log odds ratio between disease and exposure;

$$\beta=\log[\{p_1/(1-p_1)\}/\{p_0/(1-p_0)\}],$$

where p_1 denotes the probability of disease for exposed individuals and p_0 denotes the probability of disease for unexposed individuals. Due to the invariance of the odds ratio to case-control studies, the same model could have been applied whether the study was conducted as a prospective cohort study or as a retrospective case-control study and the interpretation of the "β" coefficient would be the same in either situation.

If the variable of interest X is continuous rather than discrete, then the interpretation of the "β" coefficient in the simple logistic regression model corresponds to the increase in the log odds that is expected when the value of X is increased by one unit. If p_x denotes the probability of disease given the variable $X=x$, then

$$\beta=\log[\{(p_{x+1})/(1-p_{x+1})\}/\{(p_x)/(1-p_x)\}].$$

That is, "β" is the log odds ratio between disease and two exposures that are one unit apart. The simple logistic regression model assumes that the logit of the probability of disease is linearly related to X. This may often be a good first order approximation in many situations, but we can't expect this to always be the case. However, with some simple data analytic techniques we can check whether the linear assumption is reasonable and we can build more flexible models if it is not. These more flexible models may include using higher order polynomial relationships, regression splines, or just breaking up a continuous variable into several categories and modelling the relationship through a set of indicator variables for each of the categories.

Not accounting for nonlinear relationships in a logistic regression model can often lead to biased results. Although this can be a problem, it is not an issue I want to focus on in this discussion. Rather, I just want to comment that one should be aware that the logistic regression model makes some simplifying assumptions that should be checked by the investigator.

CONTROL FOR CONFOUNDING

The popularity of the logistic regression model in epidemiological research is primarily due to the fact that it can be used to model the probability of disease to many variables simultaneously. Since most epidemiological studies involve observational data bases of disease and exposure rather than controlled intervention through randomization, one must be concerned that other variables may confound the relationship between disease and exposure. In a multivariate logistic regression model, by accounting simultaneously for the effect of exposure as well as other potential confounding variables, the effect that each of these have on the probability of disease can be separated out. Therefore, the logistic regression model can be used to control for the effect of confounding.

If we consider, say, a typical multivariate logistic regression model

$$\log\{p/(1-p)\} = \alpha + \beta_1 X_1 + \beta_2 X_2 + \ldots + \beta_k X_k,$$

where X_1 is the exposure of interest and X_2 through X_k may be potential confounding variables, then the interpretation of β_1 would correspond to the log odds ratio between disease and exposure for individuals with values X_2 through X_k remaining fixed. By including the variables $X_2, \ldots, X_k$ in the model, we have controlled for their effect. In contrast, a model that did not control for these other variables and only considered the relationship between disease and exposure,

$$\log\{p/(1-p)\} = \alpha + \beta X_1,$$

could lead to misleading inference if the other variables were related to both disease and exposure.

Although multivariate regression modelling can be very useful in epidemiological research, it is not a panacea. It also has potential problems in both implementation and interpretation. The problems and possible misleading conclusions that may result from the use of multiple logistic regression modelling in acquired immunodeficiency syndrome (AIDS) epidemiological research have been discussed by Vandenbroucke and Pardoel (1). In their paper, they discuss how logistic regression analysis led investigators to believe that the use of "amyl nitrite" was a causative factor in the transmission of AIDS. In particular, they refer to a study by Marmor et al. (2) who published results of a case-control study in 1982. In it, the crude odds ratio for 542 or more lifetime uses of amyl nitrite (the median level in cases) versus 0 was 8.6. An odds ratio of 4.9 was found for having more than 10 sexual partners (median level in cases) in the year preceding the illness versus 0 sexual partners. When these variables were entered simultaneously into a logistic regression model to correct for possible confounding, the odds ratio for amyl nitrite became 12.3 and that for promiscuity became 2.0. This is the reverse of what should have happened, given our present knowledge.

Much discussion followed regarding the appropriateness of the logistic regression model to control for confounding and identifying causal effects. With this as a backdrop, I would like to discuss some of the problems that may occur when using multiple logistic regression analysis. This will include issues of multicollinearity, use of surrogate markers, and measurement error and the effects of these on the estimates in a logistic regression model.

SURROGATE MARKERS, CONFOUNDING, AND MULTICOLLINEARITY

In this section, let us denote by X the variable that is really the cause of disease. For example, the amount of high-risk sexual activity may be the variable "X" that relates to "p" the probability of getting AIDS. Say, that the relationship follows a logistic regression model, i.e.,

$$\log\{p/(1-p)\}=\alpha+\beta X.$$

In order that we don't get confused with issues of scaling, it will be assumed that all our variables have been scaled so that they have variance 1.

Suppose, however, instead of X we consider a variable Y that is a surrogate for X. A surrogate variable for X in this context is a variable that is correlated to X, but adds no additional prognostic information. That is, Y is a surrogate for X if

$$\rho(X,Y) > 0 \qquad \text{[i]}$$

where $\rho(X,Y)$ denotes the correlation of X and Y, and

$$P(D=1|X,Y)=P(D=1|X), \qquad \text{[ii]}$$

where $P(D=1|X,Y)$ denotes the probability of getting disease given X and Y. Again, Y is assumed to be scaled so that the variance of Y is 1.

For example, Y might correspond to the amount of amyl nitrite that may be correlated to the amount of high-risk sexual activity. If we modelled the probability of getting AIDS to Y, i.e.,

$$\log\{p/(1-p)\}=\alpha+\gamma Y,$$

then the estimate for γ, which we denote by $\hat{\gamma}$, resulting from such a logistic regression analysis would on the average equal $\beta\rho(X,Y)$.

The calculations that will be given here and in the remainder of the discussion will assume that the random variables are all normally distributed. Also, in order to get exact simple expressions, we assume that the probability follows a probit relationship. However, since the logit and probit relationships are close, the differences will be inconsequential.

Therefore, if we use a surrogate for X in the model, we see an effect on the average equal to $\beta\rho(X,Y)$, which is diminished (the amount depends on the correlation of X and Y) but still positive.

Let us continue with this line of thinking. We modelled the probability of getting AIDS to the amount of amyl nitrite "Y" and found a significant relationship. We suspect, however, that Y is confounded with "X" the amount of high-risk sexual activity. The next step may be to control for the confounding by introducing both Y and X into the model. That is, we consider the model

$$\log\{p/(1-p)\} = \alpha + \beta_1 X + \beta_2 Y.$$

According to the assumptions that were made, the estimate $\hat{\beta}_1$ will on the average be close to β and the estimate $\hat{\beta}_2$ will on the average be close to 0. This is exactly what we want to happen for this problem.

There is, however, a problem that does occur with regards to the precision of these estimates when they are highly correlated. This problem of collinearity is often not discussed in the epidemiological literature. If the standard error of the estimate for β is denoted by $se(\beta)$, in the model where X is the only term in the model, then the standard error of the estimate of $\hat{\beta}_1$ and $\hat{\beta}_2$ in the model that contains both X and Y is given by $se(\beta)/(1-\rho^2(X, Y))^{1/2}$. That is, the standard error is inflated more and more as the correlation of X and Y increases. For example, if the correlation between X and Y is 95%, then the standard error is increased by $(1-(0.95)^2)^{-1/2} = 3.2$-fold. This results in a loss of efficiency of $(3.2)^2 = 10.26$. That is, if we introduce both X and Y into the model, which we may need to do to sort out the confounding effect, then we need 10.3 times the sample size to get the same precision as having the model with only X.

Of course, I used 95% correlation to get my point across. In most problems the correlation is not that large; however, we see that trying to sort out the effect of possible confounders will also lead to estimates that are less reliable.

MEASUREMENT ERROR AND CONFOUNDING

In this section I would like to discuss the problem of measurement error. As before, let the variable X correspond to the amount of high-risk sexual activity (this is the factor that for simplicity we assume is directly related to the transmission of AIDS). In a survey we may ask the participants in the study how many sexual partners they have on the average. The answer they give will not necessarily be equal to X but rather it will correspond to another variable, say W, which we may think of as being equal to $X+$ error. The variable W may be imprecise because individuals may not be able to recollect exactly or the question did not focus on the specific high-risk activity. In any case, if we analyzed the data using a logistic regression analysis with W (the variable measured with error), say,

$$\log\{p/(1-p)\} = \alpha + \gamma W,$$

then the estimate of $\hat{\gamma}$ would be on the average close to $\beta\ [1/(1 + \sigma_e^2)]$, where σ_e^2 is the variance of the measurement error. We note that the estimate $\hat{\gamma}$

resulting from measurement error is attenuated toward 0, with greater attenuation as the measurement error gets larger.

I also want to note that not only does the estimate of the effect get attenuated with measurement error, but so does the efficiency to detect significant differences. The efficiency is also equal to $[1/(1 + \sigma_e^2)]$. For example, if the measurement error is equal to the variance of X (which we standardized to be 1), then $[1/(1 + \sigma_e^2)] = 1/2$. In such a case, the estimate of the log odds ratio will be decreased by half, and we would need twice the sample size to detect significant differences.

Finally, let us consider the situation where we conduct a logistic regression analysis with both Y (a surrogate for X, i.e., amount of amyl nitrite) and W (variable measured with error, i.e., number of sexual partners);

$$\log\{p/(1-p)\} = \alpha + \beta_1 Y + \beta_2 W.$$

In such a case the estimate $\hat{\beta}_1$ will be centered about

$$\frac{\beta\sigma_e^2\rho(X,Y)}{1-\rho^2(X,Y)) + \sigma_e^2}$$

and $\hat{\beta}_2$ will be centered at

$$\frac{\beta(1-\rho^2(X,Y))}{1-\rho^2(X,Y)) + \sigma_e^2}.$$

Unfortunately, in such a case the estimates are very unstable (large variance) and can change substantially depending on the relative value of the correlation $\rho(X,Y)$ and the measurement error σ_e^2. This becomes especially problematic when the correlation is high and the measurement error is small. For example, we have tabulated what the average value of $\hat{\beta}_1$ and $\hat{\beta}_2$ will be for different combinations of $\rho(X,Y)$ and σ_e^2:

		Average value of	
$\rho(X,Y)$	σ_e^2	$\hat{\beta}_1$	$\hat{\beta}_2$
0.99	0.20	0.90 β	0.09 β
0.95	0.10	0.48 β	0.49 β
0.90	0.01	0.05 β	0.91 β

Clearly, in the case where we include two variables in the model that are highly correlated with the true causal variable, we get very unstable estimates that can change magnitude drastically with very small perturbations.

CONCLUSION

Logistic regression analysis is a primary tool for the analysis of observational epidemiological studies for both cohort studies and case-control studies. The strength of the logistic regression model is that many variables can be analyzed simultaneously enabling us to sort the different individual effects on the probability of disease. This allows us to control for confounding. However, one must be careful not to overinterpret results from a logistic regression analysis. As we all know, statistical modelling results in statistical associations. Whether these associations are indeed causal or not is very difficult to establish based only on results from statistical modelling.

The perceived strength of logistic regression modelling in epidemiological research—the ability to control for confounding—is also a weakness of the methodology. The greater the confounding of variables, the greater the multicollinearity. This, plus the fact that variables may be measured with error, may result in estimates from a logistic regression model that are unstable and imprecise.

This is not to say that logistic regression modelling should not be used. Quite the contrary, I believe this is a very powerful tool for establishing relationships. My only caution is that we should not expect too much from statistical methods when trying to establish cause and effect relationships, especially for diseases about which very little is known.

REFERENCES

1. Vandenbroucke JP, Pardoel UPAM. An autopsy of epidemiological methods: the case of "poppers" in the early epidemic of the acquired immunodeficiency syndrome (AIDS). *Am J Epidemiol* 1989;129:455–457.
2. Marmor M, Friedman-Kien A, Laubenstein L, et al. Risk factors for Kaposi's sarcoma in homosexual men. *Lancet* 1982;1:1083–1086.

DISCUSSION

Dr. Friedman: During the break, Beth and I discussed the differences between doing research at a stage when it is pretty clear what is going on and doing research when things are still very muddled. Looking back, one of the uses of surrogate markers raises an important issue in terms of logistic regression and statistical research in general. When you use some of Beth's concepts to bounce back the use of the surrogate marker in Michael Marmor's paper, we have to ask ourselves which of the other parameters it may be a surrogate for. My suspicion is that poppers are probably a surrogate marker for a network variable (the percentage of contacts who are likely to be infected), which in Beth's symbolism is called beta. Although the technical/statistical thing is very clear, part of the process of the interpretation of logistic regression is to think through what surrogate processes might be occurring.

Dr. Tsiatis: I completely agree, but, as a statistician, I have the job of logistic regression clear in my head. The job of logistic regression is to try to model the relationship of the probability of something with the variables that you suggest, and to do that as best you can. What you're getting at is what it may mean: I can do a good job, but have meaningless results. It's up to someone else to understand what it means when I run the model. That's where you need a combination of understanding what comes out of the statistics as well as an understanding of the process as a whole. I agree that you can't do it in the absence of that.

Dr. Des Jarlais: Mike's paper has received a lot of criticism, much of which is deserved. But having talked to him about this at some length, rather than thinking about surrogate markers and such, the truth was the presence of some form of high-risk sexual activity. Another way of looking at these data is that asking about popper use and splitting it yes/no may be the truth plus measurement error; asking about total number of sexual partners and splitting it at the median of 10 may also be truth plus measurement error, but you have more measurement error with that second question about lifetime sexual partners than you have with the popper question. This means that neither is really a surrogate.

Dr. Tsiatis: I don't know about this issue, so I'm being a little unfair because I took these discussions and used them as examples. In reality, I haven't seen the data analysis and I don't know exactly what was done.

Second, I don't think they split it at those levels. I think they actually used linear models and just used predictive values at the 10 or the 542 subjects and then worked out what the predicted odds ratio would have been according to this data x term I talked about. If you work out x at 542, and you multiply beta by x, that's the result you would get. The actual numbers are not very important.

Dr. Gail: In Mike's 1982 paper, I think he raised the possibility that drug use was a surrogate for something else, even though he may not have emphasized it. And in a follow-up paper, when the biology became a little clearer and he included more detailed questioning about anal-related sex, things started to change. This may suggest that we should be using as much biological information as possible when we set up these regression models. I though this was a very elegant discussion of the combination of errors and variables with the surrogate notion that I'd never seen before, even though the book by Mosteller and Tukey on general regression methods talks an awful lot about multicollinearity and the interpretation of regression models.

But, was this done for normal linear models, and not exactly for logistics?

Dr. Tsiatis: I actually assumed a probit relationship that assumes underlying normality and that the variables were normal. That way, I could get exact calculations. But given the models' similarity, the results would probably be indistinguishable.

Dr. Nicolosi: I want to thank you for the interesting lecture you gave us. You demonstrated that the magnitude of the biasing effects that misclassification has on logistic regression in the presence of multicollinearity is beyond what most people would expect.

This could explain a certain pattern we can notice in the literature. In epidemiological research on human immunodeficiency virus (HIV), the investigations of sexual transmission have generally provided sharper and higher estimates of different risk factors than those studying intravenous drug users, and almost consistent findings across different studies. In fact with the problem of misclassification set aside, the risk factors of sexual transmission are multiple and independent. The clinical stage of the HIV-infected partner doesn't have any relation to, say, a positive history of sexually transmitted diseases in the other partner.

On the contrary, the investigations of intravenous drug users generally provide small risk estimates and wide differences across studies. Here, we have at least four problems. First, the extent of exposure's misclassification is obviously great, especially in cross-sectional studies. Second, there is the confounding effect of sexual exposure. Then, the models used in the analysis do not include all the control variables (think of the powerful effect of HIV prevalence). Finally, the principal risk factor (syringe sharing) is strongly correlated to a series of other behavioral, socioeconomical, and/or racial factors.

It was interesting to see that contrasting results are now emerging from studies of sexual transmission when they face similar problems such as the correlations among oral contraceptives, frequency of sexual intercourse, condom use, prostitution, and HIV infection.

HIV Epidemiology: Models and Methods, edited by Alfredo Nicolosi. Raven Press, Ltd., New York © 1994.

18

The Contributions of Cohort Studies to Understanding the Natural History of HIV Infection

Roger Detels

Department of Epidemiology, University of California Los Angeles School of Public Health, Los Angeles, California 90024

Cohort studies have provided much of the basic information that has led to our understanding of the natural history of human immunodeficiency virus (HIV) infection (Table 1). The original cohort studies on HIV/acquired immunodeficiency syndrome (AIDS) were in homosexual/bisexual men primarily because this was the group with the highest rate of infection and because of their courageous willingness to participate in research on this disease that was killing their friends and colleagues. Although the Multicenter AIDS Cohort Study (MACS) was one of the first collaborative cohort studies established specifically to study AIDS, earlier cohorts formed to study hepatitis vaccine in the late 1980s were re-established to study this new disease. More recently, cohort studies of intravenous drug users, women, discordant couples, and pregnant women and their offspring have been established to identify those characteristics of the natural history of HIV infection that may be unique to these groups.

Although cohort studies are an epidemiologic study design, cohort studies of HIV/AIDS, in particular, have provided far more than descriptive information about the infection, modes of transmission, and clinical characteristics of HIV infection and disease. HIV/AIDS cohort studies have provided essential information about the response of the human body to viral exposure and infection, the process of infection, the changes in the virus population within the body associated with disease progression, the processes by which HIV causes destruction of the host defense system, and the effect of treatment on both the virus and the restoration of immune function.

I would like to present some examples of the contributions of cohort studies to our understanding of the natural history of HIV disease in terms of the three major stages of HIV infection: (1) establishment of HIV infection,

TABLE 1. *The contribution of cohort studies to understanding the natural history of HIV[a] infection*

- Establishment of HIV infection
  - Susceptibility/resistance to HIV infection (genetic/environmental)
  - Relative risk of specific activities for infection
  - Characteristics of successfully infecting HIV strains
  - Early response of the human immune system to HIV
  - Promoters/cofactors for infection
- Progression of HIV infection to AIDS[b]
  - Rate of HIV progression to disease (proportion of HIV infection progressing to AIDS and dementia)
  - Immunologic and clinical predictors/markers of disease progression
  - Immune response to persisting HIV infection
    - Levels of immune components (e.g., CD4 and CD8 cells)
    - Changes in immune function
  - Viral changes associated with disease progression
    - Strain proliferation
    - Specific strains
    - Viral load
  - Genetic factors influencing disease progression
  - Clinical outcomes of HIV infection
    - Frequency of specific outcome
    - Determinants of specific clinical outcomes
  - Temporal and functional relationships among viral, immune, and clinical factors
  - Impact of treatment on AIDS-free period
- Survival after AIDS
  - Survival time in the absence of treatment
  - Immunologic and virologic factors influencing survival
  - Impact of treatment on survival
  - Response of immune and virologic parameters to various treatments and relationship to survival

[a]HIV, human immunodeficiency virus.
[b]AIDS, acquired immunodeficiency syndrome.

(2) progression of HIV infection to AIDS, and (3) survival after the AIDS diagnosis.

In addition, there are special cohort studies to evaluate factors associated with vertical transmission and discordant couples, clinical trials to evaluate efficacy of drugs, and vaccine trials to prevent both infection and disease. I apologize that I will present a majority of examples from the MACS primarily because it is one of the largest and longest running cohort studies specifically designed to study the natural history of AIDS, it has resulted in over 200 research publications on a variety of topics, and it is the cohort study with which I am most familiar.

ESTABLISHMENT OF HIV INFECTION

The difficulty in producing a vaccine for this complex disease has provided the opportunity to study the process of infection of the cell by HIV

TABLE 2. *Seroconversion to HIV-1[a] antibody seropositivity, intervals V_1–V_5*

Anal–genital intercourse reported in previous two intervals	Number seroconverting	Number of person-intervals[b]	Estimated incidence	Ratio[c]	Median number of partners in previous two intervals
Both receptive and insertive	190	5,009	0.038	31.6 (8.7, 263.0)	33
Receptive, *no* insertive	14	765	0.018	15.3 (3.5, 138.5)	13
Insertive, *no* receptive	10	1,886	0.005	4.4 (0.94–41.5)	50
No anal–genital	2	1,670	0.001	1.0[d]	8

Adapted from Detels R, English P, Visscher BR, et al., ref. 1.
[a]HIV, human immunodeficiency virus.
[b]Number of men in the exposure category in each interval time among those seroconverting.
[c]Numbers in parentheses are confidence limits.
[d]Reference category.

TABLE 3. *HIV[a] seroconversion rates by reported condom use and number of partners in previous two intervals*

Reported condom use	Number seroconverting	Number of person-intervals	Estimated incidence	Incidence ratio (no. of partners)	Incidence ratio (use of condoms)
No partners used condoms					
$n \leqslant 2$	7	855	0.008	1.0[b]	
$n = 3–8$	25	1,509	0.017	2.0 (0.9, 5.5)[c]	
$n \geqslant 9$	65	1,719	0.038	4.7 (1.2, 11.9)	
Total	97	4,083	0.024		3.3 (1.6, 8.4)[c]
Some partners used condoms					
$n \leqslant 2$	2	195	0.010	1.0[b]	
$n = 3–8$	30	829	0.036	3.6 (0.9, 30.5)	
$n \geqslant 9$	79	1,576	0.050	5.0 (1.3, 41.1)	
Total	111	2,600	0.043		6.0 (2.8, 8.3)
All partners used condoms					
$n \leqslant 2$	1	264	0.004	1.0[b]	
$n = 3–8$	5	450	0.011	2.9 (0.3, 138.5)	
$n \geqslant 9$	1	263	0.004	1.0 (0.0, 78.0)	
Total	7	977	0.007		1.0[b]

Adapted from Detels R, English P, Visscher BR, et al., ref. 1.
[a]HIV, human immunodeficiency virus.
[b]Reference category.
[c]95% confidence limits.

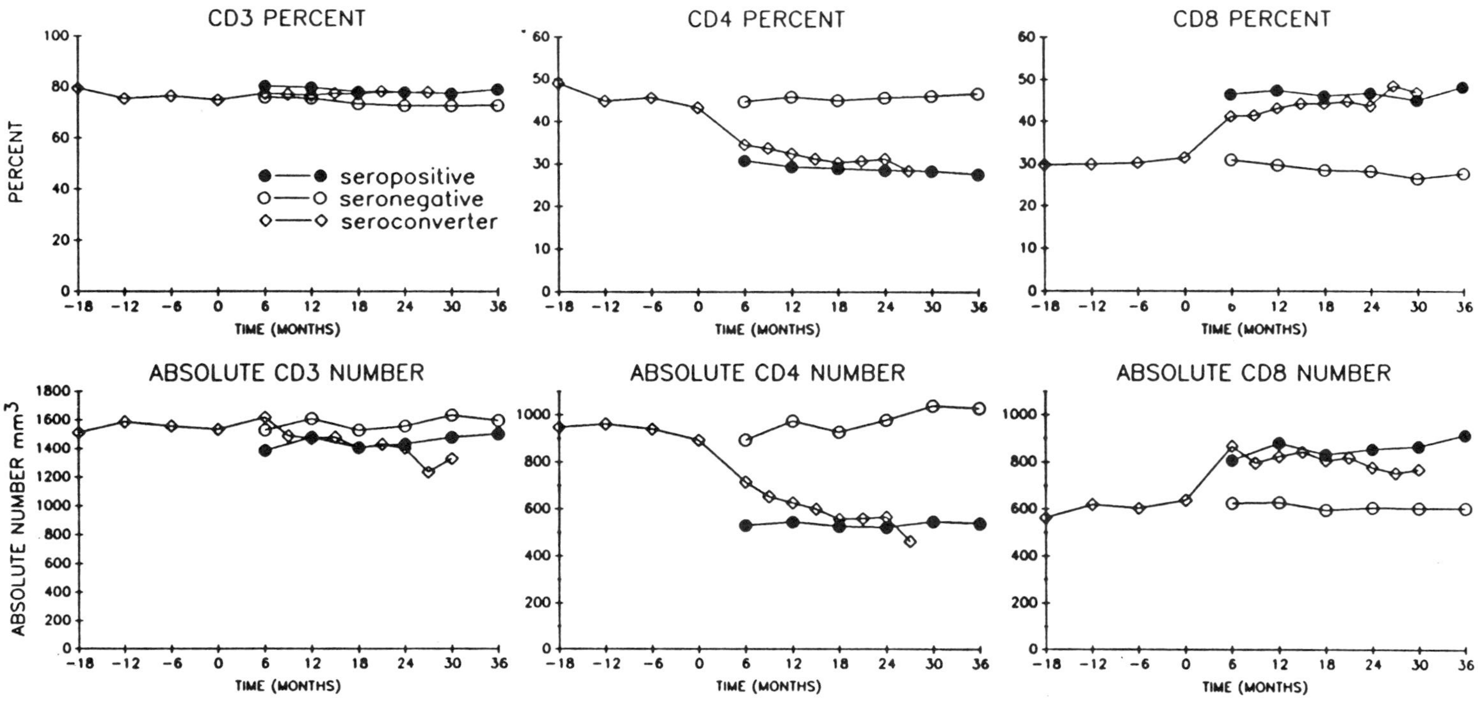

FIG. 1. Percentages and absolute CD3, CD4, and CD8 numbers in three groups of active homosexual men. There were approximately 600 seropositive men, 600 seronegative men, and 72 seroconverters. Time is presented in months. The first observations for the seropositive and seronegative groups are placed at the 6-month time point. Time = 0 for the seroconverters represents the last time these men were antibody negative for HIV. Time = 6 months represents the value when they were first antibody positive for HIV-1. Adapted from Giorgi and Detels (3).

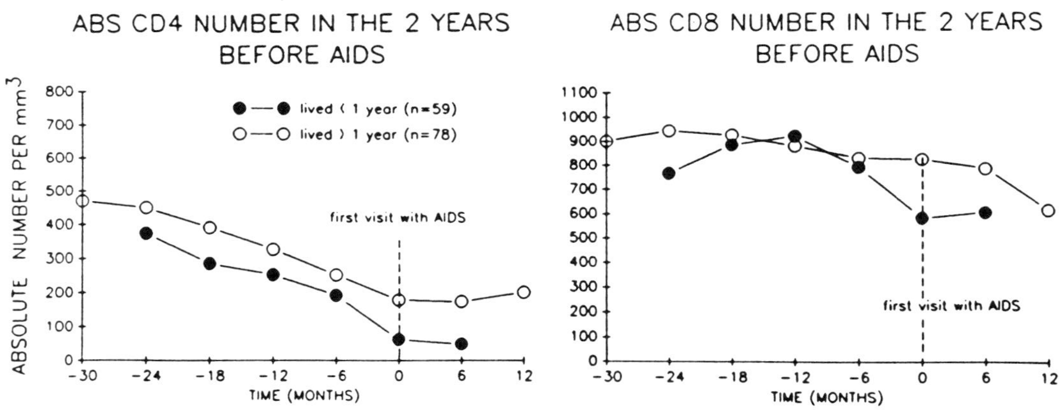

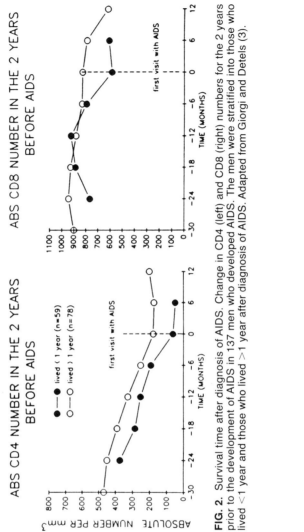

FIG. 2. Survival time after diagnosis of AIDS. Change in CD4 (left) and CD8 (right) numbers for the 2 years prior to the development of AIDS in 137 men who developed AIDS. The men were stratified into those who lived <1 year and those who lived >1 year after diagnosis of AIDS. Adapted from Giorgi and Detels (3).

more carefully using modern techniques of molecular biology than for any prior disease.

Cohort studies have established the major mode of transmission among homosexual men and the relative efficiency of each mode, as well as the effectiveness of condoms used by homosexual men in preventing transmission through anal intercourse (Tables 2 and 3) (1,2).

The initial responses to HIV infection—a drop in the level of CD4 cells, a rise in the level of CD8 cells, and parallel increases in cytokines which reflect cell activation—have been established by investigators in the MACS as well as in other cohorts (Figs. 1 and 2) (3,4).

Investigators in cohort studies have also looked for factors that may promote infection of an individual. These have included consideration of genetic factors as well as other infectious agents such as hepatitis, cytomegalovirus, herpesvirus, and Epstein-Barr virus (5–7).

Despite the information we have already obtained on transmission of HIV, it is clear that the process of infection is very complex. Follow-up of cohorts of high-risk individuals should elucidate the factors that determine successful establishment of infection.

PROGRESSION OF HIV INFECTION TO AIDS

There are two major questions regarding the progression of HIV infection to AIDS. The first of these is what proportion of individuals who are infected with HIV will eventually develop AIDS? Considering the observation that the rate of progression to AIDS may vary from as short as 1 year to over 15 years, the second question is what factors determine or promote the likelihood that an HIV-infected individual will progress to AIDS and what factors influence the rate of progression towards AIDS? Cohort studies have been particularly useful for obtaining information essential to answering these two questions that, nonetheless, still remain largely unanswered.

Studies of the reconstituted cohort of homosexual men participating in the hepatitis vaccine trials of the late 1970s by Rutherford et al. have indicated that 36% of infected men will develop AIDS within 9 years after infection (8,9). Projections of cumulative incidence in the MACS cohort and other studies have suggested that similar rates of progression are occurring in those cohorts as well (Fig. 3).

The association of HIV with persistent decline in the level of CD4 cells and elevation in markers of activation such as neopterin, beta-2-microglobulin, soluble IL-2 receptor, and IgA has been documented by Fahey et al. and others (Table 4) (10).

Studies of the MACS cohort have suggested that genetic factors may influence the rate of progression to AIDS. A rapid decline in the number of CD4 cells among the men in the MACS was more common in men with the

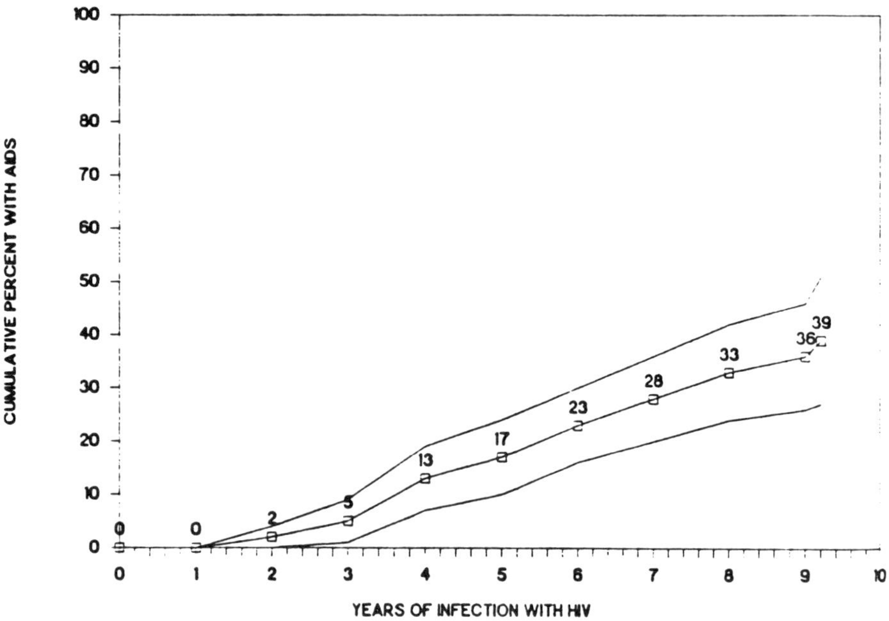

FIG. 3. Kaplan–Meier survival curve of the cumulative proportion of men with AIDS by duration of HIV infection among 135 hepatitis B vaccine trial participants (San Francisco, 1978–1988). The upper and lower lines represent the upper and lower 95% confidence intervals, respectively. Adapted from Hessol et al. (9).

A1, Cw7, B8, DR3 HLA antigen combination than in men who did not have this combination (11).

A number of immunologic and viral factors have been shown to be associated with more rapid progression to AIDS. Phair et al. observed that men who developed AIDS within 5 years of infection had a greater number of sexual partners and episodes of sexually transmitted diseases both before seroconversion and in the interval between seroconversion and AIDS, suggesting that continued repeated exposure to agents transmitted sexually may promote the rate of progression to HIV (Table 5) (12). On the other hand, those who developed AIDS within 5 years of seroconversion were also more likely to have had one or more symptoms within 6 months of seroconversion, suggesting that events occurring at the time of seroconversion, such as the strain of HIV that established infection in them, may also have played a role in determining the rate of progression to infection.

Studies conducted by Ho et al. and confirmed by others have indicated that the amount of HIV in the infected host also plays a role in progression to infection (13).

Autopsy studies have indicated that a high proportion of men with AIDS have evidence of infection of the nervous system, raising the issue of

TABLE 4. *Multivariate analysis of the relation of markers of progression to AIDS*[a]

Marker	Hazard ratio[b]	Log likelihood[c]
Number of CD4 cells	8:1	−457
Neopterin	9:1	−458
β2M	6:1	−464
CD4 cell number + neopterin	12:1	−448
CD4 cell number + β2M	12:1	−449
CD4 cell number + neopterin + sIL-2R + IgA + p24 antigen	22:1	−432

Adapted from Fahey JL, Taylor JMG, Detels R, et al., ref. 10.
[a]AIDS, acquired immunodeficiency syndrome.
[b]Ratio of highest risk group to lowest risk group.
[c]The log likelihood refers to a proportional hazards model in which each variable is continuous. The *smaller* the negative value, the greater the predictive value (e.g., −432 is more predictive than −464).

whether to bar HIV-infected individuals from jobs requiring judgment and rapid decision making. The MACS and other cohort studies have also provided important information about the timing of the development of impairment of mental processes in HIV-infected men. Serial administration of tests measuring neuropsychological performance in HIV antibody-positive men by Miller et al. and others in the MACS has demonstrated that evidence of dementia does not usually appear until 1 year or less prior to the diagnosis of AIDS and is usually accompanied by other symptoms of HIV infection (14,15).

Clinical trials, a variant of cohort studies, conducted by the collaborative AIDS Clinical Trials Group have indicated that treatment of individuals after compromise of the immune system, but before onset of AIDS, will prolong the AIDS-free interval (16). Studies by Graham et al. from the MACS have

TABLE 5. *Factors associated with rapid progression to AIDS*[a]

Factor	Ratio of cases to controls	P value
Anal receptive number of partners		
Prior to seroconversion	2.0	0.003
6 months after seroconversion	1.7	0.013
12 months after seroconversion	2.3	0.002
24 months after seroconversion	2.6	0.004
Anal insertive number of partners		
Prior to seroconversion	1.2	—
6 months after seroconversion	1.1	—
12 months after seroconversion	1.5	—
24 months after seroconversion	2.0	0.04
Percent reporting rectal gonorrhea		
Prior to seroconversion	1.6	0.06
After seroconversion	3.1	0.06

Adapted from Phair J, Jacobson L, Detels R, et al., ref. 12.
[a]AIDS, acquired immunodeficiency syndrome.

confirmed this observation and suggested that early treatment before diagnosis of AIDS also increased survival (17).

Many questions, however, remain to be answered. Although markers of disease progression have been identified, the specific changes in the function of the immune system and the temporal correlation of these to the levels and variants of HIV present in the body have not yet been elucidated. Further, the correlation of these viral and immunologic parameters to the clinical course of HIV disease has not been documented. Cohort studies are most likely to provide this essential biologic and clinical information.

SURVIVAL AFTER AIDS

Cohort studies of AIDS patients, of course, established the usual survival after disease onset. Clinical trials such as those being conducted by the AIDS Clinical Trials Group have provided the basic information about efficacy of zidovudine and other drugs (18). However, cohort studies such as the MACS have also provided confirmation of these clinical trials based on individuals followed prior to the onset of AIDS being treated in the community rather than under rigidly controlled trial conditions that select for compliant individuals (19). Other factors may enhance survival with or without treatment. These should be the subject of future research as well as the search for more effective treatments.

IMPORTANT SUBPOPULATIONS OF COHORTS

Four subpopulations that may provide important information to answer the remaining unanswered questions in the natural history of HIV infection and AIDS have been identified in the MACS (Table 6):

uninfected men who appear to be resistant to infection,
HIV-infected men who maintain an adequate level of immune function (CD4 cell level),
HIV-infected men who progress rapidly to AIDS, and, finally,
HIV-infected men with low levels of CD4 cells who do not get AIDS.

There is a subgroup of individuals who are repeatedly exposed to HIV-infected individuals either through repeated, receptive sexual intercourse with an infected partner, or through frequent, unprotected, receptive anal intercourse with many men in urban areas with a high prevalence of HIV-infected men (20). Yet, even after years of documented exposure to many infected partners, these individuals remain antibody free. Studies by Imagawa et al. have suggested that HIV may actually have entered the cells of some of these individuals without establishing infection (21,22). Studies of T cells by Shearer and Clerici and Clerici et al. and of B cells by Jehuda-

TABLE 6. *Four cohorts of particular interest to the study of HIV[a] in humans*

Persons with **repeated exposure** to many different partners or to a long-term HIV-infected partner who appears to be **resistant** to HIV infection (i.e., remain **antibody negative**)
HIV-infected persons who **maintain** a high level of **CD4 cells** (i.e., those who appear to have established a successful **equilibrium** with the virus)
HIV-infected persons with **rapid progression** to AIDS[b] (i.e., those who have failed to establish a successful equilibrium with the virus)
HIV-infected persons who **remain AIDS-free** despite having low levels of CD4 cells

[a]HIV, human immunodeficiency virus.
[b]AIDS, acquired immunodeficiency syndrome.

Cohen et al. have suggested that many of these high exposure, antibody-negative men have had prior exposure to HIV, presumably without establishment of HIV infection (23–25).

Thus, cohort studies have provided epidemiologic evidence that exposure to HIV is probably insufficient to assure infection. Cohort studies now need to focus on the process of infection of the cell itself. "Resistance" to HIV infection may be due to host factors or to characteristics of the virus to which the individuals are exposed. Investigation of early events following exposure to HIV may provide information about differences in the host response to the virus that play a role in determining whether an exposure to HIV results in infection. If investigators can identify the immunologic and virologic correlates of this "resistance," we may be able to develop alternative methods to induce relative resistance to infection.

It is not known why some individuals are able to maintain adequate levels of CD4 cells and remain symptom-free years after infection. Clearly, these individuals are coping successfully with HIV infection. If investigators can elucidate those characteristics of the individual or of the infecting HIV that prevent progression of HIV disease, they may be able to induce similar resistance to deterioration of the immune system in other infected individuals.

The other side of the coin is those individuals who progress rapidly to AIDS after a relatively short incubation period. Although some of the behavioral factors associated with rapid progression to AIDS have been elucidated, most of the biologic and virologic factors have not. Knowledge of what these factors are may permit us to develop more specific intervention strategies to enhance survival in the many individuals worldwide who are infected with HIV.

Finally, there is a particularly interesting group of individuals who are able to survive without development of AIDS despite having very low levels of CD4 cells, the major marker of immune function deterioration. This ability to withstand further progression of HIV disease in the apparent absence of an effective immune system is particularly interesting since it suggests that mechanisms not dependent on CD4 number may be involved in progression to AIDS or, conversely, in delaying progression to AIDS. Knowledge of these factors could provide an alternative strategy for interrupting progression of HIV infection, even in individuals who appear to have late stage disease with severe impairment of the immune system. Further, these investigations are likely to provide basic information about mechanisms of disease defense that may be useful in managing other diseases involving immune deterioration.

Finally, cohort studies of HIV/AIDS have demonstrated how productive collaboration by epidemiologists, immunologists, virologists, other basic scientists, and clinical investigators can be. Continued collaboration in cohort studies will answer many of the remaining important questions on the natural history of HIV/AIDS.

REFERENCES

1. Detels R, English P, Visscher BR, et al. Seroconversion, sexual activity, and condom use among 2915 HIV seronegative men followed for up to 2 years. *J AIDS* 1989;2:77–83.
2. Kingsley LA, Detels R, Kaslow R, et al. Risk factors for seroconversion to human immunodeficiency virus among male homosexuals: results from the Multicenter AIDS Cohort Study. *Lancet* 1987;1(8529):345–349.
3. Giorgi JV, Detels R. T-cell subset alterations in HIV-infected homosexual men: NIAID Multicenter AIDS Cohort Study. *Clin Immunol Immunopathol* 1989;52:10–18.
4. Lang W, Perkins H, Anderson RE, et al. Patterns of T lymphocyte changes with immunodeficiency virus infection: from seroconversion to the development of AIDS. *J AIDS* 1989;2:63–69.
5. Twu SJ, Detels R, Nelson K, et al. The relationship of hepatitis B viral infection to HIV-1 seroconversion. *J Infect Dis* [in press].
6. Ferbas J, Rahman MA, Kingsley LA, et al. Frequent oropharyngeal shedding of Epstein-Barr virus in homosexual men during early human immunodeficiency virus infection. *AIDS* [in press].
7. Levy E, Margalith M, Sarov B, et al. Cytomegalovirus IgG and IgA serum antibodies in a study of HIV infection and HIV related diseases in homosexual men. *J Med Virol* 1991;35:174–179.
8. Rutherford GW, Lifson AR, Hessol NA, et al. Course of HIV-1 infection in a cohort of homosexual and bisexual men: an 11 year follow up study. *Br Med J [Clin Res]* 1990;301:1183–1188.
9. Hessol NA, Lifson AR, O'Malley PM, et al. Prevalence, incidence, and progression of human immunodeficiency virus infection in homosexual and bisexual men in hepatitis B vaccine trials, 1978-1988. *Am J Epidemiol* 1989;130:1167–1175.
10. Fahey JL, Taylor JMG, Detels R, et al. The prognostic value of cellular and serologic markers in infection with human immunodeficiency virus type 1. *N Engl J Med* 1990;332:166–172.
11. Kaslow RA, Duquesnoy R, VanRaden M, et al. A1, Cw7, B8, DR3 HLA antigen combination associated with rapid decline of T-helper lymphocytes in HIV-1 infection: a report from the Multicenter AIDS Cohort Study. *Lancet* 1990;335:927–930.
12. Phair J, Jacobson L, Detels R, et al. Acquired immune deficiency syndrome occurring within five years of infection with human immunodeficiency virus type-1: the Multicenter AIDS Cohort Study. *J AIDS* 1992;5:490–496.
13. Ho DD, Moudgil T, Alam M. Quantitation of human immunodeficiency virus type 1 in the blood of infected persons. *N Engl J Med* 1989;321:1621–1625.
14. Miller EN, Selnes OA, Mc Arthur JC, et al. Neuropsychological performance in HIV-1-infected homosexual men: the Multicenter AIDS Cohort Study (MACS). *Neurology* 1990;40:197–203.

15. Miller EN, Selnes OA, Visscher B, et al. Changes in performance on the Trail-Making Test before and after HIV-1 seroconversion and diagnosis of AIDS: the Multicenter AIDS Cohort Study (MACS) (abstract). International Conference of AIDS, 1989: 464.
16. Volberding PA, Lagakos SW, Koch MA, et al. Zidovudine in asymptomatic human immunodeficiency virus infection: a controlled trial in persons with fewer than 500 CD4-positive cells per cubic millimeter. *N Engl J Med* 1990;322:941–949.
17. Graham NMH, Zeger SL, Park LP, et al. The effects on survival of early treatment of human immunodeficiency virus infection. *N Engl J Med* 1992;326:1037–1042.
18. Fischl MA, Parker CB, Pettinelli C, et al. AIDS Clinical Trials Group: a randomized controlled trial of a reduced daily dose of zidovudine in patients with acquired immunodeficiency syndrome. *N Engl J Med* 1990;323:1009–1014.
19. Graham NMH, Zeger SL, Saah AJ, et al. Effect of zidovudine and *Pneumocystis carinii* pneumonia prophylaxis on progression of HIV-1 infection to AIDS. *Lancet* 1991; 338(8762):265–269.
20. Detels R, Visscher B, Lee M, et al. Levels of blood cells in men relatively resistant to completed HIV infection (WeA 1048). VIII International Conference on AIDS, Amsterdam, July 1992.
21. Imagawa DT, Lee MH, Wolinsky SM, et al. Human immunodeficiency virus type 1 infection in homosexual men who remain seronegative for prolonged periods. *N Engl J Med* 1989;320:1458–1462.
22. Imagawa D, Detels R. HIV-1 in seronegative homosexual men [Letter]. *N Engl J Med* 1991;325(17):1250–1251.
23. Shearer G, Clerici M. TH1 and TH2 cytokine production in HIV infection (WeA 1047). VIII International Conference on AIDS, Amsterdam, July 1992.
24. Clerici M, Giorgi JV, Chou CC, et al. Cell-mediated immune response to human immunodeficiency virus (HIV) type 1 in seronegative homosexual men with recent sexual exposure to HIV-1. *J Infect Dis* 1992;165:1012–1019.
25. Jehuda-Cohen T, Slade BA, Powell JD, et al. Polyclonal B-cell activation reveals antibodies against human immunodeficiency virus type 1 (HIV-1) in HIV-1 seronegative individuals. *Proc Natl Acad Sci U S A* 1990;87:3972–3976.

DISCUSSION

Dr. Padian: Your whole talk was geared towards biological factors and you didn't look at behavioral factors over time. In cohort studies, where you run the risk of people telling you what you want to hear, how do you deal with getting behavioral responses over time?

Dr. Detels: This is a point that concerns me. The slides I showed you on the factors associated with infection were done in 1987, and there is some interest in updating them, particularly in relation to the issue of oro-genital intercourse, which remains a very important question in the gay community. If you take away all their activities, you're going to get less compliance than if you take away only a few of those activities.

The problem is that the personal cost of admitting that you do anal intercourse becomes higher each year. In 1985, 1986, and 1987, it was perhaps indiscreet to admit that you practiced anal intercourse; in 1991, it was downright stupid. We have had a marked increase in what I call immaculate infections not associated with reported sexual activities, and inside the MACS, we have debated how to get around the problem. In the late 1980s, it was sufficient to go back to these guys and say, "Is it possible you did a little anal?" The majority said "yes." That's now getting to be impossible, so what we do at UCLA is go back to them (we have to tell them if they've seroconverted) and ask them whether it's possible that we hadn't understood them at the time of the last questionnaire. If they say, "That's probably true, you didn't." I leave it at that. We have relatively few individuals who absolutely maintain that we got it right.

Dr. Nicolosi: If I remember correctly, you said that not everybody who is infected gets the disease. But the San Francisco cohort study shows that, 11 years after the first detected case of seropositivity, 50% of seropositive cases develop AIDS. If this were a normal distribution, you would expect the other 50% to develop AIDS over the next 11 years. Of course, if the distribution is not normal, things will be different. But at this point, given the aging effect (because the investigator gets older along with his study), how can we say that not everybody who is infected gets the disease or dies? It seems to me to be premature from a theoretical point of view.

Dr. Detels: If you look at Hessel's paper and the rate of progression to AIDS by each succeeding year, you see that the rate is actually going down. It is not a smooth upwards curve, but a curve that is beginning to change its slope. The assumption that everybody is going to get AIDS is based on the assumption that the slope of the curve to the progression to AIDS will remain steady, whereas the evidence from the San Francisco cohort shows that the slope is decreasing. What it will do in the end, I don't know. I can't predict whether it will level off, or whether it will peak and then decline. But when I looked at it, it was not a straight line: there was a reduction in the number of individuals. If you look at the survivors, and then look at the rate of AIDS among the survivors in each succeeding year, you see that the rate is changing.

The other thing I'd like to emphasize is that the argument that everybody is going to get AIDS has been used to suggest that there are no such things as promoters or cofactors. I don't think that argument holds. Otherwise, why does one individual get AIDS within 1 year (and that has been clearly documented in a lot of cohort studies), and some individuals don't get it for 15 or 20 years? I don't think that argument is a reasonable argument against promoters or cofactors.

Dr. Gail: Another advantage of some of these cohort studies has to do with estimating the absolute rate of infection in the cohort as opposed to the factors that influence who gets infected. There is some nice work by Peter Bacchetti, for example, showing what happened in San Francisco, and there's work in the MACS and work in the hemophiliac cohort showing how the wave of infection passed through the cohort. This is something you can only get from cohort studies; you can't get it from case-control studies.

As to what is happening to incubation distribution as you go into longer periods of time, we'll be talking about the possible effects of treatment later this afternoon. It is certainly true that the San Francisco study shows us that the potential for treatment has to be taken into account as you go beyond 6 or 7 years. I wonder whether people are interested in trying to re-establish what the incubation distribution is these days, based on following new seroconverters in the current climate of treatment.

Dr. Detels: Alvaro, didn't we do some of that in the MACS recently—changes in the incubation period associated with treatment?

Dr. Muñoz: There's the work by Neil Graham and Scott Zeger showing the effect of treatment on extension of AIDS-free time. There are some nontrivial issues related to the selection bias of those receiving treatment in a cohort study.

Dr. Des Jarlais: When you were considering what can be learned about behavior through cohort participation, you didn't address the question as to how the participation in itself might affect behavior and how that may affect the chances of infection or the chances of these behavioral co-factors, including the case of vaccine trials.

Dr. Detels: We have discussed with Sten Vermund the possibility that the MACS might be a potential vaccine trial group, although I feel very strongly that it is an inappropriate group. When we started with HIV infection in 1985 and 1986, we had a seroconversion rate of about 15% per year; it had fallen to less than 1% by 1987 and stayed at less than 1% during the year, although in two centers there does seem to be a slight increase to as high as 2%. So, behavior does change over time.

I don't think that the MACS is a particularly good cohort because what we now have left are individuals who are relatively unlikely to be infected just because we have followed them for so long. We have a lot of resistant individuals and we have also trained them to reduce their risk of becoming infected. I think it was "Stoney" Stallones who made the statement that the best way of stopping an epidemic was to study it.

HIV Epidemiology: Models and Methods, edited by Alfredo Nicolosi. Raven Press, Ltd., New York 1994.

19

Trends in the Incidence of AIDS-Defining Outcomes in the Multicenter AIDS Cohort Study, 1985–1991

*Alvaro Muñoz, †Lewis K. Schrager, *Helena Bacellar, *Ilene Speizer, †Sten H. Vermund, ‡Roger Detels, *Alfred J. Saah, §Lawrence A. Kingsley, ||Daniela Seminara, and ¶John P. Phair

**Department of Epidemiology, The Johns Hopkins School of Public Health, Baltimore, Maryland 21205; †Epidemiology Branch, Division of AIDS, National Institute of Allergy and Infectious Diseases, Bethesda, Maryland 20892; ‡School of Public Health, University of California, Los Angeles, California 90024; §School of Public Health, University of Pittsburgh, Pittsburgh, Pennsylvania; ||Division of Cancer Etiology, National Cancer Institute, Bethesda, Maryland 20892; ¶School of Medicine, Northwestern University, Chicago, Illinois*

Most studies that have described the occurrence of different clinical events defining AIDS have been limited to cross-sectional data on individuals diagnosed with AIDS (1). To estimate the incidence of AIDS, one needs to follow HIV seropositive individuals over time to determine the incidence of the different clinical outcomes that define AIDS among the persons-time at risk. Cohort studies have been ongoing since the early 1980s and only recently have collected sufficient data to study different HIV-related clinical outcomes. Accurate determination of disease incidence is particularly important with the advent of pre-AIDS interventions to prevent or delay specific HIV-1 related outcomes (2). Clinical trials have demonstrated the efficacy of zidovudine administered prior to AIDS onset in delaying the progression to AIDS (3,4). Studies are ongoing to assess the ability of dideoxyinosine to delay progression to AIDS. Pre-AIDS administration of anti-*Pneumocystis carinii* pneumonia chemotherapy, such as aerosolized pentamidine (5), trimethoprim-sulfamethoxazole (6), and dapsone (7,8), can delay or prevent the development of *Pneumocystis carinii* pneumonia in HIV-1–infected persons. As the use of these therapies becomes more widespread, determinations of the incidence of AIDS-defining clinical events among larger numbers of HIV-infected individuals will be necessary to provide a broader assessment of the impact of such interventions. Furthermore, it is important to determine which diagnoses become more frequent once others have been curtailed by the use of therapy or once certain diagnoses requiring cofactors (e.g., a coinfection) are less common due to changes in behavior (e.g., frequency of anal receptive intercourse) influencing the prevalence and transmission of the cofactor.

The purpose of this study was to examine trends in the incidence of the initial and secondary AIDS-defining illnesses that have developed among seropositive participants in the Multicenter AIDS Cohort Study (MACS) from 1985 through 1991. Although recruitment started in the second semester of 1984, we restricted this analysis to 1985 on because the number of person-years for the second semester of 1984 was low relative to the other years due to incomplete recruiting of the cohort early in the study. Well-documented clinical outcomes and precise data on the number of at-risk persons in this cohort provided reliable information on trends in the incidence of AIDS-defining illnesses over the period in which antiretroviral and anti-*Pneumocystis carinii* pneumonia prophylaxis became available. Explanations for the trends described were sought, particularly as they related to the receipt of pre-AIDS therapy, the CD4 helper/inducer T lymphocyte (CD4+ cell) count, and the calendar time at which the AIDS-defining condition presented.

MATERIALS AND METHODS

Study Population

Homosexual and bisexual men compose the study population of the MACS, a prospective study of the transmission and progression of HIV infection. Design and methods of the MACS have been described elsewhere (9). From April, 1984, to March, 1985, a total of 4,954 AIDS-free men were enrolled in four sites in the United States: Baltimore, Pittsburgh, Chicago, and Los Angeles. These men returned semiannually for follow-up visits. At each follow-up visit the participants responded to a standard questionnaire on sexual history and clinical symptomatology, underwent a physical examination, and provided clinical specimens for laboratory evaluation and specimen banking. In April, 1987, three of the four centers began recruiting new participants into their cohorts with the goal of increasing the number of seropositive, nonwhite, homosexual and bisexual men in the MACS. As of the time of analysis (December, 1991), a total of 624 new recruits, mostly black men, were enrolled.

For the purpose of describing the time trend for the incidence of AIDS in the MACS cohort, we used data for those men who were seropositive for HIV-1 at entry or who were observed to seroconvert during the study period. Among the 4,954 in the original cohort, 1,809 (36%) of the men were seropositive at entry. For this analysis, the seroprevalent men contributed to the time at risk for developing an initial AIDS-defining diagnosis from the initial entry date until a first AIDS diagnosis, a non-AIDS death, or withdrawal from the study. At the time of analysis, 418 (13%) members of the original seronegative cohort had seroconverted. These men began contributing to the analysis of AIDS-defining illness incidence when they seroconverted. The seroconversion time of these men was taken as the midpoint of the date of the last negative HIV-1 visit and the date of the first positive HIV-1 visit.

Among the new recruits, 381 (61%) men entered the study seropositive, and 19 (8% of the seronegative) seroconverted since entry. Their contribution to the amount of person-time at risk for developing an initial AIDS-defining diagnosis was analogous to that of the original cohort. Thus, a total of 2,627 HIV-1 infected men from the cohort of 5,578 men have contributed to this analysis.

For the incidence of secondary diagnoses and death after an initial AIDS diagnosis, the population of interest was composed of the 847 who had developed AIDS between 1985 and 1991, and the contribution of time at risk was computed from the date of the initial diagnosis.

Variables and Laboratory Studies

Serostatus was determined by enzyme-linked immunosorbent assay (ELISA). Results that were positive on two ELISA tests were confirmed by Western blot. The centers reported AIDS on a continuous basis as the diagnoses were reported by the treating physicians (i.e., not only at the times of scheduled visits). Diagnoses considered AIDS defining were those listed in the 1987 revision of the Centers for Disease Control AIDS case definition (10). To maintain consistency over the time of this analysis, the 1987 CDC AIDS definition was applied to all subjects, whether their initial AIDS-defining event occurred before or after the revised classification. For the analysis and comparison of trends, AIDS-defining diagnoses were analyzed in six categories: (i) *Pneumocystis carinii* pneumonia, (ii) "other" opportunistic infections, which encompassed bacterial (atypical mycobacteria, tuberculosis, salmonella, shigella), fungal (candidiasis, histoplasmosis), and protozoal (cryptosporidiosis, isosporiasis) infections and wasting syndrome; (iii) Kaposi's sarcoma; (iv) lymphoma (non-Hodgkin's, brain); (v) neurologic diseases (cryptococcal meningitis, toxoplasmosis, encephalopathy, leukoencephalopathy); and (vi) cytomegalovirus and herpes simplex virus (CMV-HSV) infections.

At each semiannual visit, T-lymphocyte subsets were determined by the whole blood lysis method (11). For the purpose of this analysis, CD4+ cell counts were grouped as 100 or less, 101 to 200, 201 to 350, 351 to 500, and more than 500 cells per mm^3.

Collection of data on the use of prophylactic chemotherapeutic agents was started in 1987, shortly following the licensing of zidovudine. A comprehensive list of questions providing information on the use of specific AIDS medications has been administered at each subsequent visit. Our analysis assessed the effect of antiretroviral therapy (zidovudine and dideoxyinosine) on the incidence of an initial diagnosis of "other" opportunistic infections, Kaposi's sarcoma, lymphoma, neurologic diseases, or CMV-HSV infections over the period of this investigation. We also assessed the effect of *Pneumocystis carinii* pneumonia prophylaxis, including pentamidine delivered via aerosol, trimethoprim-sulfamethoxazole, and dapsone, on influencing the incidence of an initial *Pneumocystis carinii* pneumonia diagnosis. These drugs were among the most common used by MACS cohort members prior to the onset of AIDS over the period of this analysis (12).

Statistical Analysis

For the analysis of the initial AIDS-defining conditions, the outcome of interest was the incidence of the specific initial AIDS-defining diagnoses among the seropositive participants free of AIDS. The analysis spanned the period from 1985 to 1991. The incidence of AIDS was estimated by the ratio of the number of initial AIDS-defining diagnoses observed to occur in a particular year to the total number of person-years contributed by AIDS-free seropositive individuals in that year. Our methods incorporated the contributions of both the seroprevalent men after entry (regardless of their date of entry) and the seroconverters after seroconversion.

To investigate the influence of progressive immunosuppression and receipt of pre-AIDS therapy on selected AIDS-defining illness rates, contributions of these independent variables were assessed. The number of AIDS cases was modeled as a Poisson variable whose mean was proportional to the number of person-years at risk and to the antilog of a linear combination of the covariates of interest (i.e., calendar time, CD4+ cell count, and receipt of pre-AIDS therapy) (13). Specifically, the number of AIDS diagnoses was assumed to follow a Poisson distribution with mean

$$PY(t;\mathbf{x}) * \lambda(t;\mathbf{x})$$

where

$$\lambda(t;\mathbf{x}) = exp(\alpha_0 + \alpha_1 t^{1/2} + \alpha_2 t + \boldsymbol{\beta}\mathbf{x}) \qquad [1]$$

and $t=0$ for 1985, 1 for 1986, . . . , 6 for 1991; $\boldsymbol{x}$ is a vector of CD4+ cell count categories and indicators for the use of PCP prophylaxis or antiretroviral therapy; $PY(t;\boldsymbol{x})$ is the number of person-years at time t with covariates $\boldsymbol{x}$. We sought to determine the significance of α_1 or α_2, or both, for the description of the time trends of AIDS diagnoses without controlling for CD4+

cell count and prophylaxis (i.e., $\boldsymbol{\beta}=0$), and after controlling for these covariates (i.e., estimating and testing the significance of $\boldsymbol{\beta}$). In the application of our model, we incorporated the changing nature of immunosuppression and receipt of pre-AIDS therapy, permitting a more accurate account of the changing risk factors among individuals at each semiannual visit. For example, if a person had a CD4+ cell count between 201 and 350 at a given time and drops to 100 or less in a later 6-month period, his contribution would change accordingly. Similar procedures were used for the handling of the changing nature of prophylactic administration. The antilog of the coefficient for a given covariate estimates the relative incidence for AIDS associated with a unit change in the covariate. Hypothesis testing was accomplished by the Wald test and the likelihood ratio test (14). Goodness of fit was assessed by the deviance of a given model from the saturated model. In addition, the depiction of the expected and the observed data provides a graphic representation of how well these Poisson regression models fit the data.

The analysis of secondary diagnoses and death after an initial AIDS diagnosis is formally equivalent to the methods described above. The person-years were computed after the initial AIDS diagnosis, and, in addition to calendar year, the main covariate of interest was the type of initial diagnosis (e.g., PCP).

RESULTS

The incidence of initial AIDS-defining diagnoses among the HIV-positive cohort members by year from 1985 to 1991 is presented in Table 1. The total number of AIDS cases was 847. Person-years at risk describes the total amount of time that seropositive AIDS-free men were at risk for developing an initial AIDS-defining event during a given year (Table 1, second column). The temporal decline in person-years at risk largely was due to the development of AIDS among HIV-1–infected study participants. Transient or permanent loss to follow-up contributed to this decline to a smaller degree, while new seroconversions and the addition of new enrollees after 1987 moderated this decline somewhat. The total number of initial AIDS-defining events occurring within each year is shown, along with the incidence of each event (Table 1, columns three through eight). Incidence is expressed as the risk of developing a given AIDS-defining event per 100 person-years at risk within each calendar year.

The trends in initial AIDS-defining diagnoses over time are plotted in Fig. 1. The data points depicted with open circles represent the observed incidences per 100 person-years, shown in parentheses in Table 1. The curves represent best-fit models using Poisson regression analyses. With the years coded 0 for 1985, 1 for 1986, 2 for 1987 and so on, the model for PCP includes

TABLE 1. *Incidence of initial AIDS-defining diagnoses among HIV seropositive gay men, 1985–1991*

		AIDS defining diagnoses[a]					
Year	Person-years	PCP	Other OI	KS	Lymphoma	Neurologic	CMV-HSV
1985	1812.8	33 (1.8)	12 (0.7)	30 (1.7)	0 (0.0)	8 (0.4)	2 (0.1)
1986	1755.7	64 (3.7)	11 (0.6)	22 (1.3)	2 (0.1)	3 (0.2)	5 (0.3)
1987	1696.7	72 (4.2)	17 (1.0)	22 (1.3)	5 (0.3)	10 (0.6)	13 (0.8)
1988	1679.7	65 (3.9)	13 (0.8)	32 (1.9)	4 (0.2)	15 (0.9)	6 (0.4)
1989	1532.6	54 (3.5)	26 (1.7)	35 (2.3)	11 (0.7)	11 (0.7)	9 (0.6)
1990	1344.8	46 (3.4)	35 (2.6)	28 (2.1)	5 (0.4)	10 (0.7)	14 (1.0)
1991	1196.6	30 (2.5)	40 (3.3)	25 (2.1)	7 (0.6)	9 (0.8)	12 (1.0)

From Muñoz, et al. (20).

[a]Incidence rates per 100 person-years, observed incidences in parentheses. PCP, *Pneumocystis carinii* pneumonia; other OI, other opportunistic infections; KS, Kaposi's sarcoma; CMV-HSV, cytomegalovirus and herpes simplex virus.

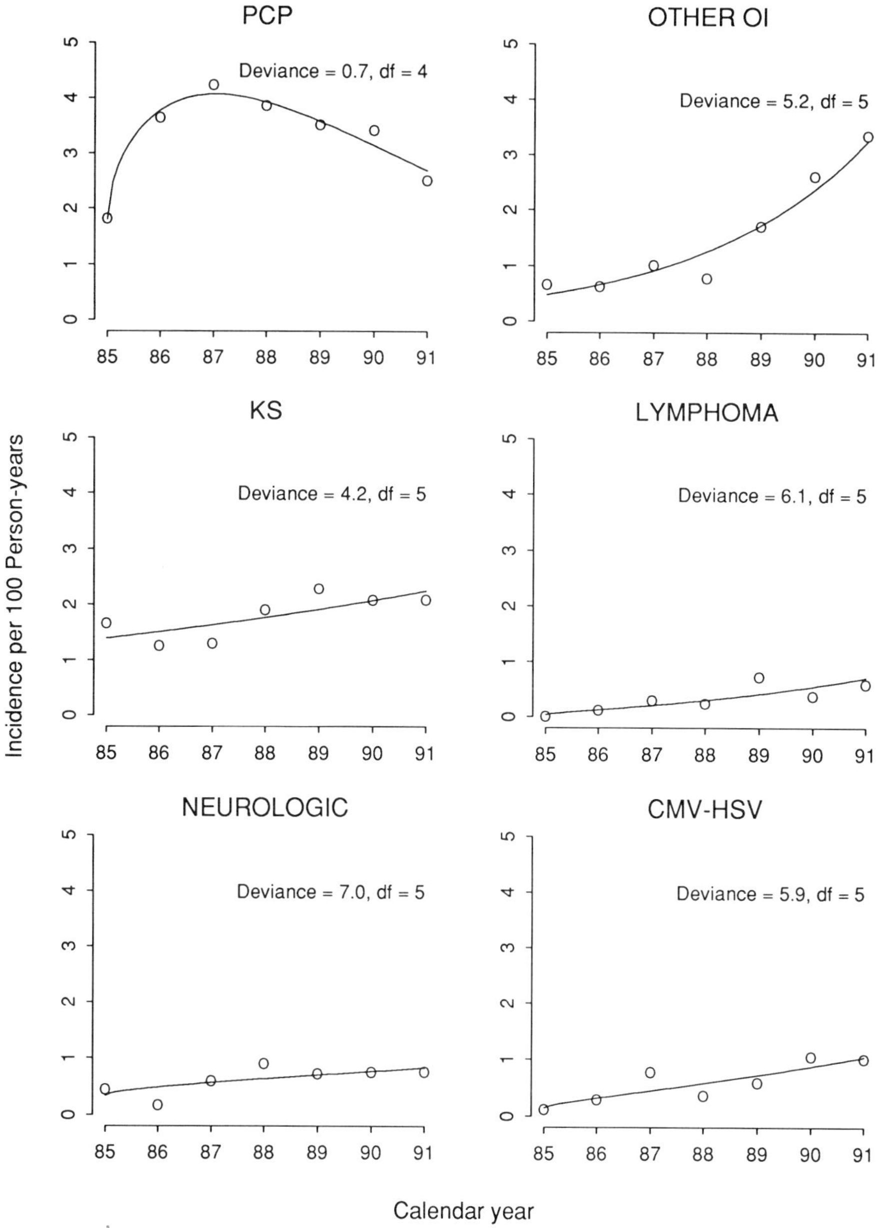

FIG. 1. Observed (*open circles*) and expected (*curves*) incidence of initial AIDS-defining diagnosis. Expected are obtained by Poisson regression methods. From Muñoz et al. (20).

a term for the square root of year and a term for year (i.e., in Eq. (1), $\alpha_1 \neq 0$ and $\alpha_2 \neq 0$); the models for "other" opportunistic infections and KS include a term for year (i.e., in Eq. (1), $\alpha_1 = 0$ and $\alpha_2 \neq 0$); and the models for lymphoma, neurologic diseases, and CMV-HSV include a term for the square root of year (i.e., in Eq. (1), $\alpha_1 \neq 0$ and $\alpha_2 = 0$). The incidence of PCP rose steeply until 1987 but has declined since then ($p < 0.001$), while "other" opportunistic infections have steadily increased ($p < 0.001$). Incidence of Kaposi's sarcoma showed an upward trend ($p = 0.028$), as did the incidence of lymphomas ($p < 0.001$). Neurologic and CMV-HSV related diseases showed slight but significant increases over time ($p = 0.039$ for neurologic and $p < 0.001$ for CMV-HSV). Figure 1 depicts the relative contribution of different diagnoses to the total incidence of AIDS over the period from 1985 to 1991. *Pneumocystis carinii* pneumonia, KS, and "other" opportunistic infections have been the three most common diagnoses during the entire period. "Other" opportunistic infections switched from being the third most common diagnosis in 1985 to being the most common in 1991, with current levels being close to those observed for PCP in 1987. Similarly, among the three remaining, less common diagnoses (i.e., lymphoma, neurologic diseases, and CMV-HSV), the viral infections switched from being the lowest in 1985 to being the highest in 1991.

The trends depicted in Fig. 1 may be explained in part by the progressive immunosuppression in infected individuals. Table 2 displays the incidence of initial AIDS-defining diagnoses among HIV seropositive MACS participants by categories of the CD4+ cell count. For example, from 1985 to 1991 we have observed 347.8 person-years of AIDS-free seropositive individuals with CD4+ cell counts below 100; 111 (31.9%) were observed to develop *Pneumocystis carinii* pneumonia within one year. For all defining conditions there was a very strong association between low CD4+ cell count and high incidence. There was positive confounding between CD4+ cell counts and calendar year (i.e., low CD4+ counts are more common in 1991 than in 1985 for individuals infected prior to 1985). Therefore, some of the upward trends in Fig. 1 may be totally explained by progressive immunosuppression. Given that incidences of PCP, "other" opportunistic infections, and KS were one percent or below when CD4+ was above 350 and incidences of lymphoma, neurologic diseases, and CMV-HSV were below one percent when CD4+ was above 200, we restricted the analysis of the joint effect of CD4+ cell count and calendar year to these categories of CD4+ cell count.

To determine the simultaneous effect of year of diagnosis and level of immunosuppression on the incidence of initial AIDS-defining events, we use Poisson regression methods. In the regression models we treated CD4+ as a categorical variable and year as a continuous variable, taking values from 0 for 1986 to 5 for 1991. The exclusion of 1985 from this analysis was due to a substantial lack of CD4+ cell counts prior to 1985. Table 3 shows two models for each of the AIDS diagnoses: one without calendar year as a co-

TABLE 2. *Incidence of initial AIDS-defining diagnoses among HIV seropositive gay men by CD4+ cell count*

CD4+ cell count	Person-years	AIDS-defining diagnoses[a]					
		PCP	Other OI	KS	Lymphoma	Neurologic	CMV-HSV
≤100	347.8	111 (31.9)	79 (22.7)	52 (15.0)	9 (2.6)	25 (7.2)	25 (7.2)
101–200	629.4	57 (9.1)	24 (3.8)	41 (6.5)	6 (1.0)	8 (1.3)	11 (1.7)
201–350	1715.7	62 (3.6)	15 (0.9)	30 (1.7)	4 (0.2)	11 (0.6)	4 (0.2)
351–500	2221.8	30 (1.4)	6 (0.3)	18 (0.8)	3 (0.1)	3 (0.1)	3 (0.1)
>500	4619.3	8 (0.2)	3 (0.1)	12 (0.3)	1 (<0.1)	2 (<0.1)	1 (<0.1)

From Muñoz, et al. (20).
[a]Incidence rates per 100 person-years, observed incidences in parentheses.

TABLE 3. *Poisson regression models for the incidence of AIDS by CD4+ cell count and calendar year, 1986–1991*

	PCP		Other OI		KS		Lymphoma		Neurologic		CMV-HSV	
Constant[a]												
CD4≤100	−1.23	−0.38	−1.53	−2.30	−2.01	−1.76	−3.59	−3.54	−2.70	−3.06	−2.57	−2.68
101≤CD4≤200	−2.45	−1.69	−3.39	−4.09	−2.78	−2.56	−4.54	−4.50	−4.39	−4.71	−3.94	−4.04
201≤CD4≤350	−3.22	−2.56	−4.74	−5.37	−4.09	−3.89	**	**	**	**	**	**
Year[b]		−0.33		0.23		−0.09		−0.02		0.11		0.04
Deviance	66.6	10.8	24.9	12.2	12.4	10.4	15.1	15.1	10.6	9.6	8.6	8.5
Degrees of freedom	15	14	15	14	15	14	10	9	10	9	10	9
Goodness of fit *p*-value[c]	<0.01	0.70	0.05	0.59	0.65	0.73	0.13	0.09	0.39	0.38	0.57	0.49

[a]First column for each diagnosis represents model without calendar year as a covariable ($\alpha_1 = 0$, $\alpha_2 = 0$), and the second column represents model with calendar year as a covariate ($\alpha_1 = 0$, $\alpha_2 \neq 0$).
[b]Year coded as, 0 = 1986, 1 = 1987, . . . , 5 = 1991.
[c]p-value = probability that chi-square with degrees of freedom will be above deviance.
**Analysis restricted to first two CD4 categories, because outcome is uncommon for CD4>200.

variate (i.e., in Eq. (1), $\alpha_1=0$ and $\alpha_2=0$) and one with calendar year as a covariate (i.e., in Eq. (1), $\alpha_1=0$ but $\alpha_2 \neq 0$). A deviance close to or below the degrees of freedom is indicative of a good fit and corresponds to a high p-value. Differences of deviances between the two models' fit for each diagnosis are the likelihood ratio statistics, which follow a chi-square distribution with one degree of freedom and whose associated p-value determines the statistical significance of calendar year after controlling for CD4+ cell count. *Pneumocystis carinii* pneumonia and "other" opportunistic infections required the inclusion of year after adjusting for CD4+ cell count, thus indicating significant residual trends: downward for PCP ($\hat{\alpha}_2 = -0.33$, likelihood ratio statistic: $55.8 = 66.6 - 10.8$, $p<0.001$) and upward for "other" opportunistic infections ($\hat{\alpha}_2=0.23$, likelihood ratio statistic: $12.7 = 24.9 - 12.2$, $p<0.001$). In contrast, the goodness of fit of the models including only CD4+ cell count for the other four diagnoses in Table 3 indicated that progressive immunosuppression explains the trends depicted in Fig. 1 for these diagnoses. The statistics for KS and lymphoma, albeit nonsignificant, suggest a downward trend ($\hat{\alpha}_2<0$), while those for neurologic diseases and CMV-HSV suggest an upward trend ($\hat{\alpha}_2>0$).

The antilogs of the coefficients presented in Table 3 are useful to estimate the expected incidence rates and relative risks of different diagnoses according to categories of CD4+ cell count and relative changes per calendar year. To quantify the relative risks and 95% confidence intervals of each diagnosis, we used the models including year in Table 3; they are displayed in Table 4. The relative risks for CD4+ categories are calculated as follows: CD4+ cell count between 101 and 200 is compared with CD4$\leq$100 using the antilog of the difference between the constant terms (e.g., for PCP, RR$=0.27$ is $exp[-1.69-(-0.38)]$; values are from Table 3). The CD4+ cell count between 201 and 350 is compared with CD4 $\leq$ 100 using the same method. The relative risks per calendar year are the antilogs of the coefficients of year in Table 3 and represent the relative incidences of a given year compared to the year before. The 95% confidence intervals are derived from the standard errors of the coefficients using maximum likelihood principles. In Table 4, the lowest relative risks for 101$\leq$CD4$\leq$200, compared with CD4$\leq$100, were those of "other" opportunistic infections (RR=0.17) and neurologic diseases (RR=0.19), followed by those of CMV-HSV (RR=0.26) and PCP (RR=0.27); and the weakest association was that of KS (RR=0.45). Lymphoma had only a marginally significant association (RR=0.38, 95% CI=0.14,1.09). The relative risks for 201$\leq$CD4$\leq$350, compared with CD4$\leq$100, were significantly lower than the previous ones, with "other" opportunistic infections showing the strongest association (RR=0.05), and PCP and KS having similar relative risks (RR=0.11 and 0.12, respectively).

The relative risks per calendar year were significantly different from one (i.e., confidence intervals do not contain one) for PCP and "other" opportunistic infections (Table 4). The 0.72 relative risk of PCP indicates that, after adjusting for CD4+ cell count, the incidence of PCP in a given year is

TABLE 4. *Relative risks and 95% confidence intervals of initial AIDS-defining diagnoses for CD4+ categories and per calendar year*

	AIDS defining diagnoses[a]					
	PCP	Other OI	KS	Lymphoma	Neurologic	CMV-HSV
$CD4 \leq 100$						
RR[b]	1.00	1.00	1.00	1.00	1.00	1.00
$101 \leq CD4 \leq 200$						
RR	0.27	0.17	0.45	0.38	0.19	0.26
(95% CI)	(0.19, 0.38)	(0.10, 0.28)	(0.29, 0.70)	(0.14, 1.09)	(0.08, 0.45)	(0.13, 0.53)
$201 \leq CD4 \leq 350$						
RR	0.11	0.05	0.12	**	**	**
(95% CI)	(0.08, 0.16)	(0.03, 0.08)	(0.07, 0.19)			
Per calendar year						
RR	0.72	1.26	0.91	0.98	1.12	1.04
(95% CI)	(0.66, 0.79)	(1.11, 1.44)	(0.81, 1.03)	(0.72, 1.35)	(0.88, 1.42)	(0.84, 1.27)

From Muñoz, et al. (20).

[a]Estimates derived from the models including year in Table 3.

[b]RR, relative risk.

**Analysis restricted to first two CD4 categories, because outcome is uncommon for $CD4 > 200$.

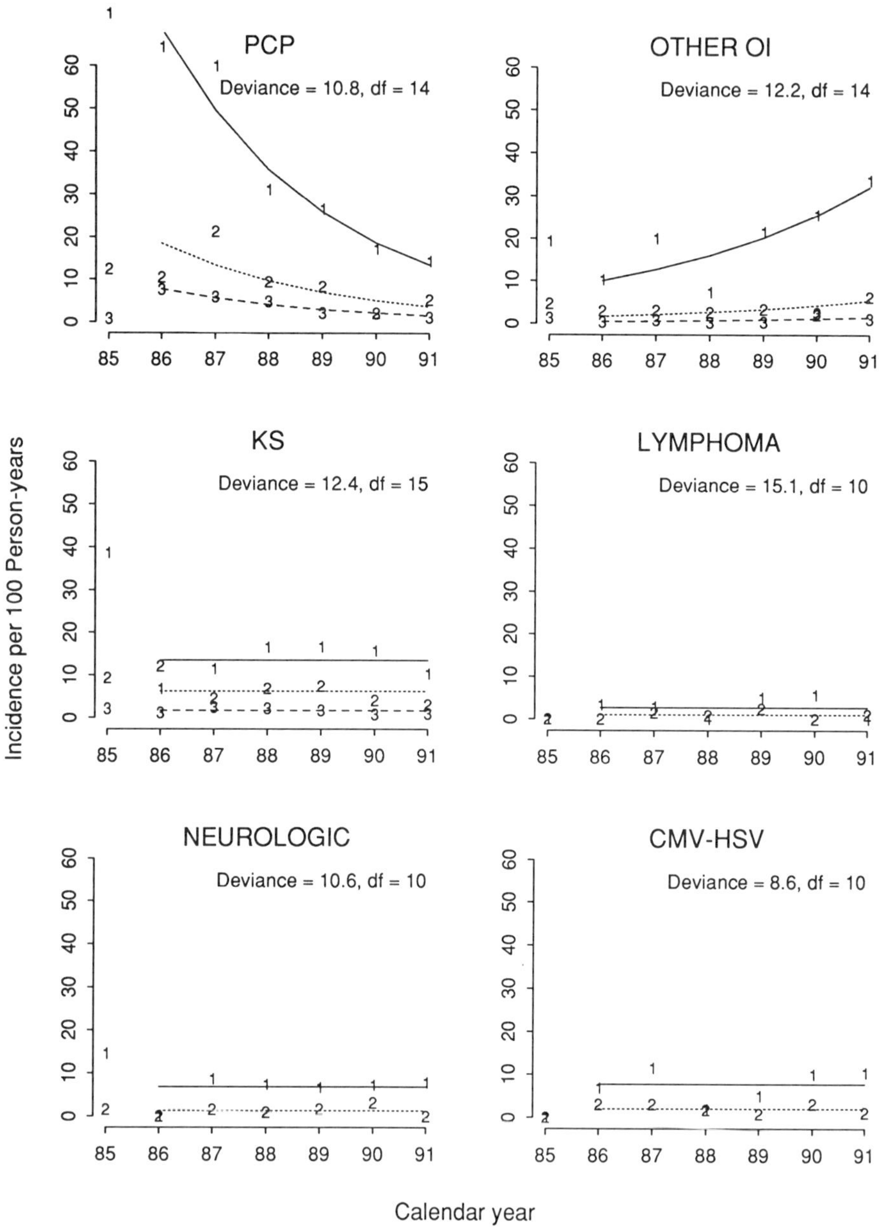

FIG. 2. Observed and expected incidence of initial AIDS-defining diagnoses. Digits in plots represent observed incidence rates for CD4+ categories as follows: 1, CD4≤100; 2, 101≤CD4≤200; 3, 201≤CD4≤350. Curves in plots represent expected incidence rates for CD4+ categories as follows: (———) for CD4≤100, (-----) for 101≤CD4≤200, (– – –) for 201≤CD4≤350; obtained using models in Table 3. From Muñoz et al. (20).

expected to be 72% of the rate in the previous year. In contrast, the incidence of "other" opportunistic infections in a given year is expected to be 126% (or 26% higher) that of a previous year. The relative risks per calendar year of KS (RR = 0.91) and lymphoma (RR = 0.98) are lower than one, suggesting a downward trend after adjusting for CD4+ cell count. In contrast, the relative risks of neurologic (RR = 1.12) and CMV-HSV (RR = 1.04) diagnoses suggest an upward trend even after adjusting for CD4+ cell count.

Figure 2 depicts the observed incidence rates of each of the AIDS-defining diagnoses according to year and CD4+ cell count. The CD4+ cell count categories are represented in the plots by 1 for $CD4 \leq 100$, 2 for $101 \leq CD4 \leq 200$, and 3 for $201 \leq CD4 \leq 350$. The expected rates were plotted as curves or lines using the most parsimonius model with appropriate fit for each diagnosis. The expected rates for PCP and "other" opportunistic infections were obtained from the models including year as a covariate. Thus, the antilog of the constant terms in Table 3 represents the expected rates in 1986, and the coefficient of year governs the significant trends. The expected rates for KS, lymphoma, neurologic diseases, and CMV-HSV were obtained from models without the year as a covariate, thus the antilog of the constant terms represents the constant expected rate for each category of CD4+ cell count. Figure 2 clearly depicts the opposite trends exhibited by PCP and "other" opportunistic infections for all categories of CD4+ cell count. Kaposi's sarcoma was strongly associated with CD4+ cell count, and although there is not a significant overall trend, a downward trend was borderline significant ($p = 0.042$) when the analysis was restricted to the period from 1988 to 1991. Associations for the remaining diagnoses were as follows: lymphoma was weakly associated with CD4+ cell count, neurologic diseases were rarely seen for CD4+ above 100, and CMV-HSV infections were strongly associated with CD4+ cell count and showed no trend over calendar time.

In addition to CD4+ cell count and year, we were interested in assessing the impact on AIDS incidence of the use of PCP prophylaxis and antiretroviral therapy. Of particular interest was the extent to which the residual downward trend of PCP (after controlling for CD4+ cell count) noted in Fig. 2 can be explained by the effect of PCP prophylaxis. Needless to say, use of medication for AIDS, immunosuppression, and calendar year were closely related. Figure 3 provides three plots summarizing the total person-years observed in AIDS-free seropositive individuals according to CD4+ cell count categories and year, and the percentages of those person-years under PCP prophylaxis and under antiretroviral therapy. Owing to the progressive immunosuppression, the person-years in the lower CD4+ categories increased over time, and the person-years in the higher CD4+ categories decreased over time. The substantial changes in person-years observed between 1987 and 1988 were partially due to the recruitment of new seropositive individuals who tended to be in the lower CD4+ categories. Per-

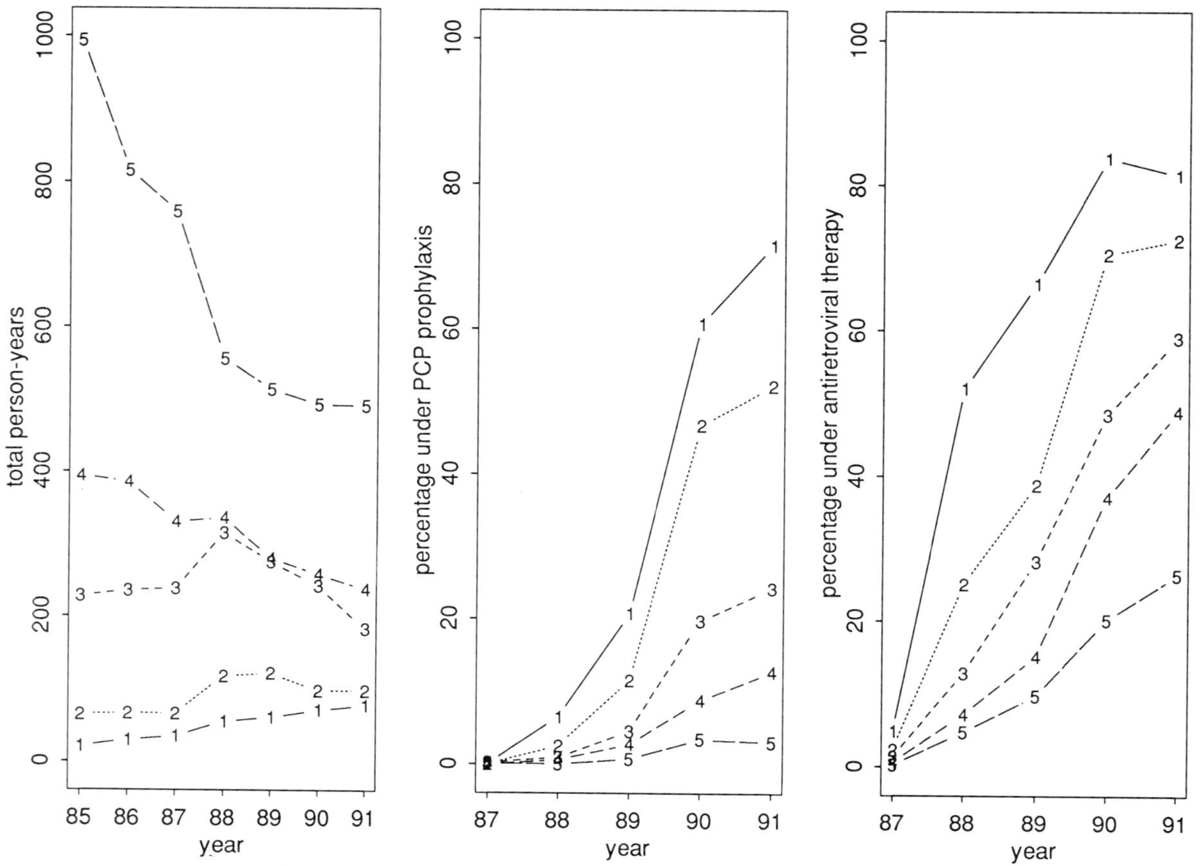

FIG. 3. Total person-years and percentages under PCP prophylaxis and antiretroviral therapy among AIDS-free HIV seropositive participants of the Multicenter AIDS Cohort Study. Digits in plots represent categories of CD4+ cell count as follows: 1, CD4≤100; 2, 101≤CD4≤200; 3, 201≤CD4≤350; 4, 351≤CD4≤500; and 5, CD4>500. No prophylaxis was licensed prior to 1987. From Muñoz, et al. (20).

centages under PCP prophylaxis or antiretroviral therapy, or both, were closely tied to progressive immunosuppression and have dramatically increased over time, with suggestions of leveling off between 1990 and 1991, but with less intensity for antiretroviral therapy when the CD4+ count is above 200 cells. The delay of the use of PCP prophylaxis relative to antiretroviral therapy is due to the later licensing of PCP prophylaxis. As expected, prophylaxis has been selectively administered to severely immunosuppressed individuals, and its use has increased sharply over time.

Table 5 shows the incidence rates for PCP according to CD4+ cell count, year, and use of PCP prophylaxis. To avoid low numbers of person-years, we combined 1986 and 1987, 1988 and 1989, and 1990 and 1991. For example, in 1986 and 1987 we observed 64.1 person-years with $CD4 \leq 100$ and under no PCP prophylaxis, while no person-years with $CD4 \leq 100$ were under PCP prophylaxis in 1986 and 1987. We restricted the analysis to CD4+ cell counts less than or equal to 200, because the use of prophylaxis and the incidence of PCP were highest for persons at these levels. Because no one reported using PCP prophylaxis prior to 1987, the adjusted relative risk for incidence of PCP was accomplished by combining years after 1988. The relative risks, which were less than one for each CD4+ category ($RR = 0.37$ for $CD4 \leq 100$ and $RR = 0.13$ for $101 \leq CD4 \leq 200$), indicate a protective effect of PCP prophylaxis. A multivariate Poisson regression including CD4+ cell count, calendar year, and PCP prophylaxis was carried out to estimate the effect of PCP prophylaxis after adjusting for the other two covariates. With simultaneous adjustment for year and CD4+ cell count, PCP prophylaxis showed a significant protective effect against the incidence of PCP ($RR = 0.32$, 95% $CI = 0.16$–0.63). Conversely, as a result of including CD4+ cell count and PCP prophylaxis, the residual downward trend with calendar year was no longer significant ($p = 0.328$). Therefore, the time-based trends of PCP incidence were explained by progressive immunosuppression and use of PCP prophylaxis.

A similar analysis to that presented in Table 5 was carried out for the effect of antiretroviral therapy on "other" opportunistic infections, KS, lymphoma, neurologic diseases, and CMV-HSV infections. Largely due to the selection bias of those receiving antiretroviral therapy (i.e., severely immunosuppressed), no significant effects of antiretroviral therapy were detected in this analysis. For KS, lymphoma, and neurologic diseases, the relative risk was less than one, suggesting a protective effect ($RR = 0.83$ for KS, $RR = 0.47$ for lymphoma, and $RR = 0.79$ for neurologic diseases). "Other" opportunistic and CMV-HSV infections were more common among those selected to receive antiretroviral therapy, suggesting a lack of effect of this type of therapy for "other" opportunistic and CMV-HSV infections, or that those receiving antiretroviral therapy were at higher risk for these infections to start with, or both.

TABLE 5. *Incidence of PCP by CD4+ cell count, calendar year, and anti-PCP prophylaxis*

		Years							
		1986–87		1988–89		1990–91			
CD4+ cell count	PCP prophylaxis	P-Y[a]	(IR)[b]	P-Y	(IR)	P-Y	(IR)	Relative risk	95% CI
≤100	no	64.1	(62.4%)	98.8	(31.4%)	49.6	(24.2%)	1.00	
	yes	0.0	(—)	15.9	(6.3%)	97.6	(10.2%)	0.37[c]	0.18–0.77
101–200	no	132.0	(15.2%)	221.2	(9.5%)	98.3	(6.1%)	1.00	
	yes	0.0	(—)	16.8	(0.0%)	96.0	(1.0%)	0.13[c]	0.02–1.02
overall	no							1.00	
	yes							0.32[d]	0.16–0.63

From Muñoz, et al. (20).
[a]P-Y, person-years.
[b]IR, incidence rate per 100 P-Y.
[c]Adjusted by calendar year, 1988 to 1991.
[d]Adjusted by calendar year (1988 to 1991) and CD4+ cell count.

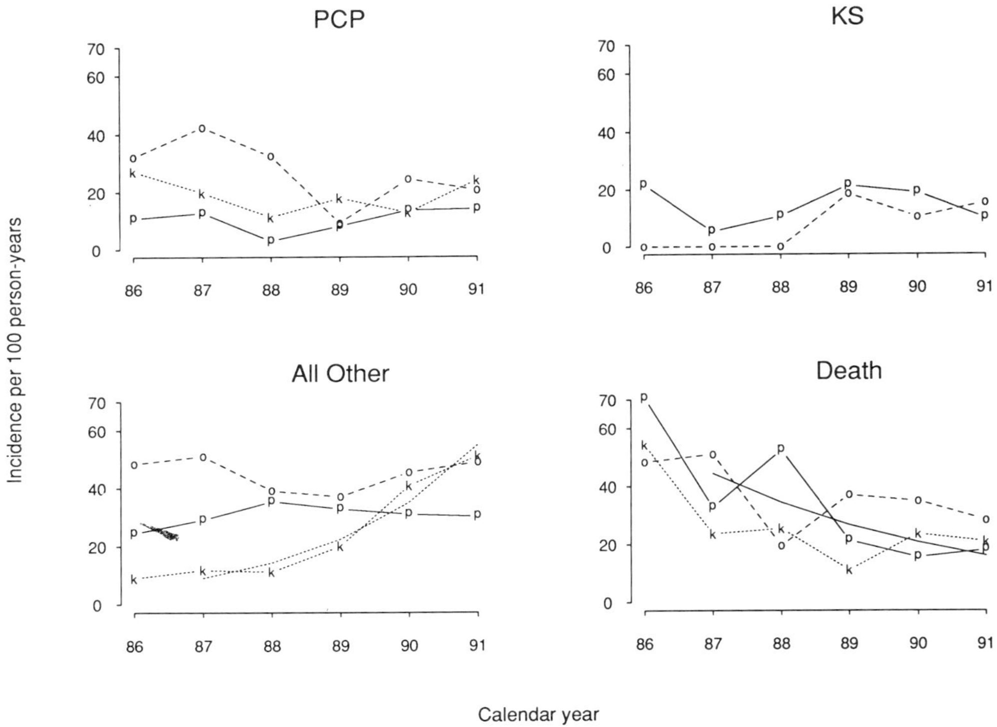

FIG. 4. Incidence of secondary diagnosis and death according to initial diagnosis (*p,* PCP; *k*, KS; *o,* opportunistic infections including bacterial, fungal, protozoal, and wasting syndrome) and year, 1986–1991. Observed incidences joined by broken lines: (———) if initial is PCP; (------) if initial is KS; (– – –) if initial is Other OI. Smooth curves are expected rates according to Poisson regression for categories with statistically significant trends. From Muñoz, et al. (20).

To complete the analysis, we undertook the description of the incidence of secondary diagnoses and death according to the initial diagnosis. Figure 4 depicts the incidence per 100 person-years of PCP, KS, all other (i.e., non-PCP, non-KS) diagnoses, and death for those having had an initial diagnosis of PCP (denoted with p in Fig. 4), KS (denoted with k), or "other" opportunistic infections (denoted by o). We restricted the analysis to these initial diagnoses because they were the most common among all diagnoses (see Fig. 1). Furthermore, given that time is needed for the initial diagnosis to be observed, we restricted the analysis to the period of 1986 on. Using Poisson regression methods, no significant trends were noted for secondary diagnosis except for an increasing trend ($p<0.001$) for non-PCP, non-KS diagnoses in those whose initial diagnosis was KS. The 1-year death rates after an AIDS diagnosis exhibited declines for the three types of initial diagnoses considered, and the trend for PCP reached statistical significance ($p=0.003$). For the two instances in which statistically significant trends were detected, we superimposed the expected curves on the depiction of the observed rates in Fig. 4.

CONCLUSION

A significant decrease in the incidence of *Pneumocystis carinii* pneumonia as the initial AIDS-defining diagnosis has been noted since 1987 within the MACS cohort. In contrast, the incidence of "other" opportunistic infections, Kaposi's sarcoma, lymphomas, neurologic diseases, and CMV-HSV infections have shown significant increases as the seropositive men in this closed cohort live longer with HIV infection. The trends of *Pneumocystis carinii* pneumonia can be explained by the progressive immunosuppression and intervention with PCP prophylaxis (Table 5). The trends of Kaposi's sarcoma, lymphoma, neurologic diseases, and CMV-HSV infections can be explained by progressive immunosuppression (Table 3). However, a residual upward trend was still present for "other" opportunistic infections after accounting for the effect of immunosuppression and pre-AIDS medications. It is interesting to note that when the relative incidence across the columns in Table 4 are compared, "other" opportunistic infections had the strongest association with low CD4+ cell counts while exhibiting no reduction with receipt of pre-AIDS prophylaxis. This underlines the need of developing new prophylaxis strategies for "other" opportunistic infections, including bacterial, fungal, and protozoal infections.

The receipt of aerosolized pentamidine, trimethoprim-sufamethoxazole, dapsone, or all three prior to the onset of AIDS significantly decreased the incidence of *Pneumocystis carinii* pneumonia (Table 5). This is not a surprising finding in light of their proven efficacy in preventing this infection when given in a prophylactic manner (5–8,15). It is also possible that antiretroviral therapy may have contributed to the reduction of the incidence of *Pneumocystis carinii* pneumonia, because most of the individuals in the MACS who received pre-AIDS prophylaxis against *Pneumocystis carinii* pneumonia also received pre-AIDS zidovudine or dideoxyinosine, or both. For example, in the first semester of 1991, 88% of those taking *Pneumocystis carinii* pneumonia prophylaxis were also taking zidovudine, dideoxyinosine, or both. Although 92 individuals in the 201≤CD4≤500 cell category developed *Pneumocystis carinii* pneumonia as their initial AIDS-defining infection, the incidence rate of this pneumonia was only one seventh the incidence occurring among individuals with CD4+ counts ≤200/mm^3.

As the incidence of PCP declined, the incidence of "other" opportunistic infections increased. These opposite trends remained after controlling for the progressive immunosuppression as measured by CD4+ cell count. In contrast to PCP prophylaxis, which showed a protective effect against the incidence of PCP, those using antiretroviral therapy exhibited higher rates, rather than showing lower rates, of "other" opportunistic infections. It has been documented (12) that those in the MACS receiving antiretroviral therapy not only are relatively more immunosuppressed but exhibited high rates of HIV-related symptoms (e.g., oral thrush). Even if antiretroviral therapy is beneficial, the selection bias present among those receiving prophylaxis may require much more complex analytical approaches to detect an effect (15). In any case, the increasing occurrence of "other" opportunistic infections should be taken into consideration for the planning and delivery of health services in populations that have high prevalence of HIV infection.

The overall incidence of Kaposi's sarcoma declined from 1985 to 1987 (Fig. 1), then it exhibited an increase to a rather constant level between 1988 and 1991. After controlling for CD4+ cell count, there was a clear association between immunosuppression and incidence of KS, but it was of a lesser magnitude than other diagnoses, except for lymphomas. The CD4+ cell count-adjusted incidence of KS showed a downward trend after 1988 (Fig. 2), which suggests a protective effect of antiretroviral therapy (RR=0.91). Alternatively, the downward trend may be related to lower prevalence of the hypothesized agent for KS (16) in individuals who have been infected for more than 5 years and have considerably reduced the sexual practices that are putatively related to the transmission of the hypothesized infectious agent.

Lymphoma showed a weak association with CD4+ cell count, but the crude upward trend with calendar year (Fig. 1) was explained by progressive immunosuppression. It has been projected that the incidence of lymphoma will rise as more persons prolong their pre-AIDS state with prophylaxis (17,18). Compared with "other" opportunistic infections, the increase of lymphomas, although present, has not been considerable.

In this cohort, the median survival time after AIDS diagnosis has increased from 12 months in 1985 to approximately 18 months in 1990 (19).

Given this relatively short survival time, there is limited power in detecting trends of secondary diagnoses. However, we found a strong upward trend of non-PCP, non-KS diagnoses in individuals initially diagnosed with KS (Fig. 4). More important was the downward trend of the 1-year death rate after most diagnoses. In consonance with the downward trend of PCP as the initial AIDS diagnosis, we found a statistically significant downward trend of the 1-year death rate after PCP.

In summary, the incidence of PCP and the hazard of death after PCP have declined significantly over time, and the decline is due to the effectiveness of PCP prophylaxis and treatment. Antiretroviral therapy, proven to be effective in clinical trials, has been selectively administered to individuals at higher risk, and although this selection bias creates analytical difficulties, one would have expected higher rates had therapy not been administered. The residual upward trends of "other" opportunistic infections underlines the need of developing and testing new strategies to curtail or delay the onset of these diseases.

ACKNOWLEDGMENTS

This study was supported by NIH research contracts AI-72634, AI-72676, AI-32535, AI-72631, AI-72632. This paper includes material from Muñoz, et al., *Am J Epidemiol* 1993;137:423–438, with permission of the publisher.

We would like to thank the following investigators and their affiliations. **Baltimore:** A Saah, H Armenian, H Farzadegan, N Graham, J Margolick, J McArthur, and J Palenicek from The Johns Hopkins School of Public Health; **Chicago:** JP Phair, JS Chmiel, B Cohen, M O'Gorman, D Variakojis, J Wesch, and S Wolinsky from the Howard Brown Memorial Clinic, Northwestern University Medical School; **Pittsburgh:** CR Rinaldo, JT Becker, P Gupta, M Ho, and LA Kingsley from the University of Pittsburgh School of Public Health; **Los Angeles:** R Detels, BR Visscher, ISY Chen, J Dudley, JL Fahey, JV Giorgi, M Lee, O Martinez-Maza, EN Miller, P Nishanian, J Taylor, and J Zack from the University of California, Los Angeles, Schools of Public Health and Medicine; **Data Coordinating Center:** A Muñoz, H Bacellar, K Chen, N Galai, Y He, DR Hoover, LP Jacobson, J Kirby, K Nelson, and I Speizer from The Johns Hopkins School of Public Health; and SH Vermund, LK Schrager, RA Kaslow, and MJ Van Raden from the *National Institute of Allergy and Infectious Diseases;* and D Seminara from the *National Cancer Institute*.

REFERENCES

1. Centers for Disease Control. HIV/AIDS surveillance report. *MMWR CDC Surveill Summ* 1992:1–18.
2. Vermund SH, Hoth DF. How can epidemiology assist in guiding interventions for the acquired immunodeficiency syndrome/human immunodeficiency virus? *Ann Epidemiol* 1990;1:141–55.

3. Fischl MA, Richman DD, Hansen N, et al. The safety and efficacy of zidovudine in the treatment of patients with mildly symptomatic HIV infection: a double blind placebo control trial. *Ann Intern Med* 1990;112:727–31.
4. Volberding PA, Lagakos SW, Koch MA, et al. Zidovudine in asymptomatic human immunodeficiency virus infection. *N Engl J Med* 1990;322:941–49.
5. Hirschel B, Lazzarin A, Chopard P, et al. A controlled study of inhaled pentamidine for primary prevention of *Pneumocystis carinii* pneumonia. *N Engl J Med* 1991;324:1079–83.
6. Fischl MA, Dickinson GM, La Voie L. Safety and efficacy of sulfamethoxazole and trimethoprim chemoprophylaxis for *Pneumocystis carinii* pneumonia in AIDS. *JAMA* 1988;259:1185–89.
7. Freedberg KA, Tosteson AN, Cohen CJ, Cotton DJ. Primary prophylaxis for *Pneumocystis carinii* pneumonia in HIV-infected people with CD4 counts below 200/mm^3: a cost-effectiveness analysis. *J Acquir Immune Defic Syndr* 1991;4:521–31.
8. Kemper CA, Tucker RM, Lang OS, et al. Low dose dapsone prophylaxis of *Pneumocystis carinii* pneumonia in AIDS and AIDS-related complex. *AIDS* 1990;4:1145–48.
9. Kaslow RA, Ostrow DG, Detels R, Phair JP, Polk BF, Rinaldo CR. The Multicenter AIDS Cohort Study: rationale, organization, and selected characteristics of the participants. *Am J Epidemiol* 1987;126:310–18.
10. Centers for Disease Control. Revision of the CDC surveillance case definition for acquired immunodeficiency syndrome. *MMWR CDC Surveill Summ* 1987;36(Suppl 1):1s–15s.
11. Giorgi JV, Cheng HL, Margolick J, et al. Quality control in the flow cytometric measurement of T-lymphocyte subsets: The Multicenter AIDS Cohort Experience. *Clin Immunol Immunopathol* 1990;55:173–86.
12. Graham NMH, Zeger SL, Kuo V, et al. Zidovudine use in AIDS-free HIV-1 seropositive homosexual men, 1987–1989: magnitude of use in pre-AIDS patients and factors associated with initiation of therapy and participation in clinical trials. *J Acquir Immune Defic Syndr* 1991;4:267–76.
13. Breslow NE, Day NE. Volume II: the design and analysis of cohort studies. In: *Statistical methods in cancer research.* Lyon, France: World Health Organization's International Agency for Research on Cancer; 1987.
14. Rao CR. *Linear statistical inference and its applications.* 2nd ed. New York: J Wiley & Sons; 1973.
15. Graham NMH, Zeger SL, Saah AJ, et al. Effect of zidovudine and *Pneumocystis carinii* pneumonia prophylaxis on progression of HIV-1 infection to AIDS. *Lancet* 1991; 338(8762):265–69.
16. Jacobson LP, Muñoz A, Fox R, et al. Incidence of Kaposi's sarcoma in a cohort of homosexual men infected with the human immunodeficiency virus type 1. *J Acquir Immun Defic Syndr* 1990;3(Suppl 1):S24–S31.
17. Gail MH, Pluda JM, Rabkin CS, et al. Projections of the incidence of non-Hodgkin's lymphoma related to acquired immunodeficiency syndrome. *J Natl Cancer Inst* 1991;83:695–701.
18. Pluda JM, Yarchoan R, Jaffe ES, et al. Development of non-Hodgkin lymphoma in a cohort of patients with severe human immunodeficiency virus (HIV) infection on long-term antiretroviral therapy. *Ann Intern Med* 1990;113:276–82.
19. Jacobson LP, Kirby J, Polk S, et al. Changes in survival rate after AIDS: 1984–1991. *Am J Epidemiol* 1993;138: (in press).
20. Muñoz A, Schrager LK, Bacellar H, et al. Trends in the incidence of outcomes defining acquired immunodeficiency syndrome (AIDS) in the Multicenter AIDS Cohort Study: 1985–1991. *Am J Epidemiol* 1993;137:423–38.

DISCUSSION

Dr. Moss: Are you saying that you didn't see any effect with antiretroviral therapy?

Dr. Muñoz: No, I didn't say that; I said that we don't see a significant effect for antiretroviral therapy using this methodology. But I did indicate that the trends for

KS and lymphoma were in the direction of protection, with a relative risk of less than one. That wasn't the case for other opportunistic infections, although I have to say that I am using an axe that may not be sharp enough to cut the tree.

Other clinical trials have shown the effectiveness of treatment; other analyses of this data using much more sophisticated techniques have shown a beneficial effect for antiretroviral therapy. But what is interesting here is that, in the presence of the same virus, with PCP prophylaxis you're able to capture the effect on PCP incidence; that wasn't the case for the others.

Dr. Detels: I'm not sure that you can look at the issue of AZT. If you look overall, you do find an AZT effect; you've got both AZT and PCP prophylaxis operating. That may be why you don't see it when you use this approach. It seems to me that you've got a therapy directly aimed at PCP and a therapy that's aimed at the underlying HIV, and you're actually looking at a combination of these two elements, not at the specific impact of AZT on HIV. If you added all of these things together, I think you would find a lower rate of going into AIDS than you did earlier, but when you parcel it out, it looks a little different.

Dr. Gail: The attempt to control for CD4 is excellent, but there is the weakness that we don't really know how long the people have been infected. I know it's not possible in this setting, but we are missing information on how long people were infected and, basically, on how sick they were, apart from what their CD4 count was telling us. Perhaps what Roger was getting at was that when you analyzed PCP prophylaxis, many of these people were probably also receiving AZT; it's perhaps a little difficult to disentangle the effects of the two drugs.

I'd like to stress the point that you made several times: the hardest thing to understand is why the people received AZT. It was perhaps the sicker ones, the ones who were most likely to be about to develop something serious or AIDS-defining who were selectively receiving it.

Just to put it into perspective, we have the results of a number of excellent clinical trials. There is the official study which shows a relative risk of about 0.3 from the time of severe immunodepression to AIDS. More recently published randomized studies show very important relative risk reductions (0.16 and 0.19) for people with less severe immune deficiencies who were given AZT. We have very strong experimental, as opposed to observational, data on this point.

Dr. Moss: Let's add that there has always been some controversy about the AZT trials; the European trials have shown no effect—no effect on mortality, and not much on progression to AIDS.

Dr. (?): [Starts answering off microphone.] . . . The VA did an analogous study to the Concord study in the USA (Protocol 298), and, again with relatively few death events, they showed that AZT did not alter survival distributions. Nevertheless, like all of the other randomized trials, they showed strong preventive effects on the development of PCP and AIDS. Consequently, it did delay the time to AIDS, although it didn't carry this through to survival. We are waiting to get more survival data from the Concord study.

Dr. Muñoz: You're absolutely right that a lot of the people taking anti-PCP prophylaxis were also on antiretroviral therapy, and that the protective effect on PCP may not only be due to pentamidine, but also to the antiretroviral drugs.

But my other comment is that I did this exercise not from the perspective of efficacy, but rather to document what has happened in this cohort given this intervention on the level of immunosuppression. That's what is interesting. It's getting close to an interventional study.

Dr. Tsiatis: I'd like to add some caution as to how we should interpret these kinds of analyses. I'm not sure that they should be taken as evidence of efficacy. I don't know much about prophylaxis, but I know a lot about the relationship of AZT and CD4 and subsequent prognosis—the time to getting AIDS, or the time to death in people with AIDS. It's a complicated picture. The treatment affects CD4 levels, and the prognosis is different between people who were on AZT and those who were not. When the treatment is affecting CD4, the fact that you're controlling for both treatment and CD4 can produce a very complicated dynamic. It's difficult to make causal statements; we are dependent on randomized clinical trials for that kind of information.

Dr. Friedman: I can think of three or four plausible variables that might affect the descriptions city by city. I wonder whether you have had a chance of stratifying your data by city to see if you were getting similar or different patterns.

Dr. Muñoz: Off the top of my head, I'd say that the progression is very similar in the four cities.

Dr. Cameron: Was the downward trend in KS between 1988 and 1991 present to the same degree and in the same direction in the original 5,000 person cohort with under 50% seropositivity, as in the subsequent cohort of 600-odd people with a seroprevalence of 61% from 1987 to 1991?

Dr. Musicco: I was wondering if Alvaro had tried a model in which he disregarded PCP prophylaxis and just looked at AZT, to see whether the two models were different in terms of trend.

In some of the analyses of observational data from various cohorts of infected people in Milan, we see clinicians with the opposite attitude; they give antiretroviral therapy to people who can tolerate it, and so we see a reverse effect. Even when controlling for such a powerful predictor as CD4, clinicians still give AZT to people with a poor prognosis. We probably need to introduce some other prognostic predictor in this kind of analysis, because clinicians are better in deciding who will go well and who will worsen.

Dr. Muñoz: First, it is very difficult (if not impossible) to disentangle PCP and AZT in this cohort; they overlap.

Number two, the cohort [members] receiving prophylaxis are not only immunodepressed, they also have more clinical symptoms. I did not have enough data to put symptoms into this analysis as well. This is a limitation.

Dr. Casabona: About the Concord study, I was talking to Dr. Weller from Middlesex 2 days ago, and it looks like the effect on survival which was shown at midterm, disappears in the long-term, probably because of resistance—although the limitation of the endpoint being death is quite obvious.

But I would like to ask Alvaro about the incidence of KS in patients who present with PCP and other opportunistic infections. Considering the effect of PCP prophylaxis, and taking into account that PCP patients may have other subsequent opportunistic infections, how do you interpret the different pattern of incidence in these two groups, if the difference is significant?

Dr. Muñoz: I didn't detect any significant trend for secondary KS, but that doesn't rule out the fact that when something decreases you need time before something else shows up.

Dr. Biggar: Do you share Roger's optimistic assessment that there will be a long-term cohort of survivors? In your data, I see nothing to be optimistic about except for the fact that we have finally got some handle on PCP; the rest of it's going down the tubes.

Dr. Muñoz: Indeed, these data show that the other trends are of concern.

Dr. Detels: You're right, I'm very optimistic. But we do have a documented subgroup in the MACS of people who have maintained a high level of CD4 cells for something like about 8 years now, although I've forgotten how many there were.

Dr. Vermund: The 67 you are talking about are people who had no net decline in at least four observations post-visit 3, as I recall. So that we have enough people in the MACS to be a little picky on a more rigid definition. But those 67 people we find very interesting. The fact that they have had no net CD4 decline since 1984 is really the edge of your bell curve, because it is really worth investigating their viral strains and their immune responses. This is a group not merely preserving CD4 count, but preserving it at a very satisfactory level.

Dr. Musicco: Do you have any data on trends of CD4 at diagnosis—calendar trend?

Dr. Vermund: You will notice that even the MACS, with 5,000 men, half of whom are infected, has very tiny cells for some of these observations. And I think that this is meeting one of Andrew Moss's earlier points about what do we do with the large gay men cohorts. We are holding a meeting in Bethesda concerning long-term survivors and getting a handle on rare events where only 2% or 3% of a cohort may be applicable to a given analysis. It is our intention to invite representatives of all of the major cohorts, given the history of the epidemic, (we're thinking of European, Canadian, and US cohorts for the most part, those that have substantial databases) with the explicit intent of sharing information and possibly doing some joint data analyses to address some of these concerns with very rare outcomes. The NCI cohorts of Vancouver, the Toronto cohort, the New York cohort; when you add them all up, there are quite a lot of studies. Also the Denmark study.

HIV Epidemiology: Models and Methods,
edited by Alfredo Nicolosi. Raven Press, Ltd.,
New York © 1994.

20

The Seroconversion Study on the Natural History of HIV Infection

G. Rezza, M. Dorrucci, P. Pezzotti, A. Lazzarin, G. Angarano, A. Sinicco, R. Zerboni, F. Aiuti, R. Pristerà, S. Gafà, F. Castelli, B. Salassa, M. Barbanera, A. Canessa, L. Ortona, E. Ricchi, P. Viale, U. Tirelli, M. Zaccarelli, and B. Alliegro

HIV-ISS (Italian Seroconversion Study), Centro Operativo AIDS—Istituto Superiore di Sanità, 00161 Rome, Italy

An understanding of the history of HIV infection is essential for physicians, health-care workers, public health officials, and HIV-infected individuals. The identification of biologic and behavioral cofactors affecting the natural history of HIV infection, as well as the identification of clinical and laboratory markers that may have prognostic significance for the development of AIDS, are important issues that may affect when therapy should be initiated. A number of characteristics (including transmission group, age, and gender) may influence the clinical progression of HIV infection (1–6). In particular, the natural history of HIV infection and factors predicting progression to AIDS among injecting drug users (IDUs) have not been adequately studied. Disease progression among IDUs may differ because of different age and sex distribution (7,8). Furthermore, continued injecting drug use appears to impair lymphocyte function, which theoretically could accelerate progression to AIDS.

To address the issues related to the unique distribution of HIV-infected subjects in Italy (9), we designed an incident cohort study of injecting drug users. Then, using the same clinical centers, we started to enroll male homosexuals and heterosexual contacts in order to compare disease progression rates among subjects belonging to different exposure categories.

MATERIALS AND METHODS

Study Population

We followed individuals recruited from 16 outpatient facilities (including AIDS or sexually transmitted disease clinics and drug dependency units)

located in general or infectious disease hospitals in several Italian cities. The subjects entering the cohort were individuals at risk for HIV infection (IDUs, male homosexuals, and heterosexual contacts) who seroconverted between 1982 and 1990. We only included subjects for whom the dates of last negative and first positive HIV tests were known.

The subjects were enrolled based on the following criteria: (i) previously enrolled in prospective studies of seronegative individuals, or (ii) incidentally detected as seroconverters (i.e., they were undergoing sequential serologic testing, or they were attending the center for other reasons, such as HIV test or viral hepatitis) with earlier sera available to document seroconversion. To reduce possible selection bias and to avoid an overestimation of the progression rate, we excluded subjects incidentally detected as seroconverters who already had AIDS-related complex (ARC) or AIDS at enrollment. Then, whether including or excluding those subjects, the results did not change significantly. Almost all the IDUs were recruited from prospective cohort studies of seronegative subjects. However, a number of IDUs was recruited because of spontaneous attendance at the clinical center.

Origin of the Study and Follow-up

We assumed that the date of seroconversion was the midpoint between the dates of last negative and first confirmed positive tests. The endpoint was the date of AIDS diagnosis according to the Centers for Disease Control and World Health Organization (CDC-WHO) case definition. The survival time was measured from the estimated date of seroconversion to the date of AIDS diagnosis, to the date of non-AIDS death, or to June, 1991. For the subjects in the last group, the outcome was considered according to the National AIDS Registry (the first name and the first letter of the family name were used for the cross-check with the Registry).

A standardized form was used to collect demographic, laboratory, and clinical information. The patients were classified using the CDC clinical classification system of HIV infection. Little information on behavioral aspects was collected and was mainly addressed to drug-injecting–related practices. Although it was recommended to repeat clinical evaluation every 6 months, the stage of the infection and other information actually were recorded at various points in time for each patient.

The data were characterized by heavy censoring, either right censoring (the follow-up was not long enough to allow all subjects to eventually reach the AIDS state) or interval censoring, attributed to the fact that seroconversion transition times could not be pinpointed to an exact date but to a time interval.

Statistical Analysis

To estimate progression rates we used the Kaplan-Meier survival method. Comparisons between progression curves were tested for statistical significance with log-rank tests. A multivariate analysis was conducted to identify independent cofactors of progression using the Cox proportional hazards model. The assumption of proportionality of the hazards for all variables was verified plotting the logarithm of the negative logarithm of the survival curves obtained by the Kaplan-Meier method. A forward purposeful selection and a stepwise selection of the covariates were used in constructing the models. The statistical criterion used to select the best models was the partial likelihood ratio test. The best scale for the continuous variables was also investigated in order to obtain the best fit for the models. Exploratory data analysis was used to monitor changes in CD4-positive (CD4+) cell number over time.

RESULTS

Nine hundred forty-two subjects were followed until December, 1991. Six hundred eighty-five (73%) of the study subjects were males, 257 (27%) were females. Five hundred sixty-four (60%) of the subjects were intravenous drug users, 229 (24%) were homosexuals, and 149 (16%) were heterosexual contacts. Among IDUs, 72% were males and 28% were females. Among heterosexual contacts, 32% were males and 68% females. Age at seroconversion ranged from 14 to 60 years, with a median of 26 years. Three hundred ninety-one subjects were less than 25 years old, 390 between 25 and 34 years old, and 150 over 35 years old. Age distribution differed in the three exposure categories. Injecting drug users were younger than heterosexual contacts, and male homosexuals were the oldest group. The mean age at seroconversion was 25 years for the IDUs, 28 for the heterosexual contacts, and 33 for the male homosexuals.

The median time between the last negative and the first positive test was 8 months, ranging between 0.5 and 24 months. The average time between the first positive test and the first visit was less than 8 months. The median follow-up time was 45 months for intravenous drug users and 41 months for homosexuals, whereas the heterosexuals were followed for a shorter period (36 months). The median intervals between visits was 6 months for IDUs (range 0.9 to 58 months), 6 months for male homosexuals (1 to 47 months), and 5 months for heterosexual contacts (1 to 47 months). The dropout rate, defined as the proportion of subjects who were not seen for a period of at least 2 years, was 12%. However, as reported before, a cross-check with the National AIDS Registry was performed for the entire cohort.

Ninety-four subjects developed AIDS as of December 31, 1991: 60 were IDUs, 27 were male homosexuals, and 7 were heterosexual contacts. The

TABLE 1. *AIDS cases: clinical characteristics*

	Injecting drug users	Male homosexuals	Hetero. contacts
AIDS cases	60 (64%)	27 (29%)	7 (7%)
Indicative disease of AIDS			
Wasting syndrome	7 (9%)	4 (12%)	0 (0%)
HIV encephalopathy	2 (3%)	0 (0%)	0 (0%)
PCP[a]	17 (23%)	6 (19%)	2 (25%)
Candidiasis	25 (33%)	4 (12%)	4 (50%)
Other opp. infections	21 (28%)	10 (30%)	2 (25%)
Kaposi's sarcoma	2 (3%)	8 (24%)	0 (0%)
Non-Hodgkin's lymphoma	1 (1%)	1 (3%)	0 (0%)

[a]*Pneumocystis carinii* pneumonia.

distribution of the diseases indicative of AIDS at diagnosis showed an excess of candidiasis in IDUs compared to the other groups. As expected, Kaposi's sarcoma was much more common among male homosexuals than among the other exposure groups (Table 1). Women were more likely to have candidiasis than men. Unfortunately, we did not look for the presence of gynecologic abnormalities on a routine basis. However, none of the women developed cervical cancer during the follow-up period. The risk of developing AIDS among IDUs was about 23% at 6 years after seroconversion. The annual incidence of AIDS increased with the duration of HIV infection; the greatest increase was observed beginning five years after HIV seroconversion. Relatively few heterosexual contacts have been enrolled so far. However, our findings show a trend similar to that of IDUs, with a low incidence of AIDS in the first 4 months, and a sharp increase from the fifth year on. Finally, among male homosexuals the increase in the incidence rate occurred earlier, during the fourth year. The Kaplan-Meier curves show that male homosexuals had a faster progression rate than IDUs; however, the differences observed in the progression rate among the different transmission categories was not significant (Fig. 1).

Age at seroconversion strongly affects the progression to AIDS. Those subjects who were under 25 years old at seroconversion progressed at the slowest rate. Subjects of 25 to 34 years progressed at a slightly more rapid pace, and subjects who were 35 and older had the most rapid progression (Fig. 2). Females appear to progress more slowly than males, but this difference is not statistically significant. However, the difference can be explained by the fact that male and female subjects also differed in their age distribution, due to the older age of homosexuals. The annual incidence rate among females showed the same pattern observed in males belonging to the same exposure category (IDUs and heterosexual contacts).

When we did a stepwise multivariate analysis (Table 2), we found that age was the only independent predictor of progression to AIDS. We can see that

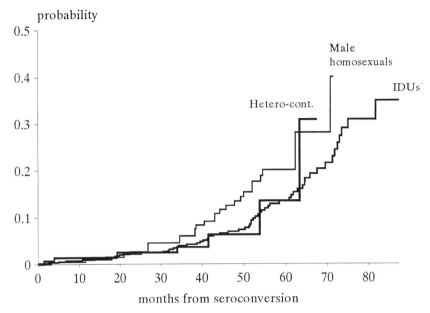

FIG. 1. Progression to AIDS according to transmission category: (———) injecting drug users, (----) male homosexuals, and (– – –) heterosexual contacts.

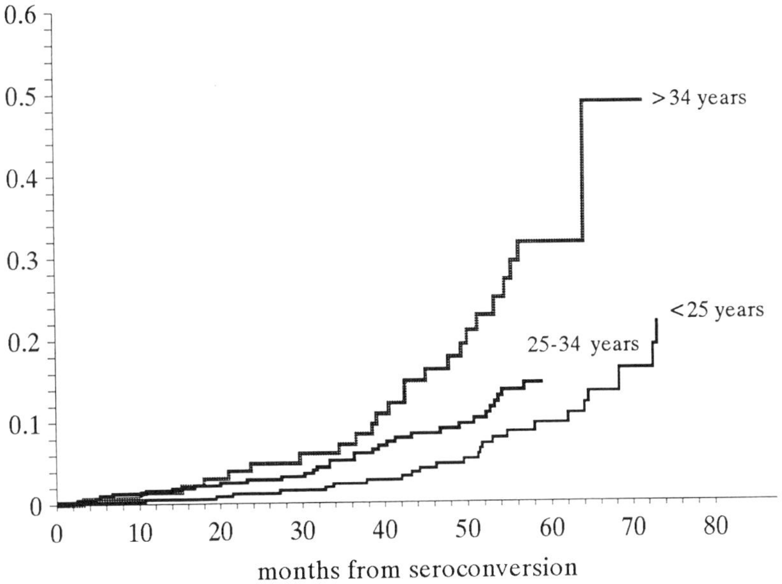

FIG. 2. Progression to AIDS by age: (———) under 25 years old, (----) 25 to 34 years old, and (– – –) over 34 years old.

TABLE 2. *Independent predictors of progression to AIDS: stratified proportional hazards model*

Variable	Relative hazard	95% CI[a]	*p*
Age			<0.001
20	1	—	
30	1.66	1.33–2.07	
40	2.75	1.77–4.28	
Sex[b]	—	—	>0.10
Type of transmission[b]	—	—	>0.10

[a]Ninety-five percent confidence intervals.
[b]Not included in the final model.

the risk of developing AIDS for individuals between 25 and 34 years was twice as high as for those under 25 years, and was four times as high for the subjects 35 years and older.

In conclusion, the time from seroconversion to AIDS was found to be strongly influenced by the age of the subjects: The risk of developing AIDS is significantly higher for subjects who were older at the time of infection. These findings confirm those from studies conducted on subjects with hemophilia, which showed that the annual risk of developing AIDS 7 years after seroconversion is about five times higher for subjects older than 25 years than for those younger than 25. In our study, the risk ratio for the same age groups was approximately three.

Injecting drug users represent the largest group in our cohort and the most important transmission category in Italy. Even if it has been postulated that drug use may accelerate HIV progression, it has never been scientifically proved. In fact, morphine has been shown to alter the function of human T lymphocytes and monocytes, promoting the growth of HIV-1 in these cells, and a deteriorating functional capacity of the T-cell system has been found to be strongly associated with the frequency of drug injection (both in HIV-positive and -negative IDUs). However, there is no definite evidence that persistent drug use may accelerate the progression of HIV infection.

In our study, we compared the risk of developing AIDS of current IDUs with that of former IDUs. Former IDUs were defined as patients who had stopped injecting drugs within the first year after HIV seroconversion. The classification was based on repeated interviews and physical examination. Current drug use was not predictive of more rapid progression. However, we had no data about the occurrence of methadone treatment or the frequency of injection and could only examine the univariate effect of any continued injection. Furthermore, because of relatively small numbers, only several events were observed in former IDUs, determining the possibility of the occurrence of a "beta" error. Analysis of other data, restricted to the

TABLE 3. *Distribution of CD4+ cell counts by transmission category*

CD4+	IDUs[a] (393)	MH[b] (197)	Hetero[c] (117)
>500	76.0%	64.5%	67.0%
200–499	23.0%	32.5%	31.0%
<200	1.0%	3.0%	2.0%

[a]Injecting drug users, number in group in parentheses.
[b]Male homosexuals, number in parentheses.
[c]Heterosexual contacts, number in parentheses.

IDUs, showed the same results reported in the total population. There was no difference between male and female IDUs in the clinical progression, and age was found to play a role as a determinant of progression.

The CD4-positive (CD4+) cell number (per μl) was identified as an early marker of clinical progression. At first visit within 1 year after seroconversion, 504 subjects had more than 500 CD4+ cells, 190 had 200 to 499 CD4+ cells, and 13 had less than 200 CD4+ cells. The distribution of CD4+ cell number at first visit varied among the three exposure categories. Overall, IDUs had higher values of CD4+ cells at first visit than subjects belonging to other exposure categories (Table 3).

CD4+ cell number had been used both as an indicator of the duration of HIV infection and a marker of disease progression. Our findings suggest that, in a limited number of subjects, the decrease of CD4+ cells to under 200 μl is not dependent on the duration of the infection, but occurred in the first year after seroconversion. As shown in Fig. 3, those subjects who have CD4+ cell counts less than 200 were more likely to develop AIDS than those who were between 200 and 500, who were more likely to develop AIDS than those over 500.

The multivariate analysis confirmed that a lower number of CD4+ cells is an independent early marker of disease. The strong association between CD4+ cell number and HIV clinical progression is found both when we treat CD4+ cells as a dichotomous variable with cutoffs of 500 and 200 and as a continuous variable.

Low CD4+ cell count at first visit was associated with age at seroconversion, suggesting a rapid decline of this lymphocyte subset in older subjects (Fig. 4). Unfortunately, information about CD4+ cell count prior to HIV seroconversion was not available for all the subjects to confirm this hypothesis. However, in a subgroup of HIV-seronegative IDUs that was followed prospectively, we observed that CD4+ cell number did not differ significantly among different age groups, suggesting that the differences in CD4+ cell count between age groups did not predate seroconversion.

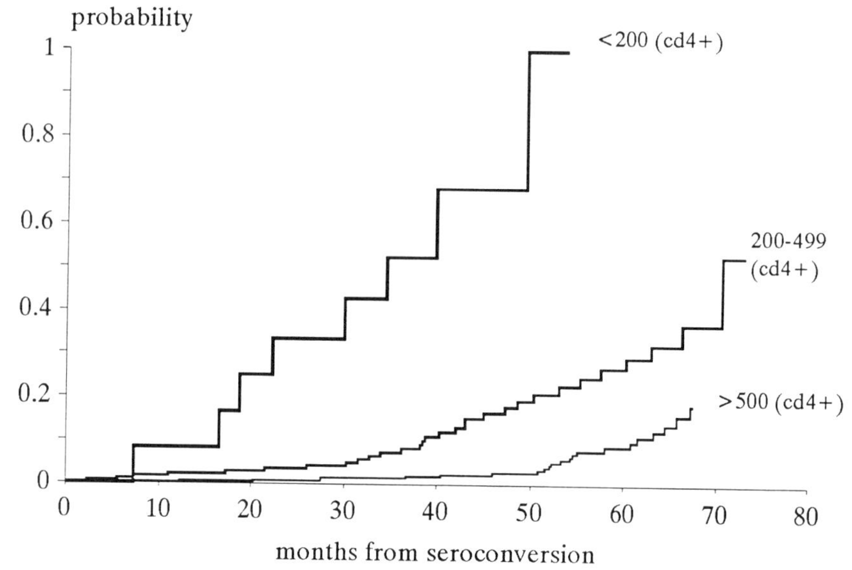

FIG. 3. Progression to AIDS according to CD4+ counts, using baseline values. CD4+ counts represented as follows: (———) less than 200 cells/μl, (----) 200 to 499 cells/μl, and (– – –) over 500 cells/μl.

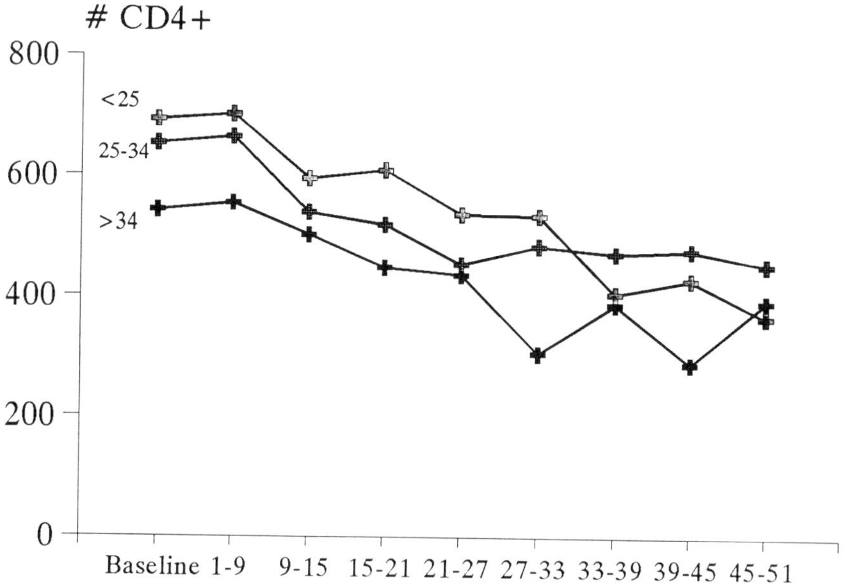

FIG. 4. Median values of CD4+ count by age at seroconversion: (———) under 25 years old, (----) 25 to 34 years old, and (– – –) over 34 years old.

CONCLUSION

Limitations and Possible Biases

A series of limitations and biases regarding the study should be pointed out. First of all, several sources of recruitment were used to enroll the subjects in the study. At the beginning of the study, in 1987, a number of subjects were enrolled retrospectively, using the look-back method. The retrospective recruitment may determine an overestimation of the progression to AIDS if subjects who were not previously followed in prospective cohort studies and were symptomatic at first visit are included in the study. In fact, those who are symptomatic may be more likely to undergo serological testing than those who have no symptoms. However, excluding these subjects may determine an underestimation of the progression rate, because in such a way all those who progress very rapidly (i.e., those who develop AIDS in the first year after seroconversion) would be excluded. This problem does not exist when all the subjects are enrolled from ongoing cohorts of seronegative subjects. However, in our study, only a small number of subjects were symptomatic at the first visit, and the results are not influenced by their inclusion in the analysis.

We considered a number of biases that could have influenced our results. First, bias could have occurred if the intervals between last negative and first positive tests were different for the various subgroups. However no differences were found in the distribution of seroconversion intervals for the different subgroups. Second, bias could have occurred if certain subgroups were more likely to receive antiviral treatment than others. We found, however, that there were no differences in use of antiviral therapy for each subgroup. Finally, bias could have occurred if there was temporary loss to follow-up among the different groups. Indeed, we found that the temporary drop out of intravenous drug users was higher than for other groups. However we tried to minimize this bias by cross-checking our files with those of the National AIDS Registry, and we feel that such a bias is unlikely to explain our observations.

Access to Care and Treatment

The interval between visits did not vary significantly between IDUs and male homosexuals. Furthermore, no difference was observed in the access to AZT treatment (10). In Italy, AZT treatment is offered, free of charge, to all subjects who are under 500 CD4+ cells per μl, irrespective of their social status; the expenses are covered by the National Health System. Equal access to treatment might rule out possible differences among groups, as is observed in the United States. Furthermore, for this reason, there is a need to compare the progression of HIV disease in IDUs of different areas of the world.

A number of conclusions can be drawn from our study:

1. Age at seroconversion strongly affects the progression to AIDS. The age effect was strong in all the transmission categories.
2. Differences between exposure groups are mainly due to the confounding effect of age. The risk of developing AIDS was higher among male homosexuals just because they were older than IDUs at seroconversion. The difference disappears after controlling for age.
3. No difference exists between males and females, especially after controlling for age. However, further studies are needed to evaluate the possible effect of gynecologic abnormalities in seropositive women.
4. The strong association between low CD4+ cell count and age can explain the more rapid progression in older subjects. Because the number of CD4+ cells did not vary among the different age classes of seronegative IDUs, it was not possible to explain why the number of CD4+ cells declines more rapidly in older subjects.
5. Persistent drug injection does not seem to play a role in accelerating HIV infection. The comparison between former and current IDUs, in our study, was limited by the small number of events; however, the similarity of the natural history of HIV infection among IDUs and the other groups seem to confirm our hypothesis.
6. A longer follow-up is needed to estimate progression rates and identify markers and determinants of HIV progression in heterosexual contacts.

In conclusion, a number of issues that have not been addressed in the paper need to be studied. First of all, we are evaluating laboratory parameters other than CD4+ cells that might be able to predict HIV disease progression in IDUs. Secondly, the protective role of antiviral treatment needs to be elucidated in IDUs in a country in which access to treatment is not selective. Third, the effect of behavioral variables and, with regard to IDUs, of drug substitutive treatment (methadone) on HIV disease should be studied. Finally, ongoing cohort studies on IDUs will provide a chance to implement vaccine trials in the near future.

ACKNOWLEDGMENT

This work has been funded with a grant of the Progetto AIDS, Ministero della Sanità-Istituto Superiore di Sanità.

REFERENCES

1. Moss A, Bacchetti P. Natural history of HIV infection. *AIDS* 1989;3:55–61.
2. Goedert JJ, Kessler CM, Aledort LM, et al. A prospective study of human immunode-

ficiency virus type I infection and the development of AIDS in subjects with hemophilia. *N Engl J Med* 1989;321:1142–1148.
3. Blaxhult A, Granath F, Lidman, Giesecke J. The influence of age on the latency period to AIDS in people infected by HIV through blood transfusion. *AIDS* 1990;4:125–129.
4. Weber R, Ledergerber B, Opravil M, et al. Progression of HIV infection in misusers of injected drugs who stop injecting or follow a programme of maintenance treatment with methadone. *BMJ* 1990;301:1362–1365.
5. Jason J, Lui K-J, Ragni MV, et al. Risk of developing AIDS in HIV-infected cohorts of hemophilic and homosexual men. *JAMA* 1989;261:725–727.
6. Giesecke J, Scalia-Tomba G, Berglund O, et al. Incidence of symptoms and AIDS in 146 Swedish haemophiliacs and blood transfusion recipients infected with human immunodeficiency virus. *BMJ* 1988;297:99–102.
7. Rezza G and The Italian Seroconversion Study. Disease progression and early predictors of AIDS in HIV-seroconverted injecting drug users. *AIDS* 1992;6:421–426.
8. Mariotto A, Mariotto S, Pezzotti P, Rezza G, Verdecchia A. Estimation of the acquired immunodeficiency syndrome incubation period in intravenous drug users: a comparison with male homosexuals. *Am J Epidemiol* 1992;135:420–437.
9. Centro Operativo AIDS. *Aggiornamento dei casi di AIDS in Italia.* Commissione Nazionale AIDS, 30 Giugno 1992.
10. Italian Seroconversion Study. Compliance to the follow-up and access to treatment for injecting drug users in an Italian cohort. Presented at the VIII International Conference on AIDS/III STD World Congress, Amsterdam, July 1992 (Abs.9007).

DISCUSSION

Dr. Moss: I think this is the only example of a study which includes both drug users and homosexual men, and it looks like it is going to dispel a lot of myths about AIDS progression. It's also a little discouraging for those who are looking for cofactors. Questions?

Dr. Biggar: The International Registry of Seroconverters now includes 2,200 seroconverters under study. Our studies have not gone past the time that they were in therapy, and, like you, we could not find any difference after taking out Kaposi's sarcoma. If you leave Kaposi's sarcoma in the model, then gay men do come down with AIDS sooner than other groups after seroconversion; but if you remove KS as a diagnostic criterion, they have basically the same trajectory as in hemophiliacs and drug abusers (although we did not have a large number of drug users).

I'd like to ask both Roger Detels and Giovanni Rezza how they feel about the role of cofactors, in particular lifestyle cofactors. I gather that the two of you have different views concerning their importance.

Dr. Detels: You're right that I'm very biased in favor of cofactors, although I have now been sufficiently chastised to call them promoters rather than cofactors, the distinction being that promoters affect the rate of progression, while cofactors are essential factors.

First of all, and just on the basis of the distribution of incubation periods, I find it inconceivable that a disease for which the incubation period goes from 1 year to probably 20 years or more does not have some other factors that influence the rate of progression.

Another thing which has always intrigued me is that every study I know which has looked at greater progression to AIDS and which has looked at the titer of CMV, for example, has come up with the fact that a high CMV titer is very predictive of the development of AIDS, although I'm not sure whether this was adjusted for age in our study.

A further reason for my belief that promoters may be involved is that I did a study in 1987 which looked at the patterns of CD4 change. We tend to take CD4 levels in a group of men or individuals, and average out slopes. If you have nobody with increasing CD4 levels (and very few people infected with HIV show an increase in the number of CD4 cells), you have a subset with decreasing levels and a majority with constant levels, which means that the slope of the mean will be negative. We did some studies to look at distributions and found that, after 2 to 3 years of follow-up, none or very few of the men (I think only one or two in the Los Angeles center) had a straight slope of CD4 decline. And that is a hypothesis which is incompatible with the absence of promoters. The majority of men maintained a plateau over that period of time, and, of the ones who showed a decline, the majority shifted from a plateau to a downward trend. I find it hard to explain those patterns, unless other factors affect the rate of deterioration.

Dr. Muñoz: The age effect that Giovanni indicated seems to me to be too strong, so I have two questions. Firstly, you mentioned that you saw an age effect which was independent of the risk group you examined. I take it that you looked at the homosexuals separately and that the strength of association was the same as in the drug users. Is that correct?

Dr. Rezza: I didn't stratify the homosexual population because of the small number of homosexual males. I made a multivariate analysis of injecting drug users, which included the risk group, transmission category, gender, and age, and I then stratified them by different age groups. I could have done the same for homosexuals, but their number seemed too small.

Dr. Muñoz: You also mentioned CD4 levels and age. When was the CD4 measurement taken for your analysis?

Dr. Rezza: The first test was done within one year of seroconversion. There was a median time interval of something less than 8 months between the estimated date of seroconversion and the date of the test.

Dr. Cameron: Concerning age as a risk factor, age was defined as age at seroconversion, but your IDU population was the youngest population under observation and also had the longest period of observation (and therefore the highest cumulative risk of AIDS). Doesn't this mean that there may be an observation bias in determining age as a risk factor for AIDS?

Dr. Rezza: The age of Italian injecting drug users is usually lower than that of injecting drug users in other countries. This population seems to be representative of the whole population of injecting drug users in Italy. I don't think that any kind of bias was introduced by an age effect.

Dr. Cameron: What I was suggesting is that you could have adjusted the risk of AIDS for the duration of observation according to age at seroconversion.

Dr. Rezza: I don't understand, because this was a time-dependent analysis.

Dr. van den Hoek: We also compared the conversion rate in our cohort of IDUs with the conversion rate in our cohort of homosexual men, and I find it very difficult to understand why there is no difference. If you see the way drug users live and what they do, this isn't possible. Furthermore, you have a high dropout rate due to mortality. Is it possible that you are dealing with the phenomenon of the survival of the fittest? That is, that the people who survive have a longer survival time that is, therefore, comparable with the survival time of homosexual men.

Dr. Rezza: That's a very good question, because injecting drug users don't always die as a result of AIDS; they also die of overdose, and there is an excess of mortality from suicide and violent causes, which needs to be taken into account. Every year, we ask for copies of the death certificates held by the municipalities in which the drug users live in an attempt to discover whether they die from other causes. In this particular cohort, we had a relatively low level of deaths for other causes, perhaps because they were routinely followed by the clinical centers and were made more aware of their clinical condition.

Nevertheless, your question remains extremely valid and I think we should try to take into account this excess of deaths in comparing drug users with other population groups.

HIV Epidemiology: Models and Methods,
edited by Alfredo Nicolosi. Raven Press, Ltd.,
New York © 1994.

21

Epidemiological Aspects of HIV Infection and Cancer

*†Jordi Casabona and *Marti Vall

**AIDS Prevention & Control Programme, Department of Health Generalitat de Catalunya, 08028 Barcelona, Catalonia, Spain; †Preventive Medicine and Public Health Department, Autonomous University of Barcelona, Hospital de la Santa Creu i de Sant Pau, Barcelona, Catalonia, Spain*

The appearance of the AIDS epidemic in 1981 led to the study of a number of questions relating to the basic pathophysiological mechanism of the disease (the immunodeficiency), as well as to the integration of basic scientific research with epidemiological studies. The association of HIV and cancer has had a great impact on current research. The purpose of this chapter is to review some of the evidence existing in the epidemiology of HIV-associated malignancies (HAM) and to comment on some of the methodological problems and limitations which may be encountered.

One of the main difficulties in studying such an association is the need to establish the criteria with which to define the broad concept of HAM. Unlike the association of HIV infection with opportunistic infections, such as tuberculosis or toxoplasmosis, where we know the etiological agents, their biological characteristics, their modes of transmission and the natural history of the baseline condition, we have very little information about most HAMs.

After the clinical observation that transplant recipients and other iatrogenic immunosuppressed patients presented a variety of cancers (1–3), it became accepted that immunosuppression itself plays an important role in cancer production. Furthermore, it quickly became clear that HIV-infected patients, like immunosuppressed patients in general, tend to present only a few types of malignancy (4–6). Although only a few biological agents have been proved to cause cancer, many viruses (other than HIV) have been associated with the production of malignancies (7; Table 1).

TABLE 1. *Viruses for which an association with cancer has been postulated*

Viruses[a]	Possible associated malignancies
HBV, HCV, HDV	hepatocellular carcinoma
HTLV-I	adult T-cell leukemia
HTLV-II	hairy cell leukemia
EBV	Burkitt's lymphoma
	nasopharyngeal carcinoma
	high-grade lymphoma
	Hodgkin's disease
HPV-16	Kaposi's sarcoma
HPV	cervical cancer
	anal carcinoma
HSV-2	cervical cancer
HIV-1	Kaposis's sarcoma
HIV-2	
Varicella zoster	childhood leukemia

From International Agency for Research on Cancer (7).
[a]HBV, hepatitis B virus; HCV, hepatitus C virus; HDV, hepatitus D virus; HTLV-I, human T-cell leukemia, type I; HTLV-II, human T-cell leukemia virus, type II; EBV, Epstein-Barr virus; HPV-16, human papilloma virus; HSV-2, herpes simplex virus, type 2; HIV-1, human immunodeficiency virus, type 1; HIV-2, human immunodeficiency virus, type 2.

From an epidemiological point of view, the most common problems in trying to establish a causal relationship between virus and cancer are

a. The usually low prevalence of the cancer to be studied leads to considerable difficulties in terms of case detection, sample size, study period, and statistical strength.
b. The incubation periods of the putative agents are usually unknown, variable, or long. This makes it difficult to establish a possible exposure sequence (and therefore design a study) or even to be sure which came first, the cancer or the exposure.
c. Important cofactors for expressing the cancer may be unknown and are usually multifactorial (i.e., factors relating to the agent, to the host, or to the medium).
d. The process of viral oncogenesis is difficult to understand.
e. There are geographical variations in both virus characteristics and cancer expression.
f. Many of the cancers lack animal models.

HIV-associated malignancies share most of these problems, and HIV-infected patients may also be infected with more than one virus, particularly those that have similar modes of transmission. In such a context, the epidemiological study of HIV infection and cancer should be based on the known pathophysiological links between HIV, immunodeficiency, and some types of cancer, as well as on empirical observations aimed at identifying and confirming specific associations. This will make it possible to gain an insight into the pathophysiology and etiology of some of these cancers (and also of the HIV infection itself), which may lead to possible cancer prevention interventions.

Given the epidemiological focus of this report, we will only mention the possible mechanisms of HIV oncogenesis that have been postulated so far (8):

a. a direct oncogenic effect of the HIV virus
b. the reactivation of a different oncogenic agent as a result of HIV-induced immunosuppression
c. the interaction of HIV with another RNA or DNA virus, leading to an oncogenic effect.

IDENTIFYING ASSOCIATIONS

In the absence of a greater understanding of the etiology and pathophysiology of most of HAM, empirical data concerning the occurrence and distribution of cancer among HIV-infected subjects, as well as the possible risk factors for such malignancies, are crucial. Various sources of information and study designs have been used for this purpose.

Case Reports and Clinical Series

Case reports and clinical series have been fundamental in associating some malignancies with HIV infection. For example, it was the earlier identification of young homosexual men with Kaposi's sarcoma (KS) and no other known causes of immunodeficiency (9,10) that led to the identification of the new syndrome (11,12).

Since then, there have been many clinical reports of an increase in the number of cases of non-Hodgkin's lymphoma (NHL; 13,14) and Hodgkin's disease (HD; 6,15) among HIV-positive patients, particularly primary lymphoma of the brain (16). The Italian Cooperative Group on AIDS-related Tumors collects data from HIV-positive cancer patients, and they have reported that about 12% of these cancers are Hodgkin's disease (HD; 17,18). A further clinical series has also confirmed an increase in HD among HIV-seropositive and AIDS patients (19).

Because the baseline condition of HIV infection is immunosuppression, information coming from congenital immunosuppressed patients, transplant recipients, and other patients treated with immunosuppressive drugs can also provide useful information that can be extrapolated in the study of HIV infection and cancer production. Several studies of iatrogenically immunosuppressed patients have shown a 35-fold increase in NHL (20), a clear increase in squamous cell carcinoma of the skin, and, to a lesser extent, of cutaneous malignant melanoma (21) and colonorectal carcinoma (22).

Registries collecting information from congenitally immunosuppressed patients, such as the Immunodeficiency Cancer Registry of the University of Minnesota, have shown that the most frequent malignancies are NHL (49% of all cases), Hodgkin's disease (9%), and gastric carcinoma (9%; 23). Since there are no reference populations in these registries to compute rates, their data has been considered as coming from clinical series. The collaborative United Kingdom-Australasian study of cancer among immunosuppressed patients (21), also found an excess of NHL, squamous cell skin carcinoma, soft tissue carcinoma, and cutaneous malignant melanoma.

In general, the inclusion criteria for case reports and clinical series involve many selection and observational biases, one of them being an intensive medical follow-up. They may therefore serve to illustrate new associations, or new characteristics of a rare condition, but their design does not allow them to be used to extrapolate occurrence measures, compute rates, or assess risk.

Population-Based Cancer Registries

The advantage of using population-based registries is that the observed cases can be refered to a given population, making it possible to compute and compare incidence rates. Since registries of AIDS cases only collect malignancies considered to be indicative of AIDS, cancer registries are the best information source to identify possible HIV-associated cancers.

In the USA, several studies using population-based data have analyzed the possible temporal trend of cancers among young, never-married men thought to be at high risk for AIDS (Table 2; 24–30). Although these studies used different methodological approaches, all agree that only the incidence of KS and NHL is increasing in this population. One of the first studies using Surveillance, Epidemiology, and End Results (SEER) data showed an increase in Hodgkin's disease in 1985, as well as an increase in both anorectal carcinoma and hepatoma. After 1985, HD decreased or was stationary in all groups, and the increase in hepatoma and anorectal carcinoma did not follow the AIDS epidemic. Moreover, a further SEER analysis did not confirm any increase in these tumors, but only in NHL and KS (25).

In Europe, cancer incidence data was used to report an increase in KS, even before the AIDS epidemic began (31).

Cohort Studies

Cohort studies allow the follow-up of a previously defined, exposed population (people at risk for HIV, HIV-infected subjects, or AIDS patients), and, although they are hospital-based studies, they represent the best design

TABLE 2. *Incidence data for HAM from population-based cancer registries*

Study	Outcome
Biggar et al, 1985[a] (1973/80–1981/82)	2.043-fold increase in KS 5-fold increase in Burkitt's lymphoma no increase in other tumors
Biggar et al, 1987[b] (1973/78–1984)	2.479-fold increase in KS 4.2 increase in NHL no increase in hepatoma or HD
Kristal et al, 1988[c] (1980/81–1984/85)	3.2-fold increase in NHL
Harnly et al, 1988[d] (1980–1985)	5.3-fold increase in NHL
Biggar et al, 1989[e] (1973/76–1985)	1.850-fold increase in KS 6.2-fold increase in NHL
Chow et al, 1989[f] (1983–1986)	similar increase in the incidence rate of KS and the annual AIDS incidence rate
Rabkin et al, 1991[g] (1973–1987)	10-fold increase in the incidence of NHL 5,000-fold increase in the incidence of KS no increase in other tumors

[a]From ref. 24.
[b]From ref. 25.
[c]From ref. 26.
[d]From ref. 27.
[e]From ref. 28.
[f]From ref. 29.
[g]From ref. 30.

for identifying associations between HIV infection and malignancies. They make it possible to compute incidence rates and relative risk for different levels of exposure (immunosuppression) and for exposure to other possible risk factors for cancer. Furthermore, depending on the studied population, the outcome may also be correlated with seroconversion. As Dr. Roger Detels explains in Chapter 18, cohort studies are also of particular interest in following the natural history of these cancers and describing incidence trends. Their main limitations are data validity (when they are done retrospectively); the need for a large sample size to detect unusual associations; and the difficulty of ensuring the follow-up of participants, particularly among intravenous drug users (IVDUs).

The National Cancer Institute (NCI) has followed a cohort of hemophiliacs since 1981 (32), and, apart from Kaposi's sarcoma and NHL, no excess of other cancers has been identified (33). In the San Francisco City Clinic Cohort Study of hepatitis B, more than 6,000 homosexual and bisexual men were recruited between 1978 and 1980. It was reported that there was a downtrend over time in the proportion of patients presenting with KS, and no specific risk factors for KS were identified (34).

The Multicenter AIDS Cohort Study (MACS) is a prospective study of homosexual and bisexual men in four metropolitan areas of the USA. A previously published study from this project (35) did not identify any particular trend in KS incidence rates, but did find an association between KS and a past history of gonorrhea and the practice of rimming with multiple partners, thus reinforcing the hypothesis of a possible sexually transmitted agent for KS (36). Similar studies carried out in Canada (37) have found a statistically significant association between the development of KS and the number of sexual contacts between 1978 and 1982 and the use of nitrite inhalants. In Chapter 19, Dr. Alvaro Muñoz et al. present a comprehensive and updated analysis of the data from the MACS. After controlling for the progressive immunosuppression of the HIV subcohort, they found that the overall incidence of KS did not show a downward trend. However, after the dissemination of antiretroviral therapy in 1988, there was a suggestion of a slight decrease of KS as the first diagnosis of AIDS in homosexual men.

In addition to occurrence measures and risk factor assessment, cohort studies have also been used to describe the natural history of HAM. It has been shown that, while annual incidence rates for KS were constant (2.3%) between 3 and 8 years after seroconversion, the rate of NHL increased from 0.3% to 2% over the same period (38). Most of the cohort studies agree that the annual incidence rate of NHL increases with time after seroconversion or AIDS diagnosis.

We have analyzed follow-up data from 2,460 AIDS cases diagnosed in Catalonia between 1981 and 1991, contributing to a total of 3,255 person-years of follow-up (38a). There were 484 cancer diagnoses (345 KS, 130 NHL, and 9 HD), 74% of them being the presenting indicative disease of AIDS. The overall incidence rates per 100 person-years were 14 for KS, 3.6 for NHL, and 0.2 for HD. Using both natural years and annual cohort of diagnosis, no trends were found for KS or NHL. It is also interesting to note that 60% of all NHLs, were diagnosed as the first manifestation of AIDS (Table 3).

On the other hand, Katz and his colleagues (39) showed that the percentage of diagnoses of NHL shortly after an AIDS diagnosis increased from 3% in 1981 through 1985 to 10% in 1988 and 1989. These studies indicating an increase in the number of NHL diagnoses soon after the first manifestation of AIDS may be an effect of the introduction of pre-AIDS chemoprophylaxis for other opportunistic infections.

Other studies have also identified a higher risk for anal epithelial abnormalities among men with HIV and human papillomavirus (HPV) than in those with only one infection (40), HPV infection being correlated with the level of immunodeficiency. Similarly, HIV-infected women tend to be at higher risk for HPV infection and cervical intraepithelial neoplasia (41).

Finally, a cohort study in a methadone maintenance treatment program (MMTP) in New York City (42) found that solid neoplasms from the lung, larynx, and cervix were associated with HIV infection and more common than KS and NHL. However, the relationship between the onset of cancer and seroconversion was unknown in this study, and the fact that it was ret-

TABLE 3. *Distribution of KS, NHL, and HD diagnoses in a cohort of AIDS patients*

	At AIDS diagnosis		Subsequent diagnosis		Total diagnoses	
NHL	79	60.7%	51	39.5%	130	100%
KS	275	79.7%	70	20.3%	345	100%
HD	5	55.5%	4	45.5%	9	100%
Total	359	74.1%	125	25.9%	484	100%

From the Catalan Study Group on AIDS and Cancer, 1981–1991.

rospective may have led to the better clinical follow-up of HIV-positive attendees, overestimating their cancer incidence.

Case-Control Studies

Case-control studies may provide the strongest results regarding the association of particular conditions and low frequency diseases. Their main difficulty is the election of controls that ensure the comparability of all of the other variables, particularly when some of the cofactors may be unknown.

Most of the HAM case-control studies have been used to identify possible risk factors. In 1981, an American case-control study of 50 KS patients showed that a larger number of sexual partners, having been exposed to feces during sex, having had syphilis and non-A, non-B hepatitis, having been treated for enteric parasites, and having used illicit drugs, were all factors associated with KS (43). At the same time, a case-control study with only 20 KS cases from NY identified the number of sexual partners, receptive anal intercourse, and the practice of "fisting" as the behavioral variables associated with KS (44). Although some of these factors have been confirmed by later series of KS, others have not.

Given the lack of consistency regarding the association of HIV infection with HD, some case-control studies have tried to assess the role of HIV among HD cases. One study from the Atlanta Tumor Registry (45) found that 16% of all of the studied patients with HD were HIV-positive, but when only the cases of HD with mixed cellularity were considered, the figure was 58%.

In summary, although we know Hodgkin's disease is related to HIV, it has still not been shown that there is an increase in the total incidence of HD in relation to the HIV epidemic. It has been hypothesized that reports showing an association between HIV and HD may be due to misclassification. Data from Roithman and colleagues (46) showing that HD is found more frequently among IVDUs indicate that this association may be real, because any misclassification error would have been homogeneous among all transmission groups (47). Hepatocellular carcinoma is primarily caused by the hepatitis B virus, and it is likely that both cervical and anal carcinoma are also primarily caused by an infectious agent (probably the human papilloma virus types 16 or 18, or both). Although it is plausible that HIV-induced immunodeficiency increases the risk of expressing or accelerating these cancers, no increase in their incidence in the general population or in the population at risk for HIV has yet been shown. Squamous cell cancer of the skin has been shown to be associated with other forms of immunosuppression, but its incidence has not increased with the AIDS epidemic.

Although their etiopathogenic mechanisms are not yet clear, KS and NHL are the only two tumors for which there is consistent epidemiological evidence of an association with HIV infection, and, since the beginning of the AIDS epidemic, they have been considered as indicative diseases in an HIV-positive subject.

EPIDEMIOLOGY OF KAPOSI'S SARCOMA AND NON-HODGKIN'S LYMPHOMA

In the epidemiological study of a disease with an unknown etiological agent or a disease whose transmission mechanisms have not been identified, the classical host-medium-agent and person-place-time models are used to generate or test hypotheses regarding its natural history and spread patterns. Some of the existing epidemiological information on KS and NHL is reviewed here using this approach.

Person or Host

Kaposi's Sarcoma

Although extensive epidemiological research has been done in an attempt to identify host, environmental, and infectious factors, the etiology of Kaposi's sarcoma remains somewhat obscure. The fact that KS in AIDS patients is ten times more common in men that have sex with other men than in other HIV transmission groups is suggestive of some specific behavioral aspect that exposes them to an agent and facilitates its transmission. An unidentified transmissible agent has long been suspected, and recent evidence suggests that KS might be caused by an infectious agent in an immunosuppressed host (48).

Because the epidemiology of this tumor indicates it develops predominantly among men, some authors have suggested that steroid hormones directly regulate KS cell growth and autocrine growth factors (49), and therefore they might indeed play a role in progression of KS in men.

Because of a reported association between human leukocyte antigen (HLA) type and the risk for KS, HLA typing has been carried out in various studies. An early study (50) found that the frequency of HLA DR5 was significantly higher ($p<0.01$) in homosexual men with AIDS-associated KS (63%) than in community controls (23%). The authors concluded that genetic predisposition or an acquired immunoregulatory defect might be involved in the etiology of KS. However, as additional and contradictory studies have been published about susceptibility risk factors for KS linked to HLA classes I and II (51,52), the evidence is still inconclusive and merits further investigation.

Non-Hodgkin's Lymphoma

Little is known about the etiology of non-Hodgkin's lymphoma. After the recognition of AIDS as a new disease, it was noted that there was a clustering of NHL in people in the same transmission groups as those infected with HIV. The majority of these tumors have high grade histological patterns occurring in extranodal sites, particularly the central nervous system (CNS; 53). Previous studies of NHL in patients with HIV infection have been relatively small in size, and the etiological aspects for this cancer have not been investigated (53,54).

The occurrence of NHL, especially diffuse large-cell (LCL) and immunoblastic lymphoma (IL), in subjects with congenital or acquired immunodeficiency has been recognized for years (55,56). The clinical course of HIV infection has been changing over time as a result of improved therapies for both HIV-associated infectious complications and HIV infection itself. Hence, the prolonged life expectancy of patients with HIV infection in the characteristic setting of profound immunosuppression is an important factor in the increased incidence of NHL. Indeed, patients with symptomatic HIV infection who survive for up to 3 years on antiretroviral therapy may have a 46% probability (95%CI = 20-76) of developing NHL (57).

In a recent epidemiological survey, the incidence of NHL appeared to vary with age and within specific groups for HIV infection (58). This extensive survey involved the descriptive analysis of the 2,824 NHL cases reported to the AIDS registry of the USA's Centers for Disease Control (CDC) up to mid-1989. Among AIDS patients, the incidence of IL progressively increased with age (up to 3.5% in those aged 50 or more years); that of primary lymphoma of the brain, as a separate entity, remained constant at 0.6% at all ages; and that of Burkitt's lymphoma (BL) increased up to a peak of 1.8% at 10 to 19 years of age. Each type of lymphoma was twice as common in whites as in blacks, and in men as in women; it was most common in patients with clotting disorders (58). This increased frequency of BL in HIV-infected patients was unexpected and does not agree with other reports (59); in fact, the principal limitation of Beral's study (58) is its probable underestimation of NHL types, because conditions occurring after the initial case report to CDC [which might account for up to one-third of all NHLs (59)] were seldom recorded (60).

Environment

Kaposi's Sarcoma

Inhaled nitrites (or "poppers") have been one of the most frequently hypothesized etiologic cofactors in the development of KS, especially before HIV was found to be the cause of AIDS (61). In addition to the frequent association between nitrite use among men who have sex with men, volatile nitrites can form carcinogenic compounds and may transform endothelial cell lines. Nevertheless, some investigators consider nitrite use a surrogate marker for high-risk behaviors, such as unprotected receptive anal intercourse, and, because the two practices are so highly correlated, standard multivariate techniques are inadequate to separate their effects (62). Because of these contradictory findings, the relationship between nitrite inhalants, high-risk sexual practices, and the risk for HIV infection has recently come under study again (63). The more conclusive results of this study of homosexual male couples in the USA suggest a strong interaction between nitrite use and unprotected receptive anal intercourse in increasing the risk for HIV infection (adjusted OR=31.8, 95%CI=12.9-76.7 versus OR=9.0, 95%CI=2.5-32.1) in men who always, in comparison with those who never, used nitrites during that sexual practice (63). Nitrites may facilitate the entry of HIV and other pathogens into the bloodstream during receptive anal intercourse through the dilation of blood vessels and the relaxation of vascular smooth muscle.

Dr. Beral and colleagues (48) have reported that a diagnosis of KS was associated with self-reported sexual activities involving contact with feces, especially insertive oral-anal contact ($p<0.001$), in 65 homosexual or bisexual men interviewed in London in 1984 to 1985. Although these findings have been supported by others through the reanalysis of former studies (64), the study merits some comment. The study population consisted of two separate groups: 45 men who were interviewed at least 5 years before AIDS developed, and 20 men who were interviewed at the time of the onset of AIDS. The authors state that the separate results of both groups were generally similar, but it is not possible to rule out biased reporting of sexual practices in the latter group. Also, the fact that each man in the study was asked about his sexual practices during the previous 5 years makes recall bias plausible. The data are certainly suggestive of the fecal-oral transmission route of a putative KS agent, but they need to be confirmed by other epidemiological and microbiological studies specifically designed to test this interesting hypothesis. On the other hand, other studies, such as a Ugandan hospital-based, case-control study by Louie et al., did not support the hypothesis that KS is caused by a sexually transmitted agent (65).

It is probable that all types of KS are associated with some type of immunosuppression. The association between immunosuppressive therapy and KS has been previously discussed.

Non-Hodgkin's Lymphoma

Unlike the case for KS, no environmental factors have been implicated in the etiology of NHL. However, because zidovudine can act as a mutagen in mice and rats, Pluda (57) has speculated that the direct oncogenic potential of zidovudine and related drugs may contribute to the development of NHL. In this controversial area, it is important to undertake further investigations designed to establish whether the experimental effects of zidovudine in animals also occur in humans.

Agent

Kaposi's Sarcoma

Since the 1970s, cytomegalovirus (CMV), a member of the herpes family of viruses, has been extensively studied as the possible causal agent of KS. Following the detection of CMV in KS cell line cultures, a number of serological studies have shown higher CMV antibody titers in KS patients than in controls in Europe and the USA (66). Although there is an ecological association between the prevalence of CMV and KS, this association is not seen in Africans with KS, and KS is infrequent in IVDUs and hemophiliacs with AIDS, who are commonly infected with CMV. In addition, more recent laboratory studies using different techniques (antigen immunohistochemistry, in situ hybridization, Southern blotting, and polymerase chain reaction test) have not found CMV in KS biopsy specimens (67). It can thus be concluded that CMV is neither a necessary nor a sufficient factor for KS and that it may be a bystander in neoplastic tissue, existing as a latent infection or reactivated by immunosuppressive therapy or HIV infection (68). The role of CMV in the semen, and the subsequent risk for KS, awaits further studies.

Other known viruses, especially DNA viruses, have also been considered to be potential KS agents. Discrepant serological data from various study designs have been reported concerning Epstein-Barr virus (EBV), herpes simplex virus (HSV)-1, HSV-2, human T-cell leukemia virus (HTLV)-I, HTLV-II, hepatitis B virus (HBV) or hepatitis A virus (HAV; 66). The presence of most of the above viruses has been unsuccessfully looked for in cell cultures derived from AIDS-related KS cells (69). The fact that the distribution of these viruses is inconsistent with the distribution of KS, and that the multiple viruses found in KS patients are suggestive of a weakened immune system, make it unlikely that many of these viruses are single causes of the development of KS. On the other hand, the temporal sequence of these viral infections remains to be elucidated. The last virus to appear on the scene was human papillomavirus (HPV). The group of Dr. Friedman-Kien (70) has recently reported the presence of HPV-16 sequences in 20% of KS samples and papilloma-related antigens in 70% of samples from both endemic and epidemic KS types. However, these findings have not been confirmed (71).

Finally, two other nonviral infectious pathogens have been associated with KS in AIDS patients. The first is an agent (which proved to be a mycoplasma) that has been isolated in the KS tissue and in many other sites of patients with AIDS (72). Secondly, because of the high-risk sexual practices of men who have sex with men involving fecal-oral contact, and the higher frequency of intestinal parasites (especially *Entamoeba* spp.) among homosexuals with HIV-related conditions (73), it has been hypothesized that KS may result from the interaction of a chronic intestinal parasitic infection and a viral agent. In fact, a history of amebiasis has been found to be associated with an increased risk for KS (relative hazard = 1.4, 95%CI = 1.1-1.9; 74).

The etiology of KS remains a puzzle, and because there is no simple way of explaining its occurrence, various causal models have been developed (66): (i) the cofactor model argues that the combined effects of numerous infectious agents, and host and environmental factors, encourage KS proliferation; (ii) the natural avian model of an hemangiomatosis of fowl induced by a sexually transmitted retrovirus highlights resemblances with the clinical and pathological features of KS; and (iii) the susceptibility model proposes the existence of just one active agent of both endemic and epidemic KS, but varying degrees of susceptibility and different routes of transmission. Support for the last two models partly derives from the hypothesized sexually transmitted route of a KS agent early in the AIDS epidemic (36), the reports of KS occurring in homosexual men who are seronegative for HIV infection (75), the transmission of the agent through oral-anal sexual practices (48), and the emergence of gay bowel syndrome associated with a high incidence of intestinal parasites in males with HIV disease (76). There is no clear definition as to what type of agent causes KS. Retroviruses (77) and other viruses, especially enteric viruses, are the most likely suspects (68). However, in addition to the development of fine molecular techniques, the search for the etiology of KS also calls for further innovative epidemiological research.

Non-Hodgkin's Lymphoma

Epstein-Barr herpesvirus (EBV) is a B lymphotropic agent that has been consistently associated with various B lymphoproliferative diseases, such as BL and posttransplant lymphomas (78). In vitro, EBV is capable of producing polyclonal B-cell activation and immortalizing normal B lymphocytes. Polyclonal B-cell proliferative lymph node expansion is present in immunosuppressed patients with HIV disease, and EBV DNA and EBV gene expression has been demonstrated in a number of NHL cases associated with AIDS (79). Although EBV has not been universally associated with NHL in patients with AIDS (80), it has been the principal suspect in this particular group of NHL patients. In addition to the complex and changing classification of lymphoma, a further drawback in the study of NHL associated with AIDS is that NHL constitutes a histologically diverse group which may be etiologically and pathogenetically distinct. In Africa, BL is almost always associated with EBV, but this is not the case in the USA (81). Burkitt's lymphoma exhibits chromosomal translocations, particularly t(8:14) within the c-myc oncogene region of chromosome 8, which also differ between Africa and the USA (80).

Probably, the report of MacMahon et al. (82) represents one of the most important contributions towards a clarification of the role played by EBV in NHL associated with AIDS. These researchers undertook a study of necropsy material from a consecutive series of 21 affected patients. Because of the highly restricted expression of EBV in malignant tissue, and the lack of a reliable technique for handling formalin-fixed archive material, the authors adopted a new strategy for the detection of latent EBV by using short, nonprotein coding EBV transcripts (EBERs) for in situ hybridization. The expression of the EBV-EBER1 transcript was present in all primary CNS lymphomas. This 100% association suggested that the pathogenesis of NHL associated with AIDS may differ from that of the systemic disease, in which only about 40% of the tumors are associated with EBV. The results of this study suggest that the pathogenesis of primary CNS lymphomas in patients with AIDS may be distinct from that of other AIDS-related lymphomas (82).

Setting aside the frequent limitations of the small number of cases studied and the technical difficulties involved in identifying EBV in previous studies (83), the lack of consistency of study results and epidemiological findings emphasizes the differences in the pathogenesis of different NHL types. Consequently, each type of NHL needs to be studied separately in investigations for causal agents. Much epidemiological research has to be done in order to identify the probable involvement of different pathogenetic stimuli in histologically diverse NHLs associated with AIDS.

Place

Kaposi's Sarcoma

In 1981, the CDC collected information on 30 cases exclusively from New York and California, all of them being homosexual or bisexual men (9). In the USA, this distribution has been constant, and homosexual men with AIDS are more likely to develop KS if they are from the areas were the epidemic started. Whereas patients from the Northeast and California have the highest percentages of KS, in the states of the Midwest this percentage is the lowest: Thirty percent of all AIDS cases among homosexual and bisexual men in California and 31% of those in New York had KS, but only 5% of those coming from Kansas did. At least in the USA, KS is the only AIDS-indicative disease with such a precise and consistent geographical distribution (36).

The geographical distribution of KS among homosexual and bisexual men is similar in other countries, but it varies a lot when heterosexual cases are analyzed, KS being much more frequent in Central America and Africa than in other, Western countries (84,85).

Among subjects acquiring HIV infection parenterally, the percentage of KS is similar in all of the countries where such information exists: 2.5% in USA (36), 2.8% in Catalonia (Spain; 86) and Italy (87). In the USA, KS in IVDUs (as in homosexual and bisexual men) is more likely in those areas where the AIDS epidemic started (36).

Given that southern European areas have a higher prevalence of endemic KS cases, we postulated that the factor(s) involved in KS among AIDS patients could be the same. If so, AIDS cases in Southern Europe should have a higher proportion of KS as their presenting indicative disease than those in Northern Europe. Overall, the proportion of KS cases in areas with a high prevalence of endemic KS was 24% among homosexual and bisexual men, and 4.3% among other transmission groups. In areas with no endemic KS cases, these proportions were not statistically different (31% and 5%, respectively; Figs. 1 and 2). The absence of any geographical distribution of KS among AIDS cases may indicate that risk factors for KS are widely distributed among the different groups at risk of HIV (88).

Non-Hodgkin's Lymphoma

Definition criteria for NHL include Burkitt's lymphoma (ICD-9-CM 200.2), immunoblastic sarcoma (ICD-9-CM 200.8), histiocytic or large cell

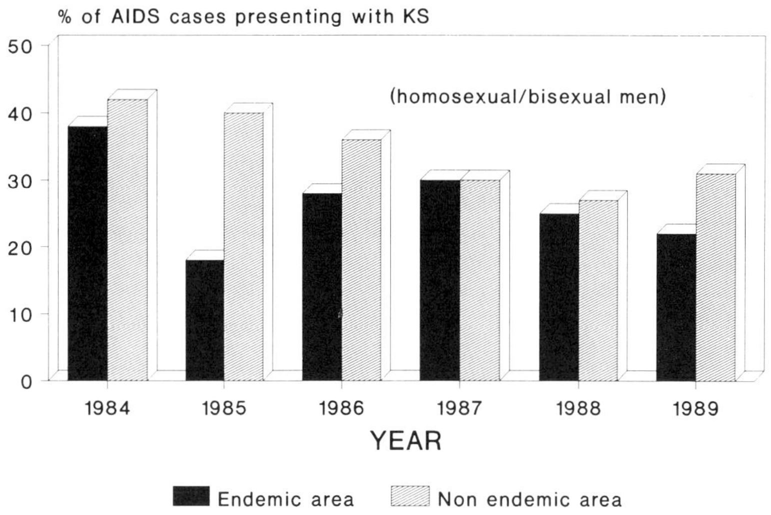

FIG. 1. Distribution by area of KS over time among homosexual and bisexual men in Europe. From Casabona et al. (88).

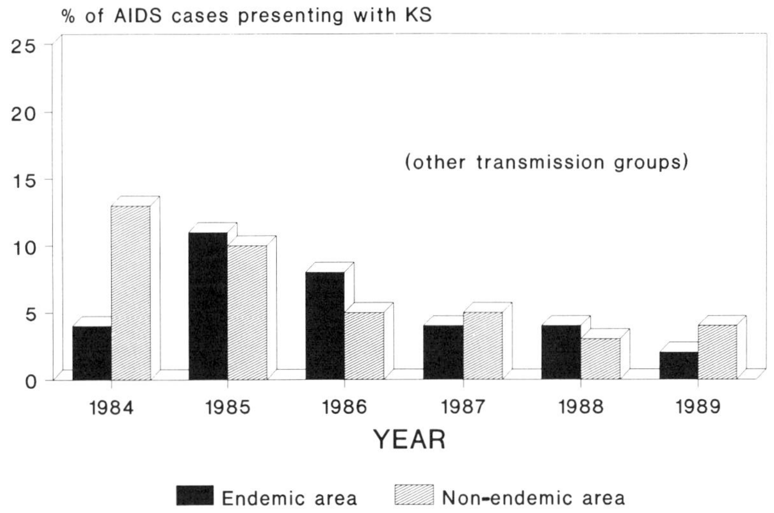

FIG. 2. Distribution by area of KS over time among other transmission groups in Europe. From Casabona et al. (88).

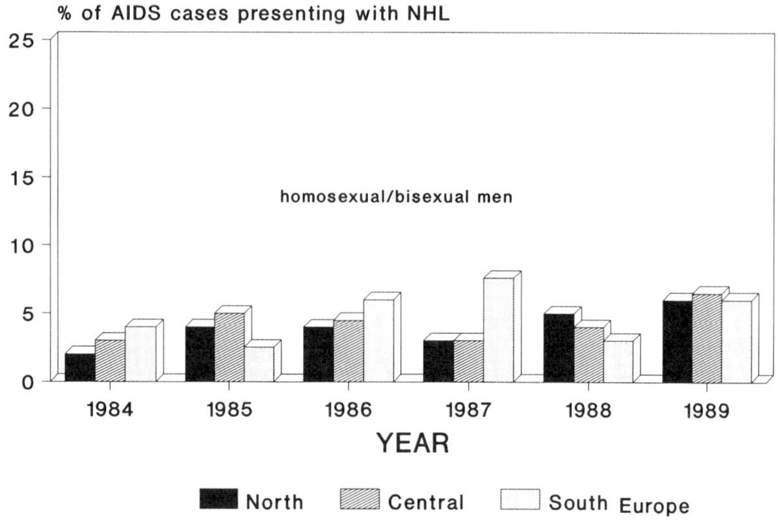

FIG. 3. Distribution by area of NHL over time among homosexual and bisexual men. From Casabona et al. (88).

lymphoma (ICD-9-CM 200.0), and primary lymphoma of the brain (ICD-9-CM 202.8; 89). Among these only Burkitt's lymphoma has a previously identified geographical pattern, being much more frequent in Africa (81). In the USA, 2.9% of all AIDS cases reported up to June 30, 1989, presented with NHL (58), this percentage being similar to the 3.3% found in Europe (88).

In the USA, the percentage of AIDS cases with NHL by state of residence at the time of diagnosis ranges from 1.2% in Kansas to 11% in Alaska. The same analysis by place of birth identified that 3% of the cases born in the USA, 3.2% of those born in Canada, and 1.2% of those born in Mexico presented with NHL. Nevertheless, the authors of this study concluded that, in general in the USA, there was no systematic variation in the risk for NHL by state of residence or place of birth (58). In Europe, a study of AIDS surveillance data failed to identify any geographical distribution of the number of cases presenting with NHL, regardless of the way in which these cases were infected (Figs. 3 and 4; 88).

Since most AIDS surveillance systems do not collect specific data by each type of NHL, some geographical patterns have not been identified. In our setting, primary lymphoma of the brain was the only NHL which showed a different distribution by transmission group, being more frequent among IVDUs (90). Therefore, primary lymphoma of the brain could be more frequent in areas where parenteral transmission is the main route of HIV infection.

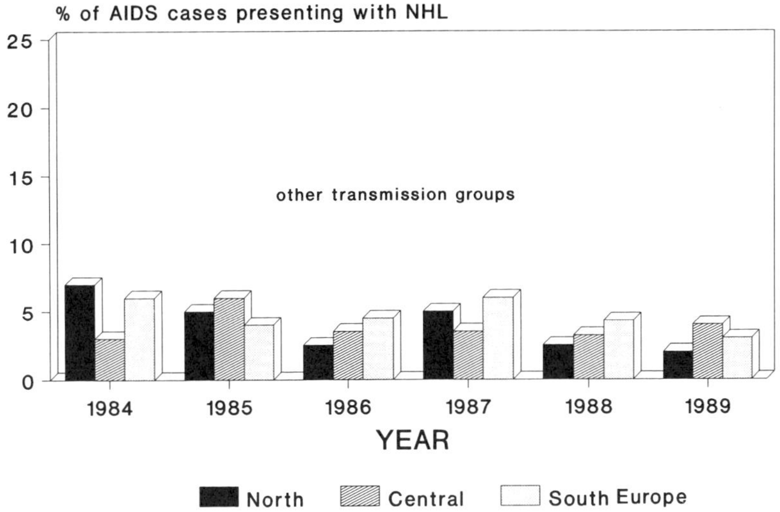

FIG. 4. Distribution by area of Europe of NHL over time among other transmission groups. From Casabona et al. (88).

Time

Kaposi's Sarcoma

As has already been said, although many population-based cancer registry studies have shown a consistent increase in the incidence of KS among the population at risk for HIV (24–26,30), one of the arguments which has been used to hypothesize that KS is caused by an agent that has been slowly removed from the population at risk is the fact that the proportion of KS among AIDS cases has been declining over the last few years (36). In the USA, the annual rate of decline has been 24% among homosexual and bisexual men, and 20% among other transmission categories (including parenteral and heterosexual transmission). This decline, which is not affected by the year of diagnosis and persists even in comparison with *Pneumocystis carinii* pneumonia cases (a disease which has been considered constant during the study period), leads Beral to argue that changes in the behavior of homosexual men over time have reduced exposure to the KS putative agent among the youngest homosexuals (36). In Europe, two studies have analyzed AIDS registry data, and both have confirmed a decline in the proportion of AIDS cases which have KS as their presenting indicative disease. Casabona and colleagues (88) have reported a decline in the proportion of AIDS cases with KS, from 40.5% in 1983 to 26% in 1988 among homosexual men, and from 12.2% to 3.2% among other transmission groups for the same

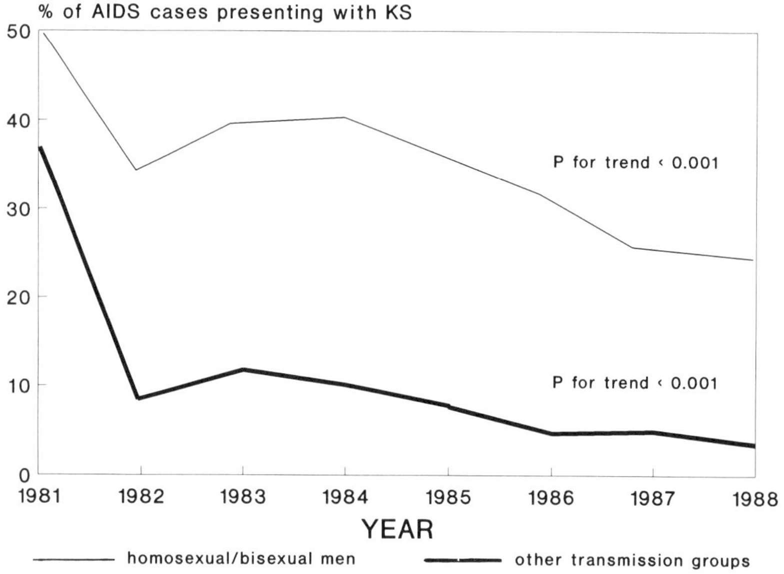

FIG. 5. Evolution of KS as a presenting indicative disease for AIDS by transmission group. From Casabona et al. (88).

period (Fig. 5). Serraino and colleagues (19) have reported that the percentage of KS cases in homosexual men was 30% for the period 1982 to 1986, and 20% in 1990; in IVDUs, the respective figures were 5% and 2.5% (91).

However, the use of AIDS surveillance data in the evaluation of trends for HAM may lead to several biases. Most AIDS registries only collect information on presenting AIDS-indicative diseases; the diseases appearing after the diagnosis are not recorded, and therefore their incidence may be underestimated. Since KS appears early in the natural history of HIV infection, this effect is probably much smaller than in the case of NHL, which is usually diagnosed later.

Other factors may also affect the distribution of the AIDS presenting disease. Since indicative diseases are a function of the underlying distribution of their associated factors, they may be affected not only by the prevalence and distribution of the infectious agents, but also by the distribution of the transmission groups in the community. Therefore, the quantification of HAMs using proportional data is also affected by possible variations in other indicative conditions.

Data from the San Francisco Clinic Cohort Study, presented at the Eighth International AIDS Conference by Dr. Katz and his colleagues (39) showed that, although the frequency of KS as a first diagnosis decreased, it slightly increased as a subsequent diagnosis. A study done in Atlanta, Georgia, showed a similar increase in age-adjusted incidence of KS among white men

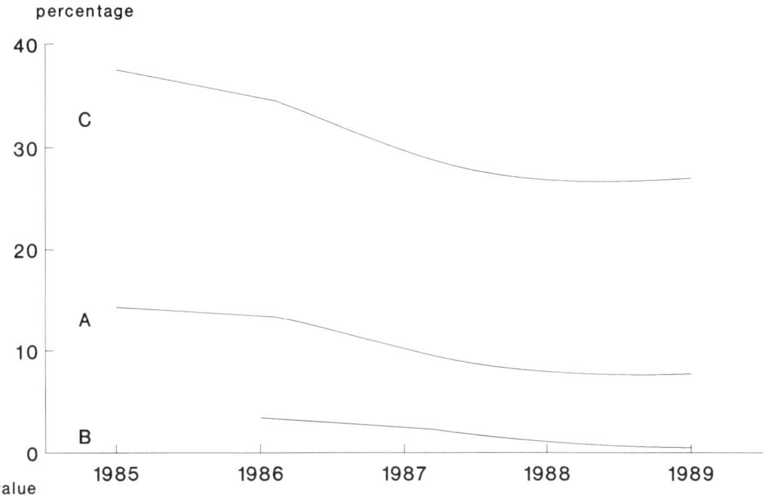

p value		1985	1986	1987	1988	1989
n.s.	A	14.3	14.4	9.74	7.3	7.7
0.04	B	-	3.4	3	0.6	0.5
n.s.	C	37.5	35.9	28.8	26	27

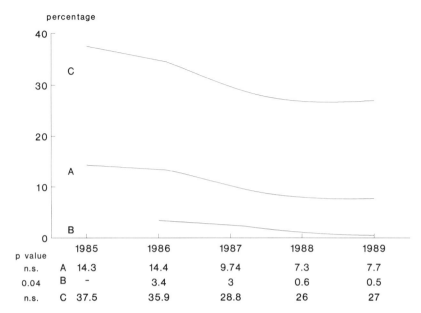

FIG. 6. Percentages of KS cases by year of diagnosis in Catalonia, computed for different groups: (A) KS among all AIDS cases (p = nonsignificant); (B) KS among intravenous drug users (IVDUs; $p = 0.04$); (C) KS among homosexual and bisexual men (p = nonsignificant). From Casabona et al. (60).

aged 25 to 49 years in comparison with the annual incidence of AIDS, and the authors suggested that this data did not support a decrease in the incidence of KS over time (29).

A study done in Catalonia, using data from 1,569 AIDS cases reported to the Catalan population-based AIDS registry between 1981 and 1990, also failed to identify any significant temporal pattern for this presenting form, but only among IVDU cases (Fig. 6; 60). In our setting, both extrapulmonary tuberculosis and toxoplasmosis are much more common among IVDUs than in other transmission groups, such as homosexuals, thus the decline in the incidence of KS among IVDUs may be partly due to the introduction of the 1987 CDC definition of AIDS; therefore, there may be regional differences in the temporal pattern of KS; any comparison should take into account possible local differences in underlying risk factors and in the characteristics and distribution of the transmission groups.

In our study, five of the KS cases were women, all of whom were IVDUs. The proportion of KS in the men and the women of this particular group was similar (1.5% and 2.7%, respectively; $p = 0.17$). Although heterosexual transmission of a putative agent for KS cannot be ruled out, parenteral transmission should also be explored further. If an infectious agent is causing KS, it is logical to expect that its increasing prevalence among different groups

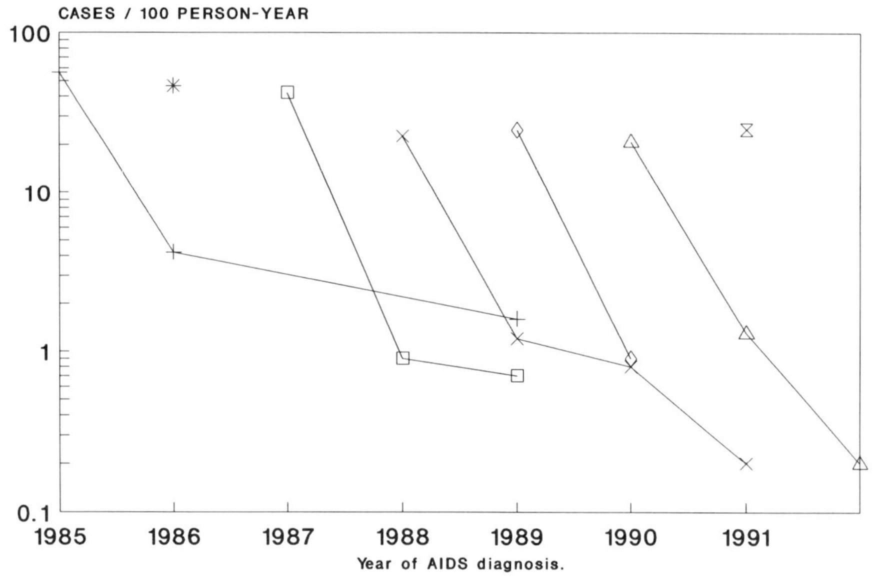

FIG. 7. Evolution of the annual incidence rate for KS in a cohort of AIDS patients. From the Catalan Study Group on AIDS and Cancer, 1981–1991.

over time will also lead to some changes in the incidence of KS. In this regard, the evolution of KS among women is of particular interest. Cancer incidence data from New York State (Rabkin CS and Biggar R, personal communication) showed that although some geographical and racial differences exist, there is a clear increase in the incidence of KS in women, which temporally and geographically follows the evolution of the AIDS epidemic in the area.

In our setting, the analysis of follow-up data from the cohort of AIDS patients reported to the Catalan AIDS Registry between 1981 and 1991 failed to identify any trend in the annual KS incidence rates measured by person-years (Fig. 7); (38a).

Sources of information other than AIDS surveillance data (particularly population-based cancer registries and cohorts of HIV-infected subjects) should be used to analyze the occurrence and distribution of KS and NHL among AIDS cases. It will also be necessary to assess the possible role of the introduction of zidovudine in the evolution of the incidence of KS among HIV-infected patients when adjusting by CDA cells (92). In Chapter 19, Dr. Muñoz has already updated some of these issues with new data from the MACS study. While a previous analysis of this cohort study failed to identify any trend in the annual incidence of KS (35), current data show a slight decrease.

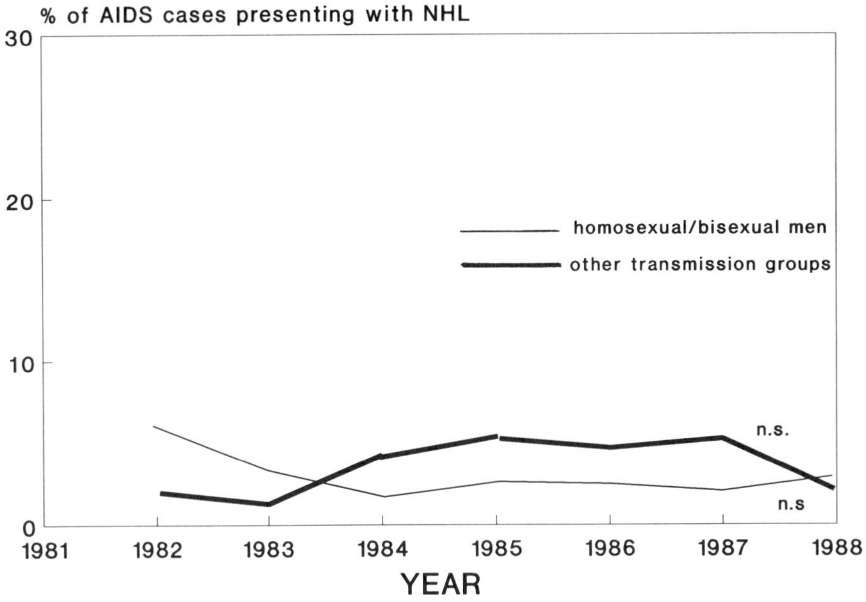

n.s. = non-significant trend

FIG. 8. Evolution of NHL as a presenting indicative disease for AIDS by transmission group. (Trends are nonsignificant.) From Casabona et al. (88).

Non-Hodgkin's Lymphoma

AIDS surveillance data from the USA shows an increase in the percentage of cases presenting with NHL (from 1.6% in 1984 to 2.9% in 1985), but this was attributed to the inclusion of immunoblastic lymphoma in the CDC reporting definition of AIDS. Since then, this percentage has remained constant at about 3% (58).

A European study using AIDS surveillance data failed to detect any temporal pattern of NHL as a presenting form for AIDS, the overall percentage being 3.3% (Fig. 8; 88), although another study suggested a slight increase in the proportion of NHL among homosexual and bisexual men (2.6% in 1986 to 3.9% in 1990) and a decrease among IVDUs (4.3% in 1986 to 2.2% in 1990; 91). As was said regarding KS, we believe that AIDS surveillance data should be complemented with other sources of information in order to identify and assess possible trends over time. It will also be necessary to analyze separately the different types of lymphoma included in this category and to adjust incidence rates for CD4+ counts to avoid the effect of changes in the occurrence of other opportunistic infections.

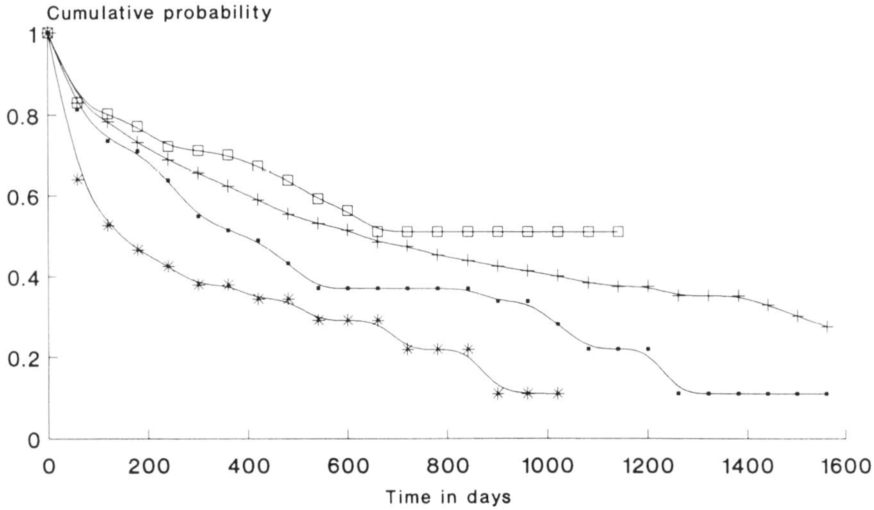

FIG. 9. Survival curves by presenting disease: (■) Kaposi's sarcoma; (+) Opportunistic infection; (✱) Non-Hodgkin's disease; (□) Other AIDS indicative diseases. From Casabona et al. (60).

Survival

While some USA studies have shown that AIDS cases with KS have a better prognosis than cases presenting with an opportunistic infection (93), others show that cases presenting with an opportunistic infection have a longer survival time (94). In our setting, patients presenting with NHL have the poorest prognosis, with a median survival time (MST) of 169 days; patients presenting with an opportunistic infection or KS have the longest survival (MST=656.7 and 423.6 days, respectively). Figure 9 shows the survival curves according to the presenting disease. While survival in KS cases did not differ from that of the rest of patients, NHL cases had a shorter survival time than any of the cases with other presenting diseases ($p<0.0001$). The high prevalence of tuberculosis infection in our community, particularly among IVDUs, may partly explain these differences (95). In any case, it is clear from our results that patients presenting with NHL have the poorest prognosis, irrespective of age, sex, or transmission group.

FUTURE CONSIDERATIONS

The future scope of HAM studies will depend not only on the prevalence and distribution of the risk factors, which are still to be identified, but also on the prevalence of the population at risk. The fact that the prevalence of HIV infection will continue to increase in most countries for at least the next 5 years will lead to an important increase in the prevalence and incidence of

HAM in the short term. Moreover, because patients with a more impaired immunological system (CD4+ cell count less than 200) are especially at risk (8), the continuous increase in the survival of AIDS patients, due to the prevention and treatment of opportunistic infections and to specific antiretroviral therapy, will particularly contribute towards this overall increase in HAM prevalence and incidence. Because NHL is the indicative disease with the poorest survival, it is also likely that NHL will be one of the leading causes of death among AIDS patients in the future.

Finally, many questions remain to be answered in the epidemiology of HAMs (particularly in the case of KS, NHL, and HD). Here, we suggest a few of them:

Is there enough data to associate the decrease in the incidence of KS reported by some studies with the removal of one or more possible putative agents from the population at risk over the last few years? What kind of data do we need to differentiate these observations from the possible effects of changes in the natural history of HIV infection due to chemoprophylaxis and antiretroviral therapy, and from regional and temporal variations in sexual behavior and in the underlying prevalence of other opportunistic agents?

If an infectious agent is associated with KS production, what indicators can be used to assess the possible incubation period of such an agent? This would be of great importance to the design of new data collection instruments aimed at identifying or confirming "exposure."

How can important methodological issues in the design of epidemiological studies (for example, the choice of controls in case-control studies aimed at determining risk factors for HAM) be resolved?

In the near future, will there be an increase in the incidence of HD and anal and cervical carcinoma in the general population of the areas with a high HIV prevalence? Will the distribution of KS change in the same way as the distribution of HIV transmission is changing in some Western countries? Is there any association between development or progression of anal or cervical cancer, with HIV infection or immunosuppression.

REFERENCES

1. Spector BD, Perry GS, Kersey JH. Genetically determined immunodeficiency disease (GDID) and malignancy: report from the immunodeficiency cancer registry. *Clin Immunol Immunopathol* 1978;11:12–29.
2. Penn I. Volume 28: tumors arising in organ transplant recipients. In Klein G, Woodhouse S, eds. *Advances in cancer research*. Orlando, FL: Academic; 1978.
3. Penn I. Depressed immunity and the development of cancer. *Clin Exp Immunol* 1981;46:459–474.
4. Levine AM, Gill PS, Meyer PR, et al. Retrovirus and malignant lymphoma in homosexual men. *JAMA* 1985;254:1921–1925.
5. Kaplan MK, Susin M, Pahwa SG, et al. Neoplastic complications of HTLV-III infection: lymphomas and solid tumors. *Am J Med* 1987;82:389–396.

6. Lowenthal DA, Straus DJ, Campbell SW, et al. AIDS-related lymphoid neoplasia: the Memorial Hospital experience. *Cancer* 1988;61:2325–2337.
7. International Agency for Research on Cancer. Report of ad-hoc IARC monographs advisory group on viruses and other biological agents such as parasites. Lyon, France: International Agency for Research on Cancer; 1991; IARC publication, no 91/001.
8. Cremer KJ, Spring SB, Gruber J. Role of human immunodeficiency virus type I and other viruses in malignancies associated with acquired immunodeficiency disease syndrome. *J Natl Cancer Inst* 1990;12:1016–1024.
9. Centers for Disease Control. Kaposis's sarcoma and Pneumocystis pneumonia among homosexual men New York City and California. *MMWR Morb Mortal Wkly Rep* 1981;30:305–308.
10. Durack DT, Phil et al. Opportunistic infections and Kaposis's sarcoma in homosexual men. *N Engl J Med* 1981;305:1465–1467.
11. Pichenik AE, Fischl MA, Dickinson GM, et al. Opportunistic infections and Kaposi's sarcoma among Haitians: evidence of a new acquired immunodeficiency state. *Ann Intern Med* 1983;98:277–284.
12. Centers for Disease Control. Task force on Kaposi's sarcoma and opportunistic infections. *N Engl J Med* 1982;306:1248–1252.
13. Doll DC, List AF. Burkitt's lymphoma in a homosexual. *Lancet* 1982;i:1026–1027.
14. Ziegler JL, Miner RC, Rosenbaum E, et al. Outbreak of Burkitt's lymphoma in a homosexual. *Lancet* 1982;ii:631–632.
15. Knowles DM, Chamulak GA, Subar M, et al. Lymphoid neoplasia associated with the acquired immunodeficiency syndrome (AIDS): the New York University Medical Center experience with 105 patients (1981–1986). *Ann Intern Med* 1988;108:744–753.
16. O'Sullivan MG, Whittle IR, Gregor A, et al. Increasing incidence of CNS primary lymphoma in South-East Scotland. *Lancet* 1991;338:895–896.
17. Tirelli U, Vaccher E, Rezza G, et al. Hodgkin's disease in association with acquired immunodeficiency syndrome (AIDS): a report on 36 patients. *Acta Oncol* 1989;28:637–639.
18. Monfardini S, Vaccher E, Lazzarin A, et al. Characterization of AIDS-associated tumors in Italy: report of 435 cases of an IVDA-based series. *Cancer Detect Prev* 1990;14:391–393.
19. Serraino M, Bellas C, Campo E, et al. Hodgkin's disease in patients with antibodies to human immunodeficiency virus: a study of 22 patients. *Cancer* 1990;65:2248–2254.
20. Hoover RH, Fraumeni JF. Risk of cancer in renal-transplant recipients. *Lancet* 1973;ii:55–57.
21. Kinlen LJ, Sheil AGR, Peto J, Doll R. Collaborative United Kingdom-Australasian study of cancer in patients treated with immunosuppressive drugs. *BMJ* 1979;2:1461–1466.
22. Blohme I, Brynger H. Malignant disease in renal transplant patients. *Transplantation* 1985;39:23–25.
23. Kersey JH, Shapiro RS, Filipvich AH. Relationship of immunodeficiency to lymphoid malignancy. *Pediatr Infect Dis J* 1988;7:S10–S12.
24. Biggar RJ, Horm J, Lubin JH, et al. Cancer trends in a population at risk of acquired immunodeficiency syndrome. *J Natl Cancer Inst* 1985;74:793–797.
25. Biggar RJ, Horm J, Goedert JJ, et al. Cancer in a group at risk of acquired immunodeficiency syndrome (AIDS) through 1984. *Am J Epidemiol* 1987;126:578–586.
26. Kristal AR, Nasca PC, Burnett WS, et al. Changes in the epidemiology of non-Hodgkin's lymphoma associated with epidemic human immunodeficiency virus (HIV) infection. *Am J Epidemiol* 1988;128:711–718.
27. Harnly ME, Swan SH, Holly EA, et al. Temporal trends in the incidence of non-Hodgkin's lymphoma and selected malignancies in a population with a high incidence of acquired immunodeficiency syndrome (AIDS). *Am J Epidemiol* 1987;128:261–267.
28. Biggar RJ, Burnett W, Mikl J, et al. Cancer among New York men at risk of acquired immunodeficiency syndrome. *Int J Cancer* 1989;43:979–985.
29. Chow WH, Liff JM, Greenberg RS, et al. A comparison of acquired immunodeficiency syndrome and Kaposi's sarcoma incidence rates, Atlanta, 1983–86. *Am J Public Health* 1989;79:503–505.
30. Rabkin CS, Biggar RJ, Horm JW. Increasing incidence of cancers associated with human immunodeficiency virus epidemic. *Int J Cancer* 1991;47:692–696.

31. Bendsoe N, Dictor M, Blomberg J, et al. Increased incidence of Kaposis's sarcoma in Sweden before the Aids epidemic. *Eur J Cancer* 1990;26:699–702.
32. Goedert JJ, Kessler CM, Aledort LM, et al. A prospective study of human immunodeficiency virus type 1 infection and the development of AIDS in subjects with hemophilia. *N Engl J Med* 1989;321:1141–1148.
33. Rabkin CS, Blattner WA. HIV Infection and cancers other than Non-Hodgkin Lymphoma and Kaposi's sarcoma. In: Beral V, Jaffe HW, Weiss RA, eds. *Cancer, HIV and AIDS*. New York: Cold Spring Harbor Laboratory Press; 1991.
34. Lifson AR, Darrow WW, Hessol NA, et al. Kaposi's sarcoma in a cohort of homosexual and bisexual men. *Am J Epidemiol* 1990;131(2):221–231.
35. Jacobson LP, Muñoz A, Fox R, et al. Incidence of Kaposi's sarcoma in a cohort of homosexual men infected with the human immunodeficiency virus type 1. *J Acquir Immune Defic Syndr* 1990;3[suppl 1]:S24.
36. Beral V, Petterman TA, Berkelman RL, et al. Kaposi's sarcoma among persons with AIDS: a sexually transmitted infection? *Lancet* 1990;335:123–128.
37. Archibald CP, Schechter MT, Le TN, et al. Evidence for a sexually transmitted cofactor for AIDS-related Kaposi's sarcoma in a cohort of homosexual men. *Epidemiology* 1992;3:203–209.
38. Rabkin CS, Goedert JJ. Risk of non-Hodgkin lymphoma and Kaposi's sarcoma in homosexual men. *Lancet* 1990;336:248–249.
38a. Casabona J, Blanc C, Vall M, et al. Incidence of Kaposi's sarcoma, Non-Hodgkin lymphomas and Hodgkin disease in a cohort of AIDS patients. IXth International Conference on AIDS, Berlin, June 1993; (Abstract vol. 2) 659.
39. Katz MH, Hessol N, Buchbinder S. Late manifestations of AIDS: temporal changes in opportunistic infections and cancers. Presented at the International Conference on AIDS, Amsterdam, The Netherlands, 1992.
40. Melbye M, Palefsky J, Gonzales J, Ryder L, Biggar RJ. Immune status as a determinant of human papilloma virus detection and its correlations with anal epithelial abnormalities. *Int J Cancer* 1990;46:203–206.
41. Feingold, Vermund SH, Burk RD, Kelley KF, et al. Cervical cytologic abnormalities and papilloma virus in women infected with human immunodeficiency virus. *J Acquir Immune Defic Syndr* 1990;3:896–903.
42. Gachupin-Garcia A, Selwyn PA, Salisbury, Budner N. Population-based study of malignancies and HIV infection among injecting drug users in a New York City methadone treatment program, 1985–1991. *AIDS* 1992;6:843–848.
43. Jaffe HW, Choi K, Thomas PA, et al. National case-control study of Kaposi's sarcoma and *Pneumocystis carinii* pneumonia in homosexual men: part 1, epidemiologic results. *Ann Intern Med* 1983;99:145–151.
44. Marmor M, Friedman-Kein AE, Zolla-Pazner S, et al. Kaposi's sarcoma in homosexual men. *Ann Intern Med* 1984;100:809–815.
45. Liff JM, Eley JW, Khabbaz RF, Selik RM, Chan WC. HIV seropositivity and Hodgkin's lymphoma. Presented at the 30th Interscience Conference on Antimicrobial Agents and Chemotherapy, Altanta, Georgia, 1990; (Abstract 1121) 273.
46. Roithmann S, Tourani JM, Andrieu JM. Hodgkin's disease in HIV-infected intravenous drug abusers. *N Engl J Med* 1990;323:275–276.
47. Beral V. The epidemiology of cancer in AIDS patients. *AIDS* 1991;5(suppl 2):S–S103.
48. Beral V, Bull D, Darby S, et al. Risk of Kaposi's sarcoma and sexual practices associated with faecal contact in homosexual or bisexual men with AIDS. *Lancet* 1992; 339:632–635.
49. Law R, Massod R, Lin G, et al. Role of steroid hormones in AIDS Kaposi's sarcoma. *AIDS Weekly* 1992 December:15.
50. Friedman-Kien AE, Laubenstein LJ, Rubinstein P, et al. Disseminated Kaposi's sarcoma in homosexual men. *Ann Intern Med* 1982;96:693–700.
51. Qunibi W, Akhtar M, Sheth K, et al. Kaposi's sarcoma: the most common tumour after renal transplantation in Saudi Arabia. *Am J Med* 1988;84:225–232.
52. Mann DL, Murray C, O'Donnell M, et al. HLA antigen frequencies in HIV-1 related Kaposi's sarcoma. *J Acquir Immune Defic Syndr* 1990;3[suppl 1]:S51–55.
53. Ziegler JL, Beckstead JA, Volberding PA, et al. Non-Hodgkin's lymphoma in 90 homosexual men: relation to generalized lymphadenopathy and the acquired immunodeficiency syndrome. *N Engl J Med* 1984;311:565–570.

54. Kaplan LD, Abrams DI, Feigal E, et al. AIDS-associated non-Hodgkin's lymphoma in San Francisco. *JAMA* 1989;261:719–724.
55. Kersey JH, Spector BD, Good RA. Primary immunodeficiency diseases and cancer: the immunodeficiency-cancer registry. *Int J Cancer* 1973;12:333–347.
56. Kinlen LJ. Immunosuppressive therapy and cancer. *Cancer Surv* 1982;1:567–583.
57. Pluda JM, Yarchoan R, Jaffe ES, et al. Development of non-Hodgkin lymphoma in a cohort of patients with severe human immunodeficiency virus (HIV) infection on long-term antiretroviral therapy. *Ann Intern Med* 1990;113:276–282.
58. Beral V, Petterman T, Berkelman, et al. AIDS-associated non-Hodgkin lymphoma. *Lancet* 1991;337:805–809.
59. Roithmann S, Tourani JM, Andrieu JM. AIDS-associated non-Hodgkin lymphoma. *Lancet* 1991;338:884–885.
60. Casabona J, Salas T, Salinas R. Trends and survival for AIDS associated malignancies. *Eur J Cancer* 1993;29:877–881.
61. Haverkos HW, Dougherty J. Health hazards of nitrite inhalants. *Am J Med* 1988;84:479–482.
62. Vandenbroucke JP, Pardoel VPAM. An autopsy of epidemiologic methods: the case of "poppers" in the early epidemic of the acquired immunodeficiency syndrome (AIDS). *Am J Epidemiol* 1989;129:455–457.
63. Seage G, Mayer KH, Horsburgh Jr CR, et al. The relation between nitrite inhalants, unprotected receptive anal intercourse, and the risk of human immunodeficiency virus infection. *Am J Epidemiol* 1992;135:1–11.
64. Darrow WW, Peterman TA, Jaffe HW, et al. Kaposi's sarcoma and exposure to faeces. *Lancet* 1992;339:685.
65. Louie L, Desmond SD, Katongole-Mbidde E, et al. Kaposi's sarcoma may not be an STD in Uganda. Presented at the VIII International Conference on AIDS, Amsterdam, The Netherlands, 1992 (PoC 4335).
66. Wahman A, Melnick SL, Rhame FS, Potter JD. The epidemiology of classic, African, and immunosuppressed Kaposi's sarcoma. *Epidemiol Rev* 1991;13:178–199.
67. van den Berg F, Schipper M, Jiwa M, et al. Implausibility of an aetological association between cytomegalovirus and Kaposi's sarcoma shown by four techniques. *J Clin Pathol* 1989;42:128–131.
68. Peterman TA, Jaffe HW, Friedman-Kien AE, Weiss RA. The aetiology of Kaposi's sarcoma. In: *Cancer Surveys Volume 10: Cancer, HIV and AIDS*. Imperial Cancer Research Fund; 1991:23–37.
69. Salahudain SZ, Nakamura S, Eiberfeld P, et al. Angiogenic properties of Kaposi's sarcoma-derived cells after long-term culture in vitro. *Science* 1988;242:430–433.
70. Huang YQ, Li JJ, Rush MG, et al. HPV-16-related DNA sequences in Kaposi's sarcoma. *Lancet* 1992;339:515–518.
71. Biggar R, Dunsmore N, Kurman RJ, et al. Failure to detect human papillomavirus in Kaposi's sarcoma. *Lancet* 1992;339:1064–1065.
72. Lo SC, Shih JW, Yang NY, et al. An infectious agent in patients with AIDS. *Am J Trop Med Hyg* 1989;40:213–226.
73. Pearce RB, Abrams DI. *Entameba histolytica* in homosexual men. *N Engl J Med* 1987;316:690–691.
74. Hessol N, Fusaro R, Bacchetti P, et al. Cofactors for HIV disease progression in homosexual men: 1978–1991. Presented at the VIII International Conference on AIDS, Amsterdam, The Netherlands, 1992.
75. Bowden FJ, McPhee DA, Deacon NJ, et al. Antibodies to gp41 and nef in otherwise HIV-negative homosexual man with Kaposi's sarcoma. *Lancet* 1991;337:1313–1314.
76. Abrams DI. The relationship between Kaposi's sarcoma and intestinal parasites among homosexual males in the United States. *J Acquir Immune Defic Syndr* 1990;3[suppl 1]:S24–31.
77. Rappersberger K, Tschachler E, Zonzitis E, et al. Endemic Kaposi's sarcoma in human immunodeficiency virus type 1-seronegative persons: demonstration of retrovirus-like particles in cutaneous lesions. *J Invest Dermatol* 1990;95:371–381.
78. Luxton JC, Thomas JA, Crawford DH. Aetiology and pathogenesis of non-Hodgkin lymphoma in AIDS. In: *Cancer Surveys Volume 10: Cancer, HIV and AIDS*. Imperial Cancer Research Fund; 1991:103–119.

79. Birx DL, Redfield RR, Tosato G. Defective regulation of Epstein-Barr virus infection in patients with acquired immunodeficiency syndrome (AIDS) or AIDS-related disorders. *N Engl J Med* 1986;314:874–879.
80. Subar M, Neri A, Inghirami G, et al. Frequent C-myc oncogene activation and infrequent presence of Epstein-Barr virus genoma in AIDS-associated lymphoma. *Blood* 1988;72:667–671.
81. Lenoir G, O'Connor G, Olweny CLM, eds. *Burkitt's lymphoma.* Lyon, France: International Agency for Research on Cancer; 1985; IARC publication no 60.
82. MacMahon EME, Glass JD, Hayward SD, et al. Epstein-Barr virus in AIDS-related primary central nervous system lymphoma. *Lancet* 1991;338:969–973.
83. Nakhleh RE, Manivel JC, Copenhaver CM, et al. In situ hybridization for the detection of Epstein-Barr virus in central nervous system lymphomas. *Cancer* 1991;67:444–448.
84. Clumeck N, Sonnet J, Taleman H, et al. Acquired immunodeficiency syndrome in African patients. *N Engl J Med* 1984;310:492–497.
85. Van De Perre P, Rouvroy D, Lepage P, et al. Acquired immunodeficiency syndrome in Rwanda. *Lancet* 1984;62–65.
86. Casabona J, Salas T, Lacasa C, et al. Kaposi's sarcoma in people with AIDS from an area in southern Europe. *J Acquir Immun Defic Syndr* 1990;9:929–930.
87. Vaccher E, Tirelli U, Lazzarin A, et al. Epidemic Kaposi's sarcoma in Italy, a country with intravenous drug abusers as the major group at risk for AIDS: report of 60 cases. *AIDS* 1989;3:321.
88. Casabona J, Melbye M, Biggar RJ, et al. Kaposis's sarcoma and non-Hodgkin's lymphoma in European AIDS cases: no excess risk of Kaposi's sarcoma in Mediterranean countries. *Int J Cancer* 1991;47:49–53.
89. Anonymous. Human immunodeficiency virus (HIV) infection codes and new codes for Kaposi's sarcoma. *MMWR Morb Mortal Wkly Rep* 1991;40:1–7.
90. Casabona J, Sanchez E, Graus F, et al. Trends and survival for AIDS patients presenting with indicative neurologic diseases. *Acta Neurol Scand* 1991;84:51–55.
91. Monfardini S, Serraino D. Epidemiology of AIDS-related tumours in Europe. *World Health Forum* 1991;1(3):234–241.
92. Muñoz A, Schrager LK, Bacellur H, et al. Trends for the incidence of AIDS defining outcomes in the multicenter AIDS Cohort Study, 1985–1991. *Am J Epidemiol* 1993; 137:423–438.
93. Lemp GF, Payne SF, Neul D, et al. Survival trends for patients with AIDS. *JAMA* 1990;263(3):402–406.
94. Batalla J, Gatell JM, Cayla JM, et al. Predictors of the survival of AIDS cases in Barcelona, Spain. *AIDS* 1989;3:355–359.
95. Casabona J, Bosch A, Salas T, et al. The effect of tuberculosis as a new AIDS definition criterion in epidemiological surveillance data from a south European area. *J Acquir Immune Defic Syndr* 1990;3:272–277.

DISCUSSION

Dr. Biggar: I would like to comment on Hodgkin's disease. Several Italian investigators have published reports that there is an excess risk of Hodgkin's in AIDS patients. Two recently published studies, by Nancy Hessol et al. and Peggy Reynolds et al., also suggest that Hodgkin's risk may be excessive in AIDS patients. I note that these two American studies were done in San Francisco and studied the same population, so they are not completely independent. While the association seen in these studies could be true, there are also problems to be considered, particularly the problem of misclassification. The frequency of non-Hodgkin's lymphoma is so high that a slight amount of misclassification of this disease could result in a spurious excess of Hodgkin's. For example, if 700 excess cases were observed, figures seen in our own studies, and 35 (5%) were misclassified as Hodgkin's disease, Hodgkin's disease would appear to be about six-fold increased. Based on other studies, five percent misclassification is about the level of misclassification one might expect in the age group getting AIDS.

I would also like to bring up a new study we are starting. We have linked cancer registry data for over 80,000 AIDS cases in California, Florida, Atlanta, and New Jersey. The objective is to sort out the AIDS-cancer associations. These studies will help to determine associations at rare sites and provide the statistical power to detect small relative risks for the more common cancers. However, the data will not resolve the problem of misclassification. To do this, we will need to review histologies on these diagnoses.

Dr. Susser: Can either of you say anything about the issue of canvases in sub-Saharan Africa, where there is this current tremendous explosion of heterosexually spread HIV disease, and where I suspect that Kaposi's sarcoma was not uncommon prior to the HIV epidemic? I am simply probing as to whether we know anything about changes or the current state of KS and its distribution in relation to the epidemic. An interesting piece of oncogenesis that one should think about is Burkitt's lymphoma, and it's relationship to EBV and malaria in the same territories. What can you say or speculate about this?

Dr. Casabona: Regarding my presentation itself, the African data refer not to HIV-related Kaposi's sarcoma, but to Kaposi's sarcoma in general. The case-control study didn't take into account the sero-status of the patients or its distribution reference to the population as a whole.

Dr. Galli: At the moment, we are analyzing the data of a seroprevalent cohort of asymptomatic subjects with a clinical picture of CDC stage II and III at enrollment in 1983. The fact is that age plays an important role in all malignancies, including Kaposi's sarcoma, but the incidence of Kaposi's sarcoma in homosexuals, which is of course higher, is the main reason for this influence of age. There is a greater frequency of Kaposi's sarcoma in women when we exclude homosexuals from the study, but there isn't any greater frequency of solid tumors in intravenous drug users.

From this point of view, our data are completely different from those of Gachupin-Garcia and colleagues, but I think that the two cohorts are not comparable for age. The age of our intravenous drug users ranges from 20 to 24 years, with a mean age at enrollment of about 23; all of the data in the study of Gachupin-Garcia came from subjects who were older than 33, with a maximum of 73 years, which is completely unusual for us.

Dr. Biggar: I have seen AIDS in a lot of different African areas, and (although I recognize that this is a purely anecdotal observation without any quantitative basis) in the areas in which Kaposi's sarcoma was endemic, it was presented as AIDS; but in those areas where it was not particularly endemic, it does not seem to have as high a frequency.

I am particularly familiar with areas of eastern Zaire, where I have done some work on pre-AIDS KS cases in particular, to try to determine whether there was any evidence of immunosuppression in these people, but we were unable to demonstrate much in the way of immunosuppression. As you know, endemic Kaposi's does look slightly different from AIDS-related Kaposi's in Africa.

With respect to Burkitt's and non-Hodgkin's lymphoma, this has been surprisingly difficult to demonstrate in Africa, which may be partially related to health-care problems. As I'm sure you know, Burkitt's lymphoma in itself is basically a children's disease, and of course children do not represent the population generally infected by

HIV; those that get it at birth die. So there isn't a large population of children at risk for Burkitt's lymphoma. In the areas I'm familiar with, we haven't seen any increase in Burkitt's in either adults or children, and even non-Hodgkin's diseases seem to be overwhelmed, or perhaps they are not fully worked up because the people are dying of other conditions (wasting disease being probably the most prominent, but there is also tuberculosis and other things). If they get these nodes, I'm not sure that anybody is very aggressive about proving it, and this goes for lymphomas of any kind. It is not hard to demonstrate the fact that they get lymph nodes, but these are not being called lymphoma of any sort.

In any case, we are not seeing much of an increase in Burkitt's lymphoma in any of the places that I am aware of, although perhaps the people in Kenya might have a more specific perspective on this.

[Question begins off microphone.] . . . male and female KS ratio in Africa, in the endemic disease? Quantitatively, I don't really know what it is in endemic disease. It is commonly cited as being ten to one; but in the studies that I have done in Africa, it has been closer to three or four to one. My impression is that it's the men who come for medical care to facilities where KS, for example, is diagnosed; women tend to stay at home, unless they're dragged in from the bushes.

I've seen cases of KS (of course not HIV-related) 27 years after they were originally diagnosed. It's a debilitating disease. These people crawl about on their hands and legs sometimes because they lose their feet, but it's not necessarily a killer as such. It's true that people occasionally die from it, but it's something they can have for a very long time and, of course, without any treatment whatsoever. It's obviously anecdotal, but if you live for 27 years, you don't have a profound immune defect.

Dr. Casabona: Our data are too few to show any trend as far as i.v. drug users are concerned. We consistently see both intravenous drug users and women with Kaposi's sarcoma. We now have 14 women with Kaposi's sarcoma, all of whom are intravenous drug users, so it is possible that we're moving towards other kinds of populations.

Dr. Vermund: I think that we are at an important point. We have a treatment effect, especially using *Pneumocystis* prophylaxis; and now that *Pneumocystis* prophylaxis is shifting towards trimethoprim-sulfamethoxazole, we have concurrent *Toxoplasma* prophylaxis. People are now working very hard on studies relating to CMV and MAC (*Mycobacterium avium* complex), and it may not be unreasonable to think that there will be screening strategies within the next 5 years and prophylaxis for these conditions, too. So, for every opportunistic infection we can prevent, we are presumably delaying the time to AIDS or the time to death in the immunosuppressed state.

I know this is the whole point of your thesis relating to non-Hodgkin's lymphoma. Those conditions which might be rare or have an even longer incubation time will be very important to survey. Two that come to mind are cervical and anal cancers, since papilloma virus is documented to be more pathogenic in some immunosuppressed patients. For example, a number of studies have shown cervical neoplasias and cancers to be more common in renal transplant patients.

I'm simply mentioning this as a phenomenon that might perhaps be more manifest in the treatment era than in the pretreatment era, since immunosuppressed HIV-infected persons may live longer and longer, permitting conditions with long latency periods to manifest.

Dr. Casabona: I think some data showing changes in the pattern over time in Kaposi's sarcoma are mainly related either to changes in the definition of inclusion or to changes in treatment. In our case, that was very clear with tuberculosis and toxoplasmosis, which is much more prevalent in Spain than in the rest of Europe. The only decrease we show here, using HIV data among intravenous drug users, occurred at the same time that we changed the inclusion criteria for AIDS cases, *Toxoplasma* being a much broader criterion in 1987, as well as tuberculosis. I think we need to be careful about interpreting these changes without considering these other kinds of issues, in particular when using AIDS registry data, which collects only the presenting indicative disease.

HIV Epidemiology: Models and Methods, edited by Alfredo Nicolosi. Raven Press, Ltd., New York © 1994.

22

Clinical Course of HIV Disease in a Large Cohort of ZDV-treated Patients

The Italian Experience with People who Acquired HIV Infection Through I.V. Drug Use

*Stefano Vella, *M. Floridia, *M.G. Agresti, *M. Giuliano, †R. Bucciardini, and †S. Mariotti

**Laboratory of Virology and †Laboratory of Epidemiology, Istituto Superiore di Sanità, Viale Regina Elena 299, 00161 Rome, Italy*

In Southern European countries, HIV infection has epidemiological characteristics that differ from those observed in other industrialized countries, where diffusion of HIV, at least at the beginning of the epidemics, involved mainly homosexual men. Conversely, in Southern Europe, including Italy, intravenous drug use is the main risk behavior associated with acquisition of HIV infection; as one of the consequences, the population affected is composed of a high percentage of women. Antiretroviral treatment has been available free of charge in Italy since 1987 for all HIV-infected persons with AIDS-related complex (ARC), AIDS, or a CD4-positive (CD4+) cell count below 200 per mm^3, in accordance with the National Protocol for Zidovudine (ZDV) Therapy. This protocol, issued by the National AIDS Committee, was updated in 1989 to include all HIV-infected subjects with a CD4+ count below 500 per mm^3. The aim of the protocol, in addition to evaluating the drug within a national program of drug surveillance, was to collect key data to assess the clinical course of HIV disease in patients treated with ZDV, including the evaluation of demographic, clinical, and laboratory markers of disease progression.

Clinical and laboratory data are included in the Italian Zidovudine Registry, which therefore represents an important source of information on the clinical course of HIV infection in a population mainly composed of intravenous drug users (IDUs) and characterized by a relatively high percentage of women. In most of the published studies, and in the main cohort groups currently under evaluation (e.g., the MACS), the population studied is in fact almost exclusively composed of homosexual men.

In this report, the currently available results will be summarized in terms of survival and progression to advanced disease (AIDS) for a cohort represented by more than 2,000 subjects. The aim of this work is to describe the clinical course of HIV disease, including the definition of possible clinical or laboratory markers associated with an increased risk of progression, in a sample closely reflecting the real world population currently in ZDV treatment in Southern Europe.

SUBJECTS AND METHODS

All the asymptomatic subjects (CDC 1987 groups II–III), ARC subjects [CDC 1987 groups IVa (wasting syndrome considered as AIDS), IVb (ADC considered as AIDS), IVc2], and AIDS patients (CDC 1987 group) enrolled within the National Protocol for Zidovudine Therapy were considered. These patients were enrolled and followed by over 100 clinical centers throughout Italy according to the protocol schedule, with periodic visits and laboratory assessments performed every 3 months. At enrollment, patients were asked the date of their first HIV-positive test and about risk behavior. Clinical evaluation included Karnofsky and weight assessments; clinical examination, with particular regard to HIV-related symptoms; and skin reactivity to recall antigens (Multitest Merieux, France). Laboratory data recorded at enrollment and at each follow-up visit were the following: hemoglobin level, leucocyte and granulocyte counts, platelet count, ASAT,

TABLE 1. *Selected baseline characteristics of asymptomatic subjects*

Characteristics	Number	(%)
Sex		
male	282	(74.6)
female	96	(25.4)
Mean CD4+ count		
all	311	
males	308	
females	319	
Mean age (years)		
all	29.5	
males	30.3	
females	27.3	
PCP prophylaxis		
yes	64	(16.9)
no	314	(83.1)
Mean daily ZDV dosage (mg)	500	

Data from the Italian Zidovudine Registry.

creatinine level, total number of lymphocytes, CD4+ cell count, and CD4+ to CD8+ ratio.

Patients were excluded from analysis if the date of the beginning of ZDV treatment was before July 1, 1987, or after January 1, 1991, or if this date was unavailable. For progression to AIDS (CDC 1987) and survival, a cross-linked analysis was performed with the Italian National AIDS Registry. All patients whose date of AIDS diagnosis was lacking or not included within the National AIDS Registry were excluded from analysis.

Analysis of survival and of progression to AIDS was performed using the Kaplan-Meier product limit method. The role of factors predictive of progression was estimated in a multivariate analysis using the Cox regression model.

RESULTS

Baseline Characteristics of the Population Studied

Asymptomatic Subjects

Asymptomatic subjects with a CD4+ cell count below 200 per mm^3 have been included since 1987; those who were asymptomatic with a CD4+ count between 200 per mm^3 and 500 per mm^3 have been included only since 1989, when the National Zidovudine Protocol was updated, according to the preliminary reports of ZDV efficacy in this subgroup. We will report some data for a selected sub-cohort of subjects from this setting (enrolled between November 1988 and September 1990) whose baseline characteristics are consistent with ACTG 019 inclusion and exclusion criteria (1). Our purpose is to evaluate the progression rate in a comparable population with regard to stage of the disease, but with a different demographic pattern. This group is represented by 378 subjects whose baseline characteristics and risk factor distribution are shown in Tables 1 and 2, respectively.

TABLE 2. *Risk behavior distribution of asymptomatic subjects*

Risk behavior	Number (%)
i.v. drug use	270 (71.4)
homo- or bisexual contacts	48 (12.7)
heterosexual contacts	40 (10.6)
hemophilia	8 (2.1)
transfusions	1 (0.3)
unspecified	11 (2.9)
Total	378 (100.0)

Data from the Italian Zidovudine Registry.

TABLE 3. *Selected baseline characteristics of ARC subjects*

Characteristics	Number (%)
Sex	
male	1287 (75.7)
female	413 (24.3)
Mean CD4+ count mm³	
all	185
males	180
females	197
Mean age (years)	
all	29.8
males	30.4
females	28.0
Mean daily ZDV dosage (mg)	970

Data from the Italian Zidovudine Registry.

ARC Subjects

A total of 1,700 subjects, 1,287 males (75.7%) and 413 females (24.3%), were studied (Table 3); mean age for the whole group was 29.8 years, and mean CD4+ cell count was 184.6 per mm^3; hemoglobin and platelet count were 13.1 g/dl and $171.4 \times 10^3/mm^3$, respectively (Table 4).

In Table 5 is shown the observed distribution of risk factors associated with HIV infection. As anticipated, intravenous drug use was the risk factor reported in the majority of the cases (72%). Homosexuality was reported by about 15% of males. Previous transfusions or use of blood products was reported less frequently (cumulatively, 3.3%). A significant percentage of the patients studied (16% of females and 8.5% of males) did not report any of the above mentioned factors, and the vast majority of them are likely to represent a subgroup who acquired HIV infection through heterosexual intercourse with HIV-positive subjects. As a whole, this distribution, similar to the one reported above for asymptomatic subjects, is comparable to the distribution of HIV risk factors among AIDS cases reported to the Italian health authorities in recent years and can therefore be assumed to be acceptably representative of the whole population affected.

TABLE 4. *Baseline hematological values for ARC subjects*

	All	Males	Females
Hemoglobin (g/dL)	13.1	13.4	12.3
Platelets[a]	171.4	164.8	189.1

[a]Number $\times$ 10^3 per mm^3.
Data from the Italian Zidovudine Registry.

TABLE 5. *Risk behavior distribution of ARC subjects*

Risk behavior	All (%)	Males (%)	Females (%)
i.v. drug use	1224 (72.0)	898 (69.8)	326 (78.9)
homo- or bisexual contacts	189 (11.2)	189 (14.7)	—
hemophilia	38 (2.2)	36 (2.8)	2 (0.5)
transfusions	19 (1.1)	10 (0.8)	9 (2.2)
other[a]	176 (10.3)	110 (8.5)	66 (16.0)
unspecified	54 (3.2)	44 (3.4)	10 (2.4)
Total	1700 (100)	1287 (100)	413 (100)

[a]Including heterosexual subjects with HIV-positive partner.
Data from the Italian Zidovudine Registry.

AIDS Patients

We previously investigated, in a nonrandomized observational study, the possible benefit of zidovudine treatment in AIDS patients, showing significantly increased survival at 1 and 2 years for treated patients over untreated, matched, contemporary patients (2). Data for this cohort of treated patients are summarized in Tables 6 and 7.

Progression to AIDS

Asymptomatic Subjects

All the patients in this group had a Karnofsky index value of 100, and 86.5% of them had CD4+ cell counts above 200 per mm^3 at enrollment. After a mean follow-up period of 118.5 weeks, 37 patients progressed to AIDS and 17 to advanced ARC. Progression rates to AIDS and to advanced ARC were 4.4 and 6.7 per 100 person-years, respectively. Differences in progression rates to AIDS at 118 weeks were evident with respect to CD4+ count at enrollment, with a three-fold higher rate (10.9 versus 3.6 per 100 person-years) in the group with lower CD4+ (less than 200 versus 200 to 499 per mm^3). In a multivariate proportional hazards regression model, low

TABLE 6. *Selected baseline characteristics of AIDS subjects*

Characteristics	Number (%)
Sex	
male	136 (86.0)
female	23 (14.0)
Mean CD4+/CD8+ ratio	0.35
Mean age (years)	31
Mean daily ZDV dosage (mg)	1000

From Vella et al. (2).

TABLE 7. *Risk behavior distribution of AIDS subjects*

Risk behavior	Number (%)
i.v. drug use	106 (66.7)
homo- or bisexual contacts	28 (17.6)
homosexual contacts and IVDU	4 (2.5)
heterosexual contacts	9 (5.7)
transfusions	2 (1.3)
unspecified	10 (6.3)

From Vella et al. (2).

CD4+ cell count, p24 antigenemia, and high ZDV dosage were the best predictors of progression to AIDS.

ARC Patients

Mean CD4+ count for ARC patients at enrollment was 185 per mm^3. The majority of the patients had lymphadenopathy (74.6%), and the Karnofsky value was 100 in 67.5% of the cases. The prevalence at enrollment of other constitutional symptoms, oral candidiasis, pulmonary tuberculosis and recurrent herpes zoster infections is shown in Table 8.

The Kaplan-Meier product limit method was used to analyze progression to AIDS. Mean follow-up was 119 weeks; the observed cumulative proportion of patients remaining AIDS-free according to age is shown in Fig. 1.

A multivariate analysis in a Cox proportional hazards regression model was performed, examining as covariates sex, age, risk factor, CD4+ count, weight loss, fever, asthenia, diarrhea, oral candidiasis, herpes zoster, oral hairy leukoplakia, and pulmonary tuberculosis. Higher age and lower CD4+ count were found to be the main variables independently associated with a higher risk of progression; also, the presence of some clinical variables defining ARC and male homosexuality were associated with a higher risk. The relative risk for some of the variables entering the model is summarized in Table 9. Of particular interest is the significant increase in relative risk for

TABLE 8. *Prevalence of constitutional symptoms and minor opportunistic infections in ARC subjects at enrollment*

Asthenia	74.0%
Oral candidiasis	45.6%
Weight loss	43.1%
Fever	29.9%
Diarrhea	10.3%
Hairy leukoplakia	4.4%
Herpes zoster[a]	3.8%
TB[b], pulmonary	0.5%

[a]Recurrent or multidermatomeric infections.
[b]Tuberculosis.
Data from the Italian Zidovudine Registry.

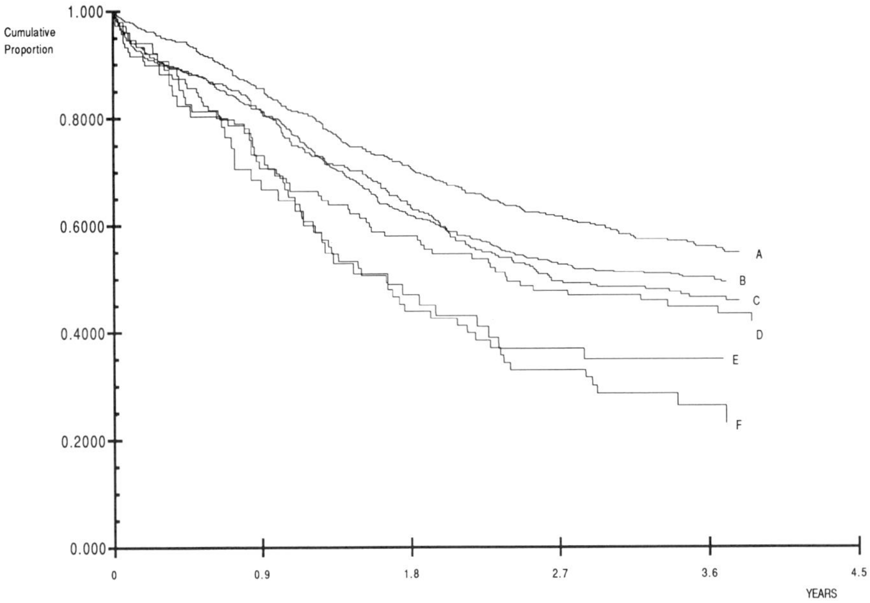

FIG. 1. Cumulative proportion of AIDS-free ARC subjects, according to age (*A*, <25 years; *B*, 26–30 years; *C*, 31–35 years; *D*, 36–40 years; *E*, 41–45 years, *F*, >45 years).

ARC patients with pulmonary tuberculosis, a disease recently included in the new AIDS case definition.

AIDS Patients and Survival Analysis

In our study comparing treated and untreated, matched, contemporary patients (2), mean CD4+ to CD8+ ratio at enrollment was 0.35 (Table 10). A Kaplan-Meier product limit method was used to estimate 1- and 2-year survival. After 1 and 2 years, the proportion of treated patients surviving

TABLE 9. *Relative risk (Cox proportional hazards method) for ARC patients' progression to AIDS*

Variable	RR[a]
Age[b]	1.02
CD4 count[c]	0.67
Weight loss	1.40
Fever	1.52
Oral candidiasis	1.38
Pulmonary TB	2.02
Homosexual males (vs. IVDU)	1.44

[a]Relative risk.
[b]Increase in risk per year added.
[c]Decrease in risk per 100 CD4/mm³ added.

TABLE 10. *Progression of disease and survival in cohorts of Italian HIV-positive, zidovudine-treated patients*

	Number	CD4 status	Progression
Asymptomatics	378	311[a]	3.4 AIDS incidence rate at 55 weeks; rate remains low at 118 weeks (4.4 events/100 person-years)
ARC	1700	185[a]	67.5% of subjects remain AIDS-free at 18 months; 50% of subjects remain AIDS-free at 36 months
AIDS	159	0.35[b]	85% surviving 12 months; 45% surviving 24 months

[a]Number of cells per mm^3.
[b]CD4+ to CD8+ ratio.
Data from the Italian Zidovudine Registry.

was 85% and 45.9%, respectively. Median survival of the whole group of treated patients with an AIDS diagnosis was 21.9 months; median survival was better in patients with a higher CD4+ to CD8+ ratio (23.2 and 20.9 months, respectively, for CD4+ to CD8+ ratio greater than 0.3 versus less than or equal to 0.3).

CONCLUSION

Zidovudine has proved effective, in controlled trials, in prolonging survival in AIDS patients (3) and in delaying progression in asymptomatic or mildly symptomatic subjects with CD4+ counts below 500 per mm^3 (1,4). Although the vast majority of patients enrolled in this study and in other cohort observational studies (5) were homosexual men, subsequent analysis indicates that, as expected, ZDV's beneficial effect can apply also to minorities and women, provided that equal access to clinical care is maintained (6,7). In Mediterranean countries, most HIV-positive subjects acquired infection through needle or syringe sharing associated with i.v. drug use; women represent a significant fraction of HIV-infected persons in all these countries.

We report progression and survival rates from a large cohort of zidovudine-treated patients in Italy. The annual progression rate observed for asymptomatic subjects is very similar to that reported in ACTG 019; progression rates to AIDS among ARC patients and survival after AIDS diagnosis are similar to those of other published studies, although they are difficult to compare because of the greater heterogeneity of subjects at enrollment and the chronological and regional differences in overall health care, including prophylaxis for opportunistic infections.

The definition of the natural history of HIV infection in zidovudine-treated cohorts in Mediterranean countries, although potentially biased by several factors linked to the observational design of these reports, may represent a useful contribution to the assessment of the expected progression rates for ZDV-treated patients in future anti-HIV drug trials and to the calculation of the impact of therapy on AIDS incidence curves.

ACKNOWLEDGMENTS

This work was supported by grants from The Italian Ministry of Health—Istituto Superiore di Sanità, AIDS Research Projects 1989, 1990, 1991.

REFERENCES

1. Volberding PA, Lagakos SW, Koch MA, et al. Zidovudine in asymptomatic human immunodeficiency infection: a controlled trial in persons with fewer than 500 CD4-positive cells per cubic millimeter. *N Engl J Med* 1990;322:941–949.
2. Vella S, Giuliano M, Pezzotti P, et al. Survival of zidovudine-treated patients with AIDS compared with that of contemporary untreated patients. *JAMA* 1992;267:1232–1236.
3. Fischl MA, Richman DD, Grieco MH, et al. The efficacy of azidothymidine (AZT) in the treatment of patients with AIDS and AIDS-related complex: a double-blind, placebo-controlled trial. *N Engl J Med* 1987;317:185–191.
4. Fischl MA, Richman DD, Hansen N, et al. The safety and efficacy of zidovudine (AZT) in the treatment of subjects with mildly symptomatic human immunodeficiency virus type 1 (HIV) infection: a double-blind, placebo-controlled trial. *Ann Intern Med* 1990; 112:727–737.
5. Graham NMH, Zeger SL, Kuo V, et al. Zidovudine use in AIDS-free HIV-1 seropositive homosexual men in the Multicenter AIDS Cohort Study (MACS), 1987–1989. *J Acquir Immune Defic Syndr* 1991;267–276.
6. Lagakos S, Fischl MA, Stein DS, et al. Effects of zidovudine therapy in minority and other subpopulations with early HIV infection. *JAMA* 1991;266:2709–2712.
7. Easterbrook PJ, Keruly JC, Creagh-Kirk T, et al. Racial and ethnic differences in outcome in zidovudine-treated patients with advanced HIV disease. *JAMA* 1991;266:2713–2718.

HIV Epidemiology: Models and Methods,
edited by Alfredo Nicolosi. Raven Press, Ltd.,
New York © 1994.

23

Antiretroviral Treatment and Sexual Infectiousness in Men Infected by Human Immunodeficiency Virus Type 1

*Adriano Lazzarin, †Massimo Musicco,
†‡Alfredo Nicolosi, †Maddalena Gasparini,
*Alberto Saracco, §Gioacchino Angarano,
for the Italian Study Group on HIV Heterosexual Transmission

**Institute of Infectious Diseases, University of Milan, IRCCS "S. Raffaele," 20132 Milan, Italy; †Institute of Advanced Biomedical Technologies, National Research Council, Department of Epidemiology and Medical Informatics, 20131 Milan, Italy; ‡Gertrude H. Sergievsky Center, Columbia University, New York, New York, 10032; §Clinic of Infectious Diseases, University of Bari, Italy*

Zidovudine has been shown to improve survival of people with AIDS (1), and one of the consequences of the treatment is an increase in the prevalence of HIV-infected people in the population. It has been estimated from mathematical models that the diffusion of antiretroviral therapy might accelerate the spread of the infection and even increase overall population mortality for AIDS (2). However, this would be possible only if the infectiousness of HIV-infected people remained unaffected by antiretroviral treatment.

Zidovudine treatment not only reduces the rate of progression to overt AIDS in patients with symptomatic HIV infections (3), it also increases the number of CD4-positive (CD4+) cells (4) and induces the disappearance of viral antigens from peripheral blood (5). For these reasons, it is possible that antiretroviral treatment may also reduce the sexual infectiousness of infected people, and Anderson et al. (6) have actually shown that zidovudine decreases viral load in the semen of treated individuals.

Several studies have reported a higher risk for HIV sexual transmission among women whose partners have AIDS, a reduced number of CD4+ cells, or who are antigen-positive (7-11). Since zidovudine is generally reserved for subjects with advanced disease (and, therefore, more infectious), the potential role of antiretroviral therapy in reducing the risk of virus transmission may be impossible to detect in cross-sectional studies based on prevalent cases. We are conducting a prospective study of HIV infection among stable monogamic couples discordant for HIV (12), in which infectiousness can be monitored over time by means of periodic assessments of the clinical and laboratory markers of disease progression (clinical evolution, the number of CD4+ cells, and the presence of viral antigens in the blood). We therefore consider this cohort a unique setting in which to study whether infected men treated with zidovudine present a reduced rate of sexual transmission of the virus to their partners.

METHODS

Studied Population

The couples were recruited in 16 participating centers: 8 hospital departments of infectious diseases, 5 intravenous drug user outpatient clinics, and 3 centers for HIV surveillance. All of the HIV-infected subjects attending the centers were asked about their stable, monogamous heterosexual partners. Each partner who was not already known to be HIV-infected was invited for an interview and screening tests for serum antibodies against HIV. The presence of antibodies was assessed by means of immunoenzymatic methods using commercially available kits; positive sera were retested with a second immunoenzymatic test and confirmed by Western blot.

Information was collected about intravenous drug use, sexual intercourse with other subjects, blood transfusions or blood-derivate therapies, and prostitution to exclude subjects with risk factors other than sexual exposure to their infected stable partner.

Between February 1, 1987, and May 30, 1992, 525 women who were seronegative at the inclusion visit were asked to return to the center at least every 6 months for interviews and HIV-antibody tests. Of these women, 436 (81%) had at least one follow-up visit and were included in the present study.

At every visit, a structured interview was administered to the participating woman by the attending physician at each center. The questionnaire elicited information about the history of sexually transmitted diseases (STDs), the frequency and type of sexual intercourse, and the contraceptive methods used since the previous follow-up visit.

Males and females were separately advised on the risk and prevention of sexual HIV transmission by the same physician. The use of condoms was strongly and repeatedly recommended. Given that the preliminary results of our study (8) had indicated an increased risk for HIV infection in women using intrauterine devices (IUDs), it was suggested that they have the device removed and abstain from sexual intercourse during 1 month after removal.

Statistical Analysis

The incidence of seroconversion was evaluated by the person-year method, and seroconversion rates were derived (13). Each visit was considered as an independent observation and person-years were calculated by summing all of the time intervals between two successive visits. Using this approach, each woman could contribute in terms of person-years to various categories of exposure if she reported different exposures at different visits. The time of seroconversion was conventionally considered as the midpoint between the first seropositive and the last seronegative test. Relative risks were estimated as incidence rate ratios, and their confidence intervals were calculated using the test-based method (14).

For the study of behavioral risk factors, the frequency of intercourse was divided into two categories: one intercourse or less per week, and more than one intercourse per week. The type of sexual intercourse was dichotomized as ever or never peno-anal. Condom use was grouped into two frequency categories: always and not always. The latest available information on the infected partner (CD4+ cell count, disease stage, p24 antigen serum positivity) was collected from the standard medical records used by all centers. Men were classified according to disease stage as symptomatic (CDC group IV) or asymptomatic (CDC groups II and III).

Zidovudine treatment was prescribed by the centers' physicians generally following common guidelines. Zidovudine was mainly reserved for individuals with a CD4+ cell count of less than 500 per mm^3, and administered at a dose of 250 mg twice daily to asymptomatic and 500 mg twice daily to symptomatic subjects. In the case of adverse events, doses were reduced by 50% and then, if necessary, withdrawn. Zidovudine treatment was stopped when the occurrence of opportunistic infections required treatments with a synergistic effect on zidovudine toxicity. In order to distinguish between men treated for a short time and those on long-term treatment, the men were divided into three groups with reference to the time of the woman's interview and testing: never treated, treated for less than six months, and treated for six months or longer.

Since condom use prevents the contact of infected semen with the genital mucosa (thereby reducing the risk of transmission), we derived relative risks by adjusting for the use of condoms. A final multivariate analysis (including all the variables considered as potential risk factors for transmission) was made using Cox's proportional hazard model to estimate the independent, unconfounded contribution of each variable to the risk of infection. Statistical analyses were carried out using the software packages SPSSPC+ and Epilog Plus.

RESULTS

We followed 436 couples whose characteristics at the time of enrollment are presented in Table 1. The mean age of the women was 26.1 years and the duration of their relationship with the infected man ranged from 1 month up to about 9 years. Fewer than 10% of the women interrupted the relationship with the infected man at the time of enrollment. Most of the men had

TABLE 1. *Characteristics of the women and the relationships*

Characteristics of women		
mean age (years)	26.1	(16–51)
mean relationship duration (months)	51.3	(1–307)
relationships interrupted at or before enrollment	39	(8.9%)
Characteristics of the infected man at enrollment		
i.v. drug user	346	(79.4%)
symptoms of AIDS	110	(25.2%)
p24-positive	85	(19.5%)
treated with zidovudine	64	(14.7%)
Sexual behavior of the couple		
more than 1 intercourse per week	233	(53.4%)
anal sex	67	(15.4%)
oral sex	210	(48.2%)
always using condoms	243	(55.7%)

acquired the infection as a result of intravenous drug use, 25% presented symptoms of AIDS, 20% were positive to p24 antigen in blood, and about 50% had CD4+ cell counts of less than 400. Fifteen per cent of the men were treated with zidovudine. More than 50% of the couples always used condoms; about half of them practiced oral sex and had more than one intercourse every week, while a minority (14%) practiced anal sex.

The women had a total of 1,095 follow-up visits (mean = 2.5) and were followed for 740 person-years (p-y). Twenty-seven women seroconverted, yielding an incidence rate of 3.7 per 100 person-years. In 164 of the 1,095 visits, the women reported that they had not had any sexual intercourse with the infected partner since the preceding visit. No seroconversions were observed during these follow-up intervals, which were excluded from the analysis. Their contribution to the follow-up of the entire cohort was 103 p-y; the incidence of seroconversion, calculated on the remaining 637 p-y, was 4.2 per 100 p-y.

Condom use reduced the risk of seroconversion, the incidence rate in couples using them during all intercourse being about six times lower than in other couples (Table 2). Men with symptoms of AIDS, a positive antigene-

TABLE 2. *Incidence of seroconversion by condom use*

	HIV+	p-y[a]	IR[b] (95% CI)	IRR[c] (95% CI)
condom use				
always	5	362.5	1.4 (0.4–3.3)	1
not always	22	275.3	8.0 (5.0–12.1)	5.8 (2.2–15.3)

[a]Person-years.
[b]Incidence rates.
[c]Incidence rate ratios.

TABLE 3. *Incidence of seroconversion of the women by disease characteristics of the infected man*

	HIV+	p-y	IR (95% CI)	IRR (95% CI)
AIDS symptoms				
absent	15	466.0	3.2 (1.8–5.3)	1
present	12	161.7	7.4 (3.8–13.0)	2.5 (1.2–5.0)
p24 antigen				
absent	19	541.8	3.5 (2.1–5.5)	1
present	8	95.9	8.4 (3.6–16.5)	2.5 (1.2–6.2)
CD4+ per mm^3				
>400	9	299.8	3.0 (1.4–5.7)	1
≤400	18	277.0	6.5 (3.8–10.3)	3.0 (1.4–5.7)

mia, or a CD4+ cell count lower than 400 per mm^3 were more likely to transmit the infection to their partners (Table 3). The partners of men treated with zidovudine for less than 6 months were twice as likely to acquire the infection than the partners of untreated men, but women partners of men treated for more than 6 months showed a 70% reduction in the risk of seroconversion (Table 4); however, these risk differences were not statistically significant.

Zidovudine was taken by men with advanced disease whose infectiousness was therefore higher. In 931 follow-up visits, we observed that treated men were more likely to have AIDS, a low CD4+ cell count, or detectable p24 antigen in blood (Table 5). The association between zidovudine treatment and advanced disease was expected to have a strong confounding effect on the crude risk associated with zidovudine treatment. We therefore carried out a multivariate analysis using Cox's proportional hazard model and adjusting the risk estimates of zidovudine treatment for symptoms of AIDS, CD4+ cell number, p24 antigen positivity, and condom use. In this analysis, the increased risk of seroconversion associated with a period of treatment of less than 6 months completely vanished, and a statistically significant 90% risk reduction was observed for a treatment duration of more than 6 months (Table 6).

Finally, we carried out a multivariate analysis adjusting for disease clinical stage, and sexual behavior. Higher risks were observed in couples whose frequency of sexual intercourse was more than twice a week (RR = 2.6;

TABLE 4. *Incidence of seroconversion of the women by zidovudine treatment of the man*

	HIV+	p-y	IR (95% CI)	IRR (95% CI)
Zidovudine treatment				
no	21	480.2	4.4 (2.6–5.7)	1
≤6 months	5	49.5	10.1 (3.2–29.8)	2.1 (0.8–5.6)
>6 months	1	108.2	1.7 (1.6–6.2)	0.3 (0.0–1.6)

TABLE 5. *Clinical and laboratory characteristics of infected men according to zidovudine treatment*

	Treatment with zidovudine[a]		
	no	≤6 mo	>6 mo
p 24 antigen			
absent	621	48 (6.2)	118 (15.0)
present	53	28 (19.6)	62 (43.4)
AIDS symptoms			
absent	558	35 (5.4)	54 (8.3)
present	116	42 (14.8)	126 (44.4)
CD4+ cell number			
>400	363	19 (4.5)	43 (10.1)
≤400	311	58 (11.5)	137 (27.1)

[a]Number of infected men, with percentage the number represents in parentheses.

95%CI = 1.0–6.7) and, although not statistically significant, also in couples practicing anal (RR = 2.0; 95%CI = 0.8–4.8) or oral sex (RR = 2.1; 95%CI = 0.8–5.4). The risk estimates associated with the clinical stage of the disease were substantially unaffected by the adjustment for sexual behavior, while the estimates of the relative risks associated with condom use (RR = 0.3; 95%CI = 0.1–0.7) and a treatment period of less than six months (RR = 1.3; 95%CI = 0.4–4.0) were slightly increased. No substantial modification was observed for the risk associated with a treatment duration of six months or longer (RR = 0.2; 95%CI = 0.0–0.9)

TABLE 6. *Multivariate analysis (proportional hazard model) of zidovudine treatment and the clinical and laboratory characteristics of the infected men*

	HR[a]	95% CI
Zidovudine treatment		
no	1	—
≤6 months	1.0	0.3–3.0
>6 months	0.1	0.0–0.8
p24 antigen		
absent	1	—
present	2.3	0.9–5.6
CD4+ cells		
>400 per mm^3	1	—
≤400 per mm^3	2.1	0.9–5.1
AIDS symptoms		
no	1	—
yes	2.0	0.8–5.1
Condom use		
not always	1	—
always	0.2	0.1–0.4

[a]Hazard ratios.

CONCLUSION

In this study, men treated with zidovudine for more than 6 months showed reduced infectiousness. The 6-month interval was chosen for the analysis partly to provide a better representation of the data and partly because of general considerations: Seroconversions detected during the first 6 months of treatment may reflect infections occurring before the start of treatment, and it is also necessary to allow enough time for zidovudine to exert its antiretroviral effect. In this respect, it should be noted that increased risk for the women partners of men treated for less than 6 months was present in the crude analysis, but that disappeared when the effect of disease stage was removed. It is therefore likely that the group treated for less than 6 months included men with advanced disease (more infectious than those on long-term treatment) who may have passed the infection on to their partners immediately before the start of treatment or shortly afterwards, before the drug's antiretroviral action had begun to work.

The protective effect of zidovudine was only evident when the markers of the high degree of infectiousness of the man (p24 antigen positivity, a low CD4+ cell count, and the presence of AIDS symptoms) were accounted for. Since zidovudine therapy is generally begun after the onset of signs of disease progression (which are also markers of increased infectiousness), men who have a higher probability of transmitting the infection to their uninfected partners are more common among treated than nontreated men. This finding parallels that found in a laboratory study on viral isolation from semen (6), where reduced viral isolation from men treated with zidovudine became fully evident only when the characteristics of disease progression were taken into account.

Among the men in our study who transmitted the infection and were not treated with zidovudine, the majority (70%) presented one or more markers of increased infectiousness, but six transmitted the infection in spite of being negative for all high infectiousness markers and having a CD4+ cell count of more than 500.

The results of our study seem to indicate that inhibiting viral replication with antiretroviral drugs might reduce the infectiousness of infected subjects. If confirmed, these results may have positive implications for the prevention of man-to-woman HIV sexual transmission. In this case, antiretroviral treatment would not only be beneficial for the patients, but might also be viewed as a tool for reducing the probability of such transmission. This could represent an incentive to HIV testing and medical care for couples in which at least one partner is at risk of HIV infection, provided they can view treatment as a means of avoiding the contagion of the uninfected partner. Our results also confirm the central role of behavioral counseling and the use of condoms in preventing sexual transmission of HIV. In conclusion, the antiretroviral treatment of infected people should be considered as a preventive measure complementing adoption of safer sexual behavior.

ACKNOWLEDGMENTS

This research was supported in part by grants from the Ministry of Health (Istituto Superiore di Sanità—Progetto AIDS) and from the National Research Council of Italy (Progetto Finalizzato CNR "FATMA").

Members of the Italian Study Group on HIV Heterosexual Transmission

Gioacchino Angarano (Bari), Claudio Arici (Bergamo), Sergio Lo Caputo (Bari), Maria Léa Corrêa Leite (Milan), Paolo Costigliola (Bologna), Sergio Gafà (Reggio Emilia), Maddalena Gasparini (Milan), Giovanna Gavazzeni (Bergamo), Cristina Gervasoni (Milan), Adriano Lazzarin (Milan), Roberto Luzzati (Verona), Giacomo Magnani (Parma), Mauro Moroni (Milan), Massimo Musicco (Milan), Alfredo Nicolosi (Milan), Raffaele Pristerà (Bolzano), Francesco Puppo (Genova), Bernardino Salassa (Turin), Alessandro Sinicco (Turin), Roberto Stellini (Brescia), Umberto Tirelli (Aviano), Giuseppe Turbessi (Rome), Gian Marco Vigevani (Milan), Roberto Zerboni (Milan).

REFERENCES

1. Fischl MA, Richman DD, Hansen N, et al. The efficacy of azidothymidine (AZT) in the treatment of patients with AIDS and AIDS-related complex: a double-blind placebo-controlled trial. *N Engl J Med* 1987;317:185–91.
2. Anderson RM, Gupta S, May RM. Potential of community-wide chemotherapy or immunotherapy to control the spread of HIV-1. *Nature* 1991;350:356–359.
3. Hamilton JD, Hartigan PM, Simberkoff MS, et al. A controlled trial of early versus late treatment with zidovudine in symptomatic human immunodeficiency virus infection: results of the Veteran Affairs Cooperative Study. *N Engl J Med* 1992;326:437–43.
4. Fischl MA, Richman DD, Hansen N, et al. The safety and efficacy of zidovudine (AZT) in the treatment of subjects with mildly symptomatic human immunodeficiency virus type 1 (HIV) infection: a double-blind, placebo-controlled trial. *Ann Intern Med* 1990;112:727–37.
5. Volberding PA, Lagakos SW, Koch MA, et al. Zidovudine in asymptomatic human immunodeficiency virus infection: a controlled trial in persons with fewer than 500 CD4-positive cells per cubic millimeter. *N Engl J Med* 1990;322:941–9.
6. Anderson DJ, O'Brien TR, Politch JA, et al. Effects of disease stage and zidovudine therapy on the detection of human immunodeficiency virus type 1 in semen. *JAMA* 1992;267:2769–2774.
7. Goedert JJ, Eyster ME, Bigger RJ, Blattner WA. Heterosexual transmission of human immunodeficiency virus: association with severe depletion of T helper lymphocytes in men with haemophilia. *AIDS Res Hum Retroviruses* 1987;3:355–60.
8. Lazzarin A, Saracco A, Musicco M, Nicolosi A. Man-to-woman sexual transmission of the human immunodeficiency virus. *Arch Intern Med* 1991;151:2411–2416.
9. Padian N, Marquis L, Francis DP, et al. Male to female transmission of immunodeficiency virus. *JAMA* 1987;258:788–90.

10. European Study Group. Risk factors for male to female transmission of HIV. *BMJ* 1989;298:411–5.
11. Holmberg SD, Horsburg CR Jr, Ward JW, Jaffe HW. Biological factors in the sexual transmission of human immunodeficiency virus. *J Infect Dis* 1989;160:116–125.
12. Saracco A, Musicco M, Nicolosi A, et al. Man-to-woman sexual transmission of HIV-1: a prospective study of 343 steady partners of infected men. *J Acquir Immune Def Syndr* 1993;5:497–502.
13. MacMahon B, Pugh TF. *Epidemiology: principles and methods*. Boston, MA: Little, Brown & Co.; 1970.
14. Rothman KJ. *Modern epidemiology*. Boston, MA: Little, Brown & Co.; 1986.

DISCUSSION

Dr. Detels: Do you have the data on the relative risks using the patients with less than 6 months treatment as your reference group?

Dr. Lazzarin: The reference category in this analysis is untreated men, so there is no risk reduction in the case of treatment lasting less than 6 months, but the treatment effect is apparent when the treatment is longer than 6 months. According to what we have seen this morning, clinicians start therapy when something is going on in the disease. So we can assume that the women partners of men treated for less than 6 months have been exposed to highly infective men who were not previously treated.

Dr. Vermund: Regarding the Lazzarin study, this must be one of the most successful discordant couple studies ever presented, with 436 discordant couples. A NIAID-sponsored study has struggled for years to get 150 couples, has had no seroconverters, and has not been able to address any of these questions. You have very important data on some of the fundamental questions related to transmission. I suppose it's reassuring that it correlates biologically, even though it's worrisome (as you might expect). But it does give us a therapy handle, and, as you say, this is the first epidemiologic data that I have seen. I would like to say that this is very important corroborative evidence to a basic science paper that Anderson, O'Brien, Padian et al. published in JAMA in May. There, the biological plausibility of your epidemiologic observations is reinforced by a dramatic decline in viral load in semen after treatment. I think we're finally breaking some ground with these heterosexual studies and getting some definitive guidance, and I give a lot of credit to Dr. Padian and her colleagues for generating the clinical specimens which made the basic science work possible. We really have biological coherence here.

Dr. Padian: From a public health point of view, I think it's important to say that, when this information gets out, it would be a mistake to interpret it as meaning that if you are on AZT you don't need to use a condom, even though it may be an independent effect.

Dr. Vermund: It's quite the contrary. What they showed is that there is no effect in short-course use.

Dr. Padian: Sten's right that we have had no seroconversions in our study and so we haven't been able to look at it prospectively, but even looking at it in a cross-sectional fashion, we found that most of the men in our study were intermittently using AZT and that they were not necessarily good compliers, which makes it difficult to categorize things. I wonder if that was an issue for you, and, if so, how you dealt with it.

Dr. Musicco: We used exposure to AZT during the interval between two subsequent visits. A woman partner of a man who was treated during the period between the first and second visit, but untreated thereafter, was considered twice: first as the partner of a treated man, and then as the partner of an untreated man.

Dr. Johnson: In view of yesterday's helpful discussion concerning multivariate models, I wonder whether you could comment about that final model and what the univariate risks were for treatment as opposed to the adjusted odds. There is clearly a colinearity. There is a very strong relationship between the probability of being on zidovudine and the probability of having advanced-stage disease.

Dr. Musicco: I think Adriano has the slide of the univariate analysis somewhere, but essentially the risk estimates show a risk ratio of 1.8 for women partners of people treated for less than 6 months and a risk of 0.2 for women partners of men treated for longer than 6 months. Neither of these risks is statistically significant. Significance becomes apparent only when you adjust for the treatment status of the man. If you also adjust for sexual behavior, there remains a 90% risk reduction for women partners of men treated for longer than 6 months, and there is a small increase in the risk for partners of men treated for less than 6 months. The risk which was 1 in that model becomes 1.5, but the difference is still not statistically significant. This may be due to the fact that women partners of treated men with advanced disease have a lower frequency of sexual intercourse.

Dr. Muñoz: Did you divide these into more than 6 months and less than 6 months because you didn't have data for 0 to 3 months, 3 to 6 months, 6 to 9 months, and 9 to 12 months? I find it a little difficult not to see that 6 months as a kind of magic number; if you flip the relative risk of 0.1, you get 10, which is huge. I think you have to be careful.

Dr. Vlahov: Is long-term AZT use a marker for reduced frequency of sexual behavior?

Dr. Lazzarin: No, it isn't. But we have also adjusted by frequency of intercourse.

Dr. Casabona: I'm not sure I remember the recall period for behavioral data, the period of time prior to the event you asked the patient about; "Have you used a condom over the last 2 months, or the last . . . ?"

Dr. Lazzarin: It was an average of 6 months, not exactly 6 months.

Dr. Des Jarlais: The magic 6 months clearly shows a tremendous drop-off, but if you look at the other clinical literature on AZT, you would expect virus resistance at 12 months. So you may be talking about another 6-month magic period between 6 months of AZT and the 12 months which other data would lead us to expect for an attenuation in the results.

My second question is what sort of counseling was being given in relation to the administration of AZT; what did the woman think about the situation. And what sort of counseling was being given in the absence of AZT, because, as Sten pointed out, the seroconversion rate in the absence of AZT is really quite high. The results of the European perinatal studies are really low, but the European heterosexual transmission rates seem to be high. Obviously, the source of sampling is a major independent variable in these outcomes, but it's certainly true that what people were thinking about sexual activity and what they were expecting might have influenced their reporting of what they were doing, and possibly also their behavior.

Dr. Vella: In reply to Dr. Muñoz, I think that also from a biological point of view there may be an immediate drop in risk because there is a sort of infectiousness which goes with the viral load, but there is also a cutoff, even if it is true that this is not linear for other diseases. When you go under a certain viral load, there is no infectiousness, even if it existed one moment before. It's not a question of a slight reduction, but the number of transmittable viruses under a certain level. It is also biologically possible that the reduction after 6 months (which is the period of major work of AZT) counteracts the fact that the patients taking AZT were sicker. If they were sicker, then they have more viral load; during the 6 months, the viral load goes down, and when it goes below a certain point, there is not just less infectiousness, but no infectiousness.

Dr. Musicco: Six months turns out to be both a magic and valid number, based on Des Jarlais and Vella's considerations and as shown by our data. In fact, of the six seroconversions which we observed in men treated with zidovudine, five occurred within 4 months from treatment initiation, and one occurred after 23 months of treatment, in a woman whose male partner was p24 antigen positive.

We can suppose that the five early seroconversions might have been due to infections that were transmitted when the man was not yet treated with zidovudine. The last one occurred after 2 years of treatment and in presence of an active viral replication, which suggests the emergence of viral strains resistant to the effect of zidovudine.

Dr. Padian: This is a question for the statisticians. I was always under the impression that, when colinearity exists and you had variables that were highly correlated, this reduced your ability to detect an independent effect. Here, it seems, perhaps, the opposite [is true].

Furthermore, I was always taught that if you had something which was not significant in a univariate analysis, but became significant in a multivariate analysis, you needed to have a certain amount of suspicion. I was wondering what the statistical wisdom was on both those points.

Dr. Tsiatis: It depends on what the relationship is, not only on the colinearity, but also on the confounding nature of the two variables. For example, it's not impossible that, because it's confounded in a negative direction, you don't see any difference in a univariate analysis even when it really exists. I haven't seen the data, and I can't comment exactly upon what's going on, but if the variance grows, the effect might also grow depending on the interrelationship. These results are possible, but one would have to study the whole thing carefully.

HIV Epidemiology: Models and Methods, edited by Alfredo Nicolosi. Raven Press, Ltd., New York 1994.

24

Back-Calculation Models That Take Treatment into Account

M. H. Gail and P. S. Rosenberg

Epidemiologic Methods Section, National Cancer Institute, Bethesda, Maryland 20892

Back calculation is a procedure for estimating the previous rates of HIV infection that best account for an observed time series of AIDS incidence counts. Back-calculated estimates of rates of HIV infection depend on knowledge of the incubation distribution that describes the time from infection to onset of clinical AIDS (1,2). Once the previous rates of HIV infection, known as the infection curve, $\nu(s)$, have been estimated, they can be used to estimate cumulative numbers of infections and to project future AIDS incidence. In this paper, we review back-calculation methods that were applied to AIDS incidence data through mid-1987. These methods assume stability of the incubation distribution in calendar time. For time periods after mid-1987, these classical back-calculation models overestimated AIDS incidence in the United States in several risk groups, including homosexual men. The hypothesis that the favorable changes in observed AIDS incidence trends resulted, in part, from the introduction of effective treatments led to the development of back-calculation models that allowed for secular changes in the incubation distribution to account for treatment effects. We describe two such models and discuss applications to the AIDS epidemic in the US and to a local epidemic in the District of Columbia. A discussion follows.

BACK CALCULATION BASED ON A STATIONARY INCUBATION DISTRIBUTION

The incubation distribution, $F(t)$, is the probability that AIDS develops within t time units of infection. If one assumes that $F(t)$ remains stationary in calendar time, then the expected number of AIDS cases in calendar interval $(T_{i-1},T_i), i=1,2, \ldots I)$, is given by

$$E(Y_i) = \int_{-\infty}^{T_i} \nu(s)[F(T_i - s) - F(T_{i-1} - s)]ds \qquad [1]$$

where Y_i is the observed AIDS incidence count in interval i. Back calculation yields an estimate of the infection curve, $\hat{\nu}(s)$, that implies good agreement between the observed AIDS incidence series $[Y_i]$ and the expected series $[E(Y_i)]$. Statistical procedures used to estimate $\nu(s)$ from Eq. 1 are described by Brookmeyer and Gail (2) and by Rosenberg and Gail (3). Estimates of $\nu(s)$ can be used to estimate cumulative numbers of HIV infections and to project AIDS incidence from an extension of Eq. 1.

The accuracy of back-calculated estimates of $\hat{\nu}(s)$ and related quantities depends on the validity of three ingredients: (i) the AIDS incidence series $[Y_i]$; (ii) the parametric or nonparametric family used to model $\nu(s)$; and (iii) the assumed incubation distribution (4–6).

Reported AIDS incidence series must be corrected for reporting delays (7,8) and for the fraction of cases that are never reported (underreporting). If the degree of underreporting decreases over time, estimates of $\hat{\nu}(s)$ may be upwardly biased near the end of the reporting period for AIDS surveillance (9).

Strongly parametric models of $\nu(s)$, such as $\nu(s) = \alpha\exp(\beta s)$, can yield misleading results. The AIDS incidence series provides more information about the infection curve in the distant past then in the recent past. Thus, this exponential model will tend to fit the early portion of the AIDS incidence series well and imply continued exponential growth of $\nu(s)$, even if later AIDS incidence data suggest less rapid growth in $\nu(s)$. For this reason, most analysts have adopted weakly parametric models for $\nu(s)$, such as step function models. Step function models with four or five steps and with long last steps (about 4 years) have been shown in simulations to yield a favorable trade-off between potential bias and variance for estimating cumulative HIV infections and for projecting AIDS incidence (10). Models with many steps yield erratic estimates of $\nu(s)$ unless smoothing constraints are imposed (11,12). Such models with smoothing constraints yield visually appealing reconstructions of $\nu(s)$, but additional work would be useful to study the performance of various smoothing procedures and methods for selecting smoothing parameters.

The greatest source of uncertainty in back calculation arises from imperfect knowledge of the incubation distribution. Back-calculated estimates of $\hat{\nu}(s)$ are very sensitive to misspecification of $F(t)$, and any realistic assessment of uncertainty must take possible systematic variations of $F(t)$ into account, in addition to the stochastic error associated with random variation in AIDS incidence. Rosenberg and Gail (9) show that the systematic uncertainty associated with lack of precise knowledge of $F(t)$ is usually larger than stochastic uncertainty for estimating cumulative numbers of infections.

Despite these uncertainties, back calculation from Eq. 1 was a useful tool for estimating seroprevalence and for projecting AIDS incidence, at least through mid-1987. Rosenberg et al. (13) used data through mid-1987 to estimate that between 435,000 and 800,000 people had been infected with HIV in the United States by January 1, 1985, and between 749,000 and 1,457,000 by July 1, 1987. These numbers were in reasonable agreement with independent estimates of between 945,000 and 1,400,000 infected as of 1987 (14), which were obtained from surveys of seroprevalence in selected risk groups.

Projections of AIDS incidence from back calculation are much more stable to choice of $F(t)$ than are estimates of the numbers infected, because a change in $F(t)$ leads to compensatory changes in the estimate of $\nu(s)$. The resulting fitted values closely track the observed AIDS incidence series and lead to similar near-term projections as the original $F(t)$.

THE NEED FOR MODELS THAT PERMIT SECULAR CHANGES IN THE INCUBATION DISTRIBUTION

Because back calculation had produced reliable projections of AIDS incidence through mid-1987 (15,16), it was surprising that, beginning in mid-1987, AIDS incidence rates in the US were noticeably lower than back-calculated projections in some transmission groups, such as homosexual or bisexual men (Fig. 1). These changes were partially obscured by the fact that the surveillance definition of AIDS was broadened in the fall of 1987 (17) to include wasting syndrome, dementia, extrapulmonary tuberculosis, and other conditions, which tended to increase AIDS incidence (18). Gail, Rosenberg, and Goedert (19) used a consistently defined AIDS incidence series, which adhered to the surveillance definition of AIDS in use before it was broadened, to show that back calculation yielded serious overestimates (solid line in Fig. 1) of AIDS incidence after mid-1987 (solid squares in Fig. 1). Even if one counted all AIDS cases under the expanded surveillance definition (solid circles in Fig. 1), the back-calculated estimates were too high.

The suddenness of the deviation of the AIDS incidence series from projections in mid-1987 could not be explained by an abrupt earlier decrease in the infection curve, because abrupt changes in $\nu(s)$ are smoothed out in the subsequent AIDS incidence series by the convolution process in Eq. 1. One possible explanation was a sudden degradation in the surveillance system that was leading to increased underreporting or reporting delays beginning in 1987. However, recent evidence (20) suggests that this did not happen.

Gail, Rosenberg, and Goedert (19) presented evidence that newly introduced treatments, such as zidovudine (AZT), which was approved by the Food and Drug Administration in March, 1987, for patients with severe immunodeficiency and for prophylaxis against *Pneumocystis carinii* pneumonia, contributed to the abrupt improvements in AIDS incidence seen in mid-1987. They reviewed the clinical trial literature showing that AZT, in combination with pentamidine, had the potential to reduce the hazard of progression to AIDS by a relative risk factor of $\theta = 0.25$ to $\theta = 0.5$ in AIDS-free patients with severe immunodeficiency. They presented data indicating that enough AZT was in use to have an important impact on national AIDS

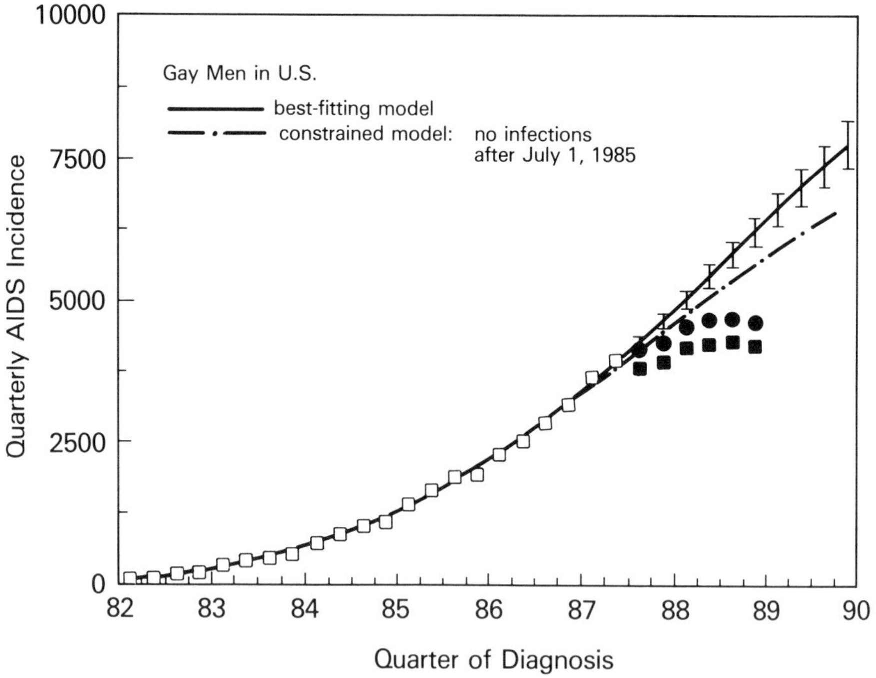

FIG. 1. Projected and observed AIDS incidence among homosexual and bisexual men in the United States. AIDS incidence (*open squares*) as defined before 1987 (consistently defined AIDS) was used in back calculations to project future consistently defined AIDS incidence (*solid line*). A 95% bootstrap confidence interval is shown about these projections. Observed consistently defined AIDS (black squares) and all AIDS (black circles) fall below the projections, beginning in mid-1987. Constraining the back-calculated infection curve to allow no infections after July 1, 1985, also leads to projections (*dot-dashed line*) that exceed the observed AIDS incidence after mid-1987. From Gail et al. (19).

incidence if it was being allocated only to patients with AIDS and to AIDS-free patients with severe immunodeficiency, who are the patients at highest risk of AIDS. The amount of AZT in use among AIDS-free homosexual men with severe immunodeficiency in the San Francisco Men's Health Study was sufficient to explain favorable changes in AIDS incidence seen in the year beginning in mid-1987, though perhaps not in the last half of 1988. The amount of AZT distributed nationally to AIDS-free homosexual men in the period from March 31, 1987, to September 18, 1987, in a program of controlled distribution was also sufficient to have had a favorable impact on AIDS incidence (21).

Another point in favor of the treatment hypothesis was that transmission groups, such as intravenous drug users and people infected by heterosexual contact, who had received relatively little AZT before developing AIDS, showed no improvements in AIDS incidence trends in mid-1987 (21).

These considerations led to attempts to incorporate treatment effects in back-calculation models. However, the uncertainties associated with such models were even greater than those faced before mid-1987. Limited information is available to characterize time trends in the extent of treatment use, treatment efficacy in the general population, and the duration of treatment efficacy. A second major uncertainty results from lack of information on the long-term natural history of HIV infection, and, in particular, on the natural history hazard function, $h_0(t)$, for the incubation distribution in the absence of treatment or changes in the surveillance definition. Because effective treatments became available in mid-1987, very little natural history information on $h_0(t)$ is available more than 5 years after infection (6). Because models that incorporate treatment do so by modulating the natural history hazard, this uncertainty has an important impact on treatment models. This is especially so because treatment models are being applied to AIDS incidence data in the 1990s, more than 10 years after some patients were infected. Bacchetti, Segal, and Jewell (22) showed that at least some of the dramatic improvements in AIDS incidence trends seen in 1987 could be explained if both the infection curve decreased sharply in 1981 and if the natural history hazard $h_0(t)$ leveled off at about 6 years. Thus the precise quantitative role of AZT and other treatments remains uncertain.

BACK-CALCULATION MODELS THAT INCORPORATE TREATMENT

Methods for the Stage Model and Time-Since-Infection Model

The introduction of AIDS-retarding treatments and the expansion of the surveillance definition of AIDS in 1987 induced secular changes in the incubation distribution. The effects of treatments that lengthen the incubation period tend to outweigh the effects of broadening the surveillance definition, which shortens incubation periods. Thus people infected in 1981 should have a less favorable incubation distribution than people infected in 1988. Brookmeyer and Liao (23) and Brookmeyer (12) suggested replacing $F(t)$ in Eq. 1 by $F(t|s)$, the probability of developing AIDS within t years of infection for a person infected at calendar time s. With this modification, back calculation that allows for secular changes in the incubation distribution still follows from Eq. 1. The challenge is to model the family of incubation distributions $F(t|s)$ indexed by s.

Brookmeyer (12) used a stage model (Fig. 2) for $F(t|s)$. In the absence of treatment, patients progress from state one (infected but AIDS-free, with CD4+ cell counts over 200 cells per μl) to state two (infected but AIDS-free with CD4+ cell counts less than or equal to 200 cells per μl) to state three (AIDS). The model is semi-Markovian. The distribution of sojourn times from state one to state two is Weibull, with hazard $h_{12}(t) = 0.0294t^{1.08}$ and

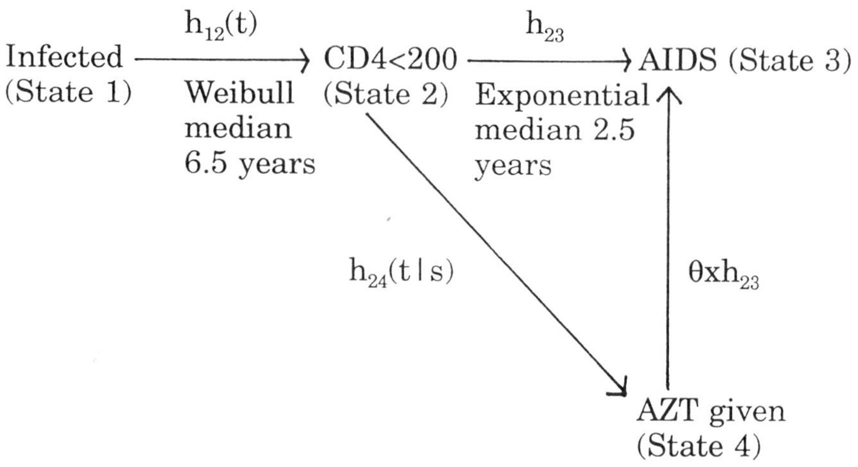

FIG. 2. Stage model of Brookmeyer (12). The functions h_{12}, h_{23}, and h_{24} are defined in the text. The hazard of transition to AIDS from stage two is reduced by treatment by the factor $\theta = 0.35$.

a median of 6.5 years. The sojourn time from state two to state three has an exponential distribution, with hazard $h_{23} = 0.277$/year and a median of 2.5 years, so that the combined incubation period has a median of 10 years. To allow for treatment, Brookmeyer introduces state four, which includes treated AIDS-free patients with CD4+ levels less than or equal to 200 cells per μl. The effect of treatment is to reduce the rate of transition to AIDS to $h_{43} = \theta h_{23} = 0.277\theta$/year, where $\theta = 0.35$ represents the relative risk reduction in AIDS hazard. The reason the stage model in Fig. 2 allows for secular change in $F(t|s)$ is that the hazard of initiating treatment, $h_{24}(t|s)$, depends on calendar time. Indeed, $h_{24}(t|s) = 0.2$/year for $t+s \geq 1987.5$ and $h_{24}(t|s) = 0$ for $t+s < 1987.5$.

Rosenberg, Gail, and Carroll (24) proposed an alternative model for taking treatment into account, called the time-since-infection (TSI) model. This model also accounts for changes in the surveillance definition of AIDS. According to the TSI model, the hazard of AIDS for a patient who was infected t time units earlier at calendar time s, and who is first given access to effective treatment at calendar time τ, is

$$\begin{aligned} h(t|s,\tau) = h_0(t)[\theta(t)\cdot I(t+s \geq \tau) + I(t+s < \tau)] \\ \times [\delta\cdot I(t+s \geq \Delta) + I(t+s < \Delta)] \end{aligned} \qquad [2]$$

where $I(A)$ is an indicator function that takes value 1 when the condition A is true and 0 otherwise.

The first term in brackets describes the effect of treatment for people at risk beyond the time, τ, when access to treatment is first available. The efficacy function, $\theta(t)$, multiplies the natural hazard, $h_0(t)$, reflecting the effect of access to treatment. The efficacy function is near 1.0 for small values of t, corresponding to short times since infection. It remains near 1.0 until about year $t=3$, when it starts to decrease to its asymptote, θ_{min}, which is reached at about year $t=7$. Values of θ_{min} equal to 0.50 and 0.35 were used. This specification of $\theta(t)$ reflects the fact that even patients with access to effective treatments will not usually receive agents like AZT or pentamidine until several years following infection.

The TSI model also makes allowance for the expanded surveillance definition of AIDS by multiplying $h_0(t)$ by a factor $\delta>1.0$ for patients at risk at or beyond $\Delta=$October 1, 1987, when the expanded definition of AIDS came into effect. The value of δ was estimated as 1.10 for homosexual men and as 1.25 for intravenous drug users. The latter group was found to have had proportionately more diagnoses from dementia and wasting syndrome after the definition of AIDS was broadened (18).

To complete the definition of the hazard in Eq. 2, one must specify a natural history hazard function. Rosenberg, Gail, and Carroll (24) obtained point estimates from the Weibull hazard $h_0(t)=0.0021\times 2.65t^{1.65}$, which corresponds to a 9 year median. Plausible ranges for estimated numbers of infections and AIDS incidence were obtained from sensitivity analyses employing different choices of $h_0(t)$ and θ_{min}. Larger functions $h_0(t)$ and values of θ_{min} tended to produce smaller estimates of cumulative HIV infections, whereas smaller natural hazards and smaller values of θ_{min} (i.e., more effective treatment) produced larger estimates of cumulative infections. To account for stochastic variability of the result for a given specification of $h_0(t)$ and θ_{min}, parametric bootstrap samples were obtained. The upper limit of the plausible range was the 97.5th percentile of the bootstrap sample based on a model with $\theta_{min}=0.35$ and with a Weibull incubation distribution with median 10 years and hazard $h_0(t)=0.0021\times 2.516\times t^{1.516}$, as in Brookmeyer and Goedert (25). The lower limit of the plausible range was the 2.5th percentile of a bootstrap sample based on a model with $\theta_{min}=0.50$ and with $h_0(t)=0.0021\times 2.65\times t^{1.65}$ until $t=8$. Beyond $t=8$, $h_0(t)$ increases linearly with a slope of 0.01.

The hazard in Eq. 2 defines $F(t|s,\tau)$, the incubation distribution for a person infected at calendar time s and first given access to treatment at calendar time τ. Rosenberg, Gail, and Carroll (24) obtained $F(t|s)$ from $\int F(t|s,\tau)dP(\tau|s)$, where $P(\tau|s)$ is the distribution of times of first access to treatment among patients infected at calendar time s. Rosenberg et al. (21) obtained empirical data on $P(\tau|s)$ based on access to AZT. For example, for homosexual men infected at $s<$April 1, 1987, $P(\tau|s)$ can be approximated by a straight line that increases from 0 at $\tau=$April 1, 1987, to 0.4 at March 31, 1990; $P(\tau|s)$ remains constant at 0.4 for $\tau>$March 31, 1990. For $s\geq$April 1, 1987, and $s<$March 31, 1990, $P(\tau|s)$ jumps from 0 to 0.4 at $\tau=$April 1, 1990, and remains constant thereafter. For $s\geq$April 1, 1990, $P(\tau|s)$ has point mass 0.4 at s. Other access distributions $P(\tau|s)$ are used for other risk groups, because, for example, intravenous drug users were slower to begin receiving

AZT treatment, and only about 10% began treatment before AIDS onset (21).

To obtain estimates of the cumulative number of people infected by HIV in the US and to make projections of AIDS incidence, Rosenberg, Gail, and Carroll (24) studied homosexual men, male homosexual intravenous drug users, male heterosexual and female intravenous drug users, and heterosexuals separately. Estimates for the US were obtained by summing over these four groups, multiplying by 1/0.94 to account for the small proportions of AIDS cases in other transmission groups, and multiplying by 1/0.85 to account for underreporting. Brookmeyer (12) estimated HIV infections in the US from an analysis of total AIDS incidence in the US, rather than by summing over subgroups. For comparison with Rosenberg, Gail, and Carroll (24), we have used the same factor 1/0.85 to adjust Brookmeyer's results for underreporting.

Comparison of Results from the Stage Model and Time-Since-Infection Model

The stage model yields higher estimates of cumulative infections than the TSI model, although there is some overlap in the plausible ranges for these two models (Table 1). The main factor accounting for this difference is that the stage model implies that more treatment was in use than the TSI model does. For example, about 25% of infected people were in treatment in January, 1989, according to the stage model, compared to 16% who had access to treatment according to data used in the TSI model. Moreover, according to the stage model, every person in treatment enjoys an immediate reduction in AIDS hazard (Fig. 2), whereas, in the TSI models, those recently infected do not benefit from an immediate reduction in hazard from access to treat-

TABLE 1. *Estimates of cumulative HIV infections and AIDS incidence in the United States*

	Stage model		Time-since-infection model	
	Point estimate	Plausible range	Point estimate	Plausible range
Estimated infections to 1990 (in thousands)		909–1,289[a]		628–988[b]
Projected AIDS incidence (in thousands)				
1991	65.0	59.0–69.6	54.7	51.4–58.8
1992	70.0	59.8–77.6	55.9	50.3–64.2
1992	72.6	58.0–84.2	54.8	47.0–68.1
1994	73.2	54.1–89.5	51.6	42.3–70.7

[a]Through April 1, 1990.
[b]Through December 31, 1990.

ment. A second factor is that the TSI model allows for expansion in the surveillance definition of AIDS (Eq. 2). This expansion partially offsets the beneficial effects of treatment on the incubation distribution, leading to lower estimates of cumulative infections.

Despite these quantitative differences, the shapes of the estimated infection curves from the TSI and stage models are similar. For example, both models indicate that the rate of HIV infections in homosexual and bisexual men peaked before 1986 and that there have been noticeable declines in HIV incidence since then.

Both the stage and TSI models project a plateau in AIDS incidence at high levels over the period 1991 to 1994 (Table 1), and there is considerable overlap in plausible ranges for these projections. However, the stage model yields somewhat higher projections, mainly because it incorporates stronger treatment effects that increase the estimated number of infections.

COMPARISONS OF HIV PREVALENCE ESTIMATED FROM THE TSI MODEL WITH SURVEY DATA IN THE DISTRICT OF COLUMBIA

Because back-calculation models that incorporate treatment are complex, it is desirable to test such models against other data sources. Recently, Rosenberg et al. (26) used the TSI model to interpret AIDS incidence trends in the District of Columbia (DC). They found evidence of a wave of infections in the last half of the 1980s among intravenous drug users (IVDUs) and among people infected through heterosexual contact. This second wave of infections was approximately equal in size to the earlier wave of infections among homosexual and bisexual men, which peaked between 1982 and 1983 (Table 2). The infections among IVDUs and people infected through heterosexual contact are projected to lead to a continuing increase of overall AIDS incidence in DC through 1995, in contrast to leveling projections for the entire US (Table 1).

To check these alarming findings from the TSI model, Rosenberg et al. (26) examined survey data on HIV prevalence. Based on a census of blood samples from newborns, it was determined that the seroprevalence percentages in black women who delivered live infants between January and June of 1991 were 1.08, 1.75, 2.49, 2.32, and 1.76, respectively, for age groups 15 to 19, 20 to 24, 25 to 29, 30 to 34, and 35 to 44 years. Multiplying these seroprevalence percentages by census-based estimates of the corresponding numbers of women in the population yielded an estimate of 1,957 infected black women, (95%CI = 1,406-2,509). This estimate can be compared with prevalences estimated from the TSI model (Table 2) by multiplying prevalence for each transmission category by the proportion of AIDS cases in that category occurring among black women. The resulting estimate is $(0.278 \times 3{,}823) + (0.583 \times 1{,}090) = 1{,}698$. However, 18.2% of black women with AIDS were in other transmission categories. An adjusted estimate of

TABLE 2. *Estimates of HIV prevalence in the District of Columbia as of 1 January, 1991, based on the TSI model*[a]

	Cumulative HIV infections as of 1 January, 1992 (plausible range)	Cumulative AIDS incidence as of 1 January, 1991	Estimated prevalence[b] (plausible range)
Transmission Category			
Homosexual/bisexual men	5,545 (5,207–12,146)	2,563	3,853 (3,515–10,454)
IVDU	4,153 (3,232–6,248)	500	3,823 (2,902–5,918)
Homosexual/bisexual male IVDU	489 (433–1,697)	218	345 (289–1,553)
Heterosexual	1,161 (630–2,219)	108	1,090 (559–2,148)
DC Total[c]	11,784 (9,867–23,167)	3,520	9,461 (7,544–20,844)

From Table 3 in Rosenberg et al. (26).

[a]A factor of 1/0.85 = 1.176 is used to account for underreporting of AIDS cases.

[b]Prevalence estimated as cumulative incidence minus 0.66 times cumulative AIDS incidence.

[c]Totals from four transmission categories multipled by 1.038 to account for other transmission categories.

prevalence is therefore 1,698/0.818 = 2,076 women. Based on national data on age at AIDS diagnosis among black women, we estimate that more than 88% of these 2,076 women were between the ages of 15 and 44 years. Thus, the back-calculated estimate is in very good agreement with the survey-based data, especially in view of the wide uncertainty associated with both procedures.

Rosenberg et al. (26) also checked back-calculated estimates of HIV prevalence in IVDUs against survey estimates. The population of IVDUs is estimated as 16,000 for DC, and survey data in 1990 indicated that 22.2% of IVDUs in treatment for drug abuse were infected, yielding an estimated prevalence of $0.222 \times 16{,}000 = 3{,}552$. This number, unlike the estimate from the census of newborns, is quite uncertain, not only because the number of intravenous drug abusers is imprecisely known, but also because the seroprevalence among those in treatment for drug abuse may differ from the seroprevalence among IVDUs not in treatment. Nonetheless, the value 3,552 is not too different from the back-calculated estimate $3{,}823 + 345 = 4{,}168$ (Table 2), with a plausible range of 3,191 to 7,471.

CONCLUSIONS

We have reviewed some of the evidence that indicates a need to incorporate treatment effects into back calculations and outlined two models that take treatment into account. Failure to account for treatment can lower estimates of cumulative HIV infections substantially. For example, Brookmeyer (12) estimated 1,050,000 infections in the US to April 1, 1990, with treatment in the model, compared to 715,000 infections if treatment effects are excluded.

Models that take treatment into account are complex. It is therefore important to test such models whenever feasible. One test is to compare results from various approaches used to incorporate treatment effects. In this regard it is encouraging that both the stage model and TSI model project a plateau in AIDS incidence in the US and yield similar estimates of when the rate of infection was greatest in various transmission categories. Most of the discrepancy between these two models arises from the greater treatment effects used in the stage model, which leads to somewhat higher estimates of cumulative HIV infections and projections of AIDS incidence (Table 1). Another model in use at the Centers for Disease Control includes six stages but estimates the amount of treatment in use in a manner similar to the TSI model (27). This model yields projections of AIDS incidence intermediate between those in Table 1. An advantage of stage models is that they permit one to estimate not only the cumulative number of HIV infections, but also the numbers in various stages of disease.

Another check on back-calculated estimates is direct comparison with survey data on seroprevalence. In this respect, the TSI model performed very well. However, the comparisons do not provide as stringent a test of the TSI model as one would like, because the epidemics among IVDUs and heterosexuals in DC are fairly recent. Thus there has been limited time for important treatment effects to appear.

Even before the introduction of effective treatments, back calculation was subject to important uncertainties, particularly in specifying the incubation distribution (9). To these uncertainties must be added our inability to predict the amount and efficacy of future treatments and how long present treatments remain effective. Furthermore, there is little information on the natural history of HIV infection beyond 5 years, and because treatment models modulate the natural history, this must be deemed a major impediment to the use of models, such as those discussed here, beyond 1995, say.

It will be helpful to estimate new baseline incubation distribution functions from empirical studies of patients receiving the current generation of treatments. This information, coupled with additional data on new trends in HIV therapeutics, may extend the time span over which back-calculation methods can be usefully applied.

ACKNOWLEDGMENT

We wish to thank Mrs. Jennifer Donaldson for assistance with graphics and for typing the manuscript.

REFERENCES

1. Brookmeyer R, Gail MH. Minimum size of the acquired immunodeficiency syndrome (AIDS) epidemic in the United States. *Lancet* 1986;2:1320–1322.
2. Brookmeyer R, Gail MH. A method for obtaining short term projections and lower bounds on the size of the AIDS epidemic. *J Am Stat Assoc* 1988;83:301–308.
3. Rosenberg PS, Gail MH. Backcalculation of flexible linear models of the human immunodeficiency virus infection curve. *Appl Stat* 1991;40:269–282.
4. Gail MH, Brookmeyer R. Methods for projecting course of acquired immunodeficiency syndrome epidemic. *J Natl Cancer Inst* 1988;80:900–911.
5. Gail MH, Brookmeyer R. Modeling the AIDS epidemic. *AIDS Update* 1990;3:1–8.
6. Gail MH, Rosenberg PS. Perspectives on using backcalculation to estimate HIV prevalence and project AIDS incidence. In: Dietz K, Farewell V, Jewell NP, eds. *AIDS epidemiology: methodologic issues*. Boston: Birkhäuser; 1992.
7. Harris JE. Reporting delays and the incidence of AIDS. *J Am Stat Assoc* 1990;85:915–924.
8. Brookmeyer R, Liao J. The analysis of delays in disease reporting: methods and results for the acquired immunodeficiency syndrome. *Am J Epidemiol* 1990;132:355–365.
9. Rosenberg PS, Gail MH. Uncertainty in estimates of HIV prevalence derived by backcalculation. *Ann Epidemiol* 1990;1:105–115.
10. Rosenberg PS, Gail MH, Pee D. Mean square error of estimates of HIV prevalence and short-term AIDS projections derived by backcalculation. *Stat Med* 1991;10:1167–1180.
11. Becker NG, Watson LF, Carlin JB. A method of nonparametric back-projection and its application to AIDS data. *Stat Med* 1991;10:1527–1542.
12. Brookmeyer R. Reconstruction and future trends of the AIDS epidemic in the United States. *Science* 1991;253:37–42.
13. Rosenberg P, Biggar RJ, Goedert JJ, Gail MH. Backcalculation of the number with human immunodeficiency virus infection in the United States. *Am J Epidemiol* 1991; 133:276–285.
14. Centers for Disease Control. Human immunodeficiency virus infection in the United States: A review of current knowledge. *MMWR Morb Mortal Wkly Rep* 1987;36:1–48.
15. Brookmeyer R, Damiano A. Statistical methods for short-term projections of AIDS incidence. *Stat Med* 1990;8:23–34.
16. Centers for Disease Control. Estimates of HIV prevalence and projected AIDS cases: summary of a workshop, October 31–November 1, 1989. *MMWR Morb Mortal Wkly Rep* 1990;39:110–119.
17. Centers for Disease Control. Revision of the CDC surveillance case definition for acquired immunodeficiency syndrome. *MMWR Morb Mortal Wkly Rep* 1987;36:3S–15S.
18. Selik RM, Buehler JW, Karon JM, Chamberland ME, et al. Impact of the 1987 revision of the case definition of acquired immune deficiency syndrome in the United States. *J Acquir Immune Defic Syndr* 1990;3:73–82.
19. Gail MH, Rosenberg PS, Goedert JJ. Therapy may explain recent deficits in AIDS incidence. *J Acquir Immune Defic Syndr* 1990;3:296–306.
20. Buehler JW, Berkelman RL, Stehr-Green JK. The completeness of AIDS surveillance data. *J Acquir Immune Defic Syndr* 1992;5:257–264.
21. Rosenberg PS, Gail MH, Schrager L, Vermund SH, et al. National AIDS incidence trends and the extent of zidovudine therapy in selected demographic and transmission groups. *J Acquir Immune Defic Syndr* 1991;4:392–401.
22. Bacchetti P, Segal M, Jewell NP. Uncertainty about the incubation period of AIDS and its impact on backcalculation. In: Jewell N, Dietz K, Farewell V, eds. *AIDS epidemiology: methodological issues*. Boston: Birkhäuser; 1992.
23. Brookmeyer R, Liao J. Statistical modelling of the AIDS epidemic for forecasting health care needs. *Biometrics* 1990;46:1151–1163.
24. Rosenberg PS, Gail MH, Carroll RJ. Estimating HIV prevalence and projecting AIDS incidence in the United States: a model that accounts for therapy and changes in the surveillance definition of AIDS. *Stat Med* 1992;11:1633–1655.
25. Brookmeyer R, Goedert JJ. Censoring in an epidemic with application to hemophilia-associated AIDS. *Biometrics* 1989;45:325–335.

26. Rosenberg PS, Levy ME, Brundage JF, et al. Population-based monitoring of an urban HIV/AIDS epidemic: magnitude and trends in the District of Columbia. *JAMA* 1992; 268:495–503.
27. Karon JM, Beuhler JW, Byers RH, et al. Projections of the numbers of persons diagnosed with AIDS and of immunosuppressed HIV-infected persons—United States, 1992–1994. *MMWR Morb Mortal Wkly Rep* 1992;41:1–29.

DISCUSSION

Dr. Des Jarlais: There's a lot of controversy as to whether the given treatments really prolong life or merely delay the onset of AIDS, and, of course, it would be unethical to do the experiments that would definitively answer that question. Have you, or has anyone else, tried using back-calculation methods to see whether the introduction of treatment led to the same dramatic change in deaths from AIDS as that which you find in relation to the incidence of AIDS, including any change in the distribution of time from AIDS to death? If treatment is having the same effect on prolonging life, you should see a similar drop in deaths among gay men as you saw in the incidence of AIDS among gay men.

Dr. Gail: What you're asking me to do is to use back calculation to go from infection to AIDS and then to death, that is, two steps. It seems to me that we have enough noise with just the first step beyond infection; I don't think that back calculation would be the right approach.

Nevertheless, there have been several observational studies in the US [Lemp et al. for San Francisco (JAMA 1990), Moore et al. for Baltimore (NEJM 1991), and Harris for the US as a whole (JAMA 1990)] suggesting that the time from AIDS diagnosis to death has been improving in the US, and that these improvements are particularly associated with a decrease in the number of PCP-associated deaths. Overall median survival has gone from something like 12 to 18 (or 20) months (depending on the study), but it is still not clear whether these figures are artificially boosted by the fact that people with AIDS are being diagnosed a little bit earlier. It is also difficult to know how complete the follow-up is in some of these studies.

If you are talking about the survival of people with advanced immunodeficiency, I think that the first clinical trial, despite some of its weaknesses, is pretty definitive in showing that AZT prolongs survival in patients with AIDS and with advanced AIDS-related complex. But I think you're referring to earlier AZT treatment.

Dr. Des Jarlais: In the gay men's group, you saw a dramatic change in the incidence curve, and you attributed that change, whether or not it is contaminated by AZT or whatever, to the provision of treatment. If treatment is really having that big an effect, I would also expect to see an equally dramatic effect (with greater confidence intervals) on the number of deaths from AIDS among gay men.

Dr. Gail: One problem is that we don't have the same access to death data as we have to incidence data. The person who has done the best job of linking death data and the incidence of AIDS is Geoffrey Harris, who followed up a set of people who developed AIDS. He found that there was a secular improvement in overall survival, mainly associated with PCP and mainly associated with gays, because they dominated the epidemic early on.

Dr. Friedman: In my talk, I spoke about arrivers and departers, and I would like to ask some questions based on those concepts. On the one hand, when you take the Washington, DC, study on child-bearing women, there is a question as to whether abortion may have had an effect on the statistics relating to the departers' children; one may have canceled out the other.

Secondly, a lot of drug injectors (and possibly members of some of the other groups, although to a much lesser degree) depart between the time of infection and the time that they become AIDS-diagnosed cases. Some of these departures are due to AIDS-related infection and some to overdoses (perhaps dramatic, as in Milan), and we know that that varies from city to city and perhaps even from county to county. I wonder how that source of noise affects this kind of analysis.

Dr. Gail: If i.v. drug users die of other causes before they have had a chance of developing AIDS, this obviously has an impact on the AIDS incidence series; we'll be seeing a smaller number of AIDS cases and back-calculating a smaller prevalence rate. It's more or less the proportion of deaths compared with the proportion of AIDS; if 10% of the people die before they have the chance of developing AIDS, there would be an inflation factor of roughly 10%.

Dr. Friedman: Fifty percent or more.

Dr. Gail: You think that 50% or more of drug users die before developing AIDS?

Dr. Friedman: It varies.

Dr. Gail: I thought it was smaller, but it's a very serious problem.

Dr. Friedman: It can be large, perhaps beyond the scale of 50%. But we know it varies a lot from city to city.

Dr. Gail: Of course, the dead people will not be attending methadone maintenance clinics . . . The abortion question is of the same type. I don't know the magnitude of the problem, but you're absolutely right; if people are lost before they can develop AIDS . . . This is a very simple model, but even so it's already too complicated; competing risks represent a very serious problem. Another risk group which is an extremely serious problem is represented by people who receive blood transfusions; they have very high mortality rates, and back calculation leads to some very confusing results.

Subject Index